AL

PRESCRIBING

SOCIAL PRESCRIBING

Paradigms, Perspectives and Practice

HEATHER HENRY
RN, BSc (Hons) Nursing, Queen's Nurse, MBA

Nurse Entrepreneur and Writer
Brightness Management Limited
Founder, BreathChamps CIC
Trustee, Being There Support for Life Limiting Illness
Greater Manchester
United Kingdom

ELSEVIER

ISBN: 978-0-443-11364-2

Content Strategist: Robert Edwards
Content Project Manager: Abdus Salam Mazumder
Design: Christian J. Bilbow
Marketing Manager: Deborah Watkins

Working together
to grow libraries in
developing countries

Printed in India
Last digit is the print number: 9 8 7 6 5 4 3 2 1

www.elsevier.com • www.bookaid.org

Contents

Foreword

It is beginning to be recognised that social prescribing can make a significant contribution to health and wellbeing. The concept, however, is not without challenges. The very term 'prescription' risks both medicalising the approach and implies something done to or given to rather than something co-created. There are also challenges around whether the focus should be on individuals or on creating more resilient communities through an asset-based approach—or both.

Not surprisingly, a recurring theme of this collection is its ability to highlight contrasting paradigms—illness treatment or health creation, individual or community orientation, transactional or relational approach, biomedical or psychosocial, the enabling or the disempowering state, centralised or participatory local control. Much of this has been around for many years. In the last 50 years in inner West Newcastle, we have had:

- Benwell Community Development Project (St James's Heritage and Environment Group, *1972–1979*), one of 12 nationally funded local projects. Staff worked directly with local residents to help them to set up tenant's associations, campaign for housing improvements, provide welfare rights advice, and support local community action in other ways.
- Newcastle City Challenge 1992 (Robinson & Townsend, 2016). A competitive nationally funded programme focused on urban regeneration and renewal of local infrastructure, including funding for the West End Health Resource Centre, now HealthWORKS Newcastle, which incidentally had link workers with European Social Fund support back in 2002.
- Newcastle New Deal for Communities 2000–2010 (Department for Communities and Local Government, DCLG 2010)—a nationally funded programme aiming to transform 39 areas with high levels of disadvantage over 10 years by achieving holistic change in relation to three place-related outcomes: crime, community, and housing and the physical environment (HPE),

and three people-related outcomes: education, health, and worklessness. The national evaluation showed some overall improvement in levelling up with more success in place-related rather than people-related outcomes. Interestingly, continuity of senior staff was associated with positive benefits. Whether the sixth of the key objectives—sustaining a local impact after the New Deal for Communities Programme funding ceases—was achieved is much more debatable. It is salutary to look at the 2019 Indices of Multiple Deprivation, which show that these areas still sit in the lowest 10–20% and this has probably deteriorated since the pandemic and the cost of living crisis.

All of the examples I give here, alongside the contributor's views in this book, illustrate how hard it is to make and sustain change in disadvantaged areas. There are residual assets from all these initiatives, but they continually struggle to survive in areas with high levels of population churn, high levels of housing insecurity and low-income, insecure jobs.

Will social prescribing have a secure and sustainable legacy? This is the crux of this book—in public health terms, we are still at the start of a process. What happens next is important and history is valuable tool for leaders to use. The 2004 rollout of NHS-funded Health Trainers is a cautionary tale. They were set up as part of the *Choosing Health* white paper (Department of Health, 2004) in response to the 2002 Wanless Report *fully engaged* scenario, which postulated that NHS long-term savings would accrue from the public becoming fully engaged in their own health. An evaluation of the Health Trainer programme (Mathers et al., 2014) concluded that over time the Health Trainer Service had shifted from a community-oriented approach to an NHS-defined priorities approach and that the shift was largely driven by the fact that '*the long-term sustainability of any new health intervention service depends on its fitting the established system's (NHS's) characteristics*'. Health Trainers have now largely been replaced by Social Prescribing Link Workers.

So a question for readers to consider as they pick and choose from the diverse range of contributions in this volume is about how do we address and balance the tensions between these contrasting paradigms without reverting to polarised perspectives. What should be the balance between emergency services (Chapter 25) and health creation (Chapter 11)? How can we best work with individuals so that they are confident to connect with their communities and at the same time ensure that gaps in community infrastructure are addressed and the existing VCSE infrastructure is sustained (Chapter 18)? Do we still need to 'prove' that social prescribing is cost effective within tightly defined criteria or should we be looking at wider cost-benefit which could include the creation of training and employment opportunities for people in communities with high levels of both disadvantage and unemployment (Chapter 6)? How do you reconcile personalised care with its intensive focus on individual needs and circumstances with a population health approach that might be about ensuring that everyone within a clearly defined group had the same level of input (Chapter 8)?

Social Prescribing Link Workers are on the front line in all of these debates. There is also much discussion about whether their future can be best assured by the development of a national regulatory framework in which they would become one of the many NHS tribes alongside doctors, nurses, health visitors and allied health professionals or whether the role would be best left to fit local contexts and circumstances. The key paradigm here is about the balance between central control and professional and local discretionary autonomy. The balance over the last 50 years has been towards an increase in regulatory frameworks in which individual professionals and organisations are held to account so that blame can be allocated when things go wrong.

The counter to this is discretionary autonomy. At an individual professional level, there is emerging evidence that this is a key issue for front-line staff. Where critical care nurses perceive they have a high degree of autonomy to do what they think is best in the circumstances, job satisfaction and collaborative approaches with less moral distress are higher than in those with less perceived autonomy (Papathanassoglou et al., 2012). More relevant to Link Workers is Understanding Street-Level Bureaucracy (Hupe et al., ed, 2016) which looks at a wide range of community public-facing roles and examines the question of how best to reconcile discretionary autonomy with hierarchical control. This is all picked up in this volume, perhaps most notably in Chapter 23 on community nursing, but it also resonates with Chapters 15, 16, 22 and 27. Similar issues arise around the degree of autonomy from central control allowed to local organisations. Clearly, VCSE organisations have a much higher degree of autonomy than NHS organisations (Chapter 18) and the NHS needs to find effective ways of working collaboratively with the VCSE. There is also a push for Place-Based Public Service Budgets (Denham and Studdart, 2024) and much of this can be found in Chapter 9. Getting the centre to cede a degree of control remains problematic and is likely to be more difficult in a time of austerity.

All of the three nationally funded local development initiatives in West Newcastle took place in happier financial times and ran into the ground when austerity began to bite. This raises bigger issues of how you invest for the long term to address inequality (Chapter 5) and create jobs and meaningful lives (Chapter 10).

If—and how—social prescribing is sustained and developed in the next 10 years in the face of increased austerity, global uncertainty and the likely impact of climate change will not be straightforward. Heather Henry has brought together a fascinating and timely collection of contributions to guide leaders at all levels in the system on this journey.

REFERENCES

Denham, J., Studdert, J., 2024. Place-Based Public Service Budgets: Making public money work better for communities. New Local. https://www.newlocal.org.uk/publications/research-reports/place-based-budgets (Accessed 12 March 2024).

Department for Communities and Local Government; 2010. The New Deal for Communities Experience: a final assessment. https://extra.shu.ac.uk/ndc/downloads/general/A%20final%20assessment.pdf (Accessed 12 March 2024).

Department of Health, 2004. Choosing Health. Making Healthier Choices Easier. https://www.yearofcare.co.uk/sites/default/files/images/DOH2.pdf (Accessed 13 March 2024).

Hupe, P., Hill, M., Buffat, A. (Eds.), 2016. Understanding Street-Level Bureaucracy. Policy Press, Bristol. https://policy.bristol-universitypress.co.uk/understanding-street-level-bureaucracy (Accessed 12 March 2024).

Mathers, J., Taylor, R., Parry, J., 2014. The challenge of implementing peer-led interventions in a professionalized health service: a case study of the national health trainers service in England. Milbank Q 92 (4), 725–753. doi:10.1111/1468-0009.12090. PMID: 25492602; PMCID: PMC4266174. https://www.ncbi.nlm.nih.gov/pmc/articles/PMC4266174/#sec-a.j.mtitle (Accessed 12 March 2024).

Papathanassoglou, ED., Karanikola, MN., Kalafati, M., Giannako-poulou, M., Lemonidou, C., Albarran, JW., 2012. Professional autonomy, collaboration with physicians, and moral distress among European intensive care nurses. Am J Crit Care 21 (2), e41–e52. doi:10.4037/ajcc2012205. PMID: 22381995. https://pubmed.ncbi.nlm.nih.gov/22381995 (Accessed 12 March 2024).

Robinson, F., Townsend, A., 2016. Benwell 40 Years On. Durham University. https://www.dur.ac.uk/media/durham-university/research-/research-centres/social-justice-amp-community-action-centre-for/documents/imagine-documents/Benwell-forty-years-on—Policy-and-change-after-the-Community-Development-Project.pdf (Accessed 12 March 2024).

St James's Heritage and Environment Group (Benwell Community Development Projects published between 1972-78). https://stjamesheritage.com/cdp-booklets (Accessed 12 March 2024).

Wanless, D., 2002. Securing our Future Health: Taking a Long-Term View. https://www.yearofcare.co.uk/sites/default/files/images/Wanless.pdf (Accessed 13 March 2023).

Chris Drinkwater, CBE, FRCGP, FFPH(Hon), FRSA
Patron
Ways to Wellness, Newcastle upon Tyne
United Kingdom
Emeritus Professor of Primary Care Development
Northumbria University, Newcastle upon Tyne
United Kingdom

Contributors

David Ashton
Practice Champion
Alvanley Family Practice
Woodley, Stockport
United Kingdom

Sue Barton, BMedSci(speech) (Hons), MSc
Deputy Director of Strategy & Change
South West Yorkshire Partnership NHS FT, Wakefield
United Kingdom

Kathryn Berzins, BA, MCC, PhD
Senior Research Fellow, IMPaCT
Applied Research Collaboration North West Coast,
    University of Central Lancashire, Preston
United Kingdom

David Buck, BSc Econ (Hons), MSc Econ (Hons), FFPH (Hons)
Senior Fellow, Public Health and Health Inequalities
The King's Fund, London
United Kingdom

Helen Christmas, BA (Hons), MA, MPH, FFPH
Public Health Consultant
Public Health
Hull City Council, Kingston upon Hull
United Kingdom

Tom Coffey, OBE
Senior Health Advisor to the Mayor of London
London, United Kingdom

Simon Cramp
Person with experience of living with a learning disability
Lifetime member of Learning Disability England
Chesterfield, United Kingdom

Chris Dabbs, BA (Hons)
Chief Executive
Unlimited Potential, Salford
United Kingdom

Gerard Patrick Devereux, MSc
Strategic Health Lead
Prevention Directorate
United Kingdom National Fire Chief Executive,
    Manchester
United Kingdom

Michael Dixon, CVO, OBE, FRCP (Hons) FRCGP
Chair College of Medicine
Brighton, United Kingdom

Bethan Griffith, MBBS, BSc, MSc
Population Health Sciences Institute
Newcastle University, Newcastle
United Kingdom

Heather Lynne Henry, RN, Bsc (Hons) Nursing, Queen's Nurse, MBA
Nurse Entrepreneur and Writer
Brightness Management Limited
Founder, BreathChamps CIC
Trustee, Being There Support for Life Limiting Illness
Greater Manchester
United Kingdom

Nancy Hey, LL.B (Hons), MSc, FRSA
Director of Evidence & Insight, Lloyd's Register
    Foundation
Formerly Executive Director
What Works Centre for Wellbeing, London
United Kingdom
Trustee
National Centre for Creative Health
United Kingdom

Linda Hindle, OBE, MSc, RD
Deputy Chief Allied Health Professions Officer for
    England
Office for Health Improvement and Disparities
Department of Health and Social Care, London
United Kingdom

Jane Horrell, BA (Hons), MSc
Research Fellow
Faculty of Health
University of Plymouth, Plymouth
United Kingdom

Michelle Howarth, MSc, PGCHE, PhD
Senior Engagement Fellow
Faculty of Health, Social Care & Medicine
Edge Hill University, Ormskirk
United Kingdom

Susanne Hughes, BA journalism and communications
Community-embedded researcher
Health and Community Sciences
University of Exeter, Exeter
United Kingdom

Paul Jarvis-Beesley, MSc
Founder, Social Prescribing Youth Network
Director of Health, StreetGames (retired)
Brighton & Hove
United Kingdom

Kate Jopling
Associate
National Voices, London
United Kingdom

Laura Lamming, BSc, Mphil
Policy Researcher
The King's Fund, London
United Kingdom

Ilse Katrina Lee, BA, MSc
Implementation Manager
Centre for Psychiatry
Queen Mary University of London, London
United Kingdom
Implementation Manager
UCLPartners, London
United Kingdom

Jacqueline Anne Leigh, RN, BSc (Hons), MSC, PhD
Professor
Nursing & Midwifery
Edge Hill University, Ormskirk, Lancashire
United Kingdom

Michael Marmot, MBBS, MPH, PhD, FRCP, FFPHM, FMedSci, FBA
Director
Institute of Health Equity
University College London, London
United Kingdom

Brendan Martin, BA (Politics)
Founder and Managing Director
Public World, London
United Kingdom

Dawn Mitchell, BSc, FRSPH
Founder, We Do Wellbeing
Fellow, Royal Society for Public Health
Consultant, StreetGames
East Yorkshire
United Kingdom

Rhian Monteith, MSc, Bsc, BEM
Director at Think Outs Limited
Fellow of College of Paramedics
Preston, United Kingdom

Gus O'Donnell, GCB, FBA, FAcSS
Crossbench peer
House of Lords, London
United Kingdom
Chairman, Frontier Economics, London
United Kingdom

Gay Palmer, RGN (adult)
Improving Health Limited
Primary Care Network
GP federation, London
United Kingdom

Marie Polley, BSc (Hons), PhD, PGCertHE
Honorary Reader
Arts and Sciences
University College London, London
United Kingdom
Director
Marie Polley Consultancy Ltd
United Kingdom

Cormac Russell, BACC Phil: BA Phil, Marte Meo Communications Therapist
Faculty
Stean Centre, DePaul, University
Asset Based Community Development Institute, Chicago
Illinois
United States

Kim Ryley, MA
Recent Past Chair of the Coalition for Personalised
   Care (C4PC)
Harrogate
United Kingdom

James Sanderson, BA (Hons)
Chair
Global Social Prescribing Alliance, Nottinghamshire
United Kingdom

Noel Sharpe, BA History and Politics
Chief Executive
Bolton at Home, Bolton
United Kingdom

Merron Simpson, BSc Biochemistry, MA Housing Studies
Chief Executive
The Health Creation Alliance, Birmingham
United Kingdom

Mark Spencer, MBBS MRCGP
GP
Mount View Practice, Fleetwood
United Kingdom
Honorary Professor
Lancaster University Faculty of Health and Medicine
Lancaster, United Kingdom
Founder and Volunteer
Healthier Fleetwood, United Kingdom
Trustee
Fleetwood Trust, United Kingdom

Justin Srivastava, BA, MSC
Retired Lancashire Police Superintendent and
   National Police Chiefs Council
Global Law Enforcement and Public Health
   Association
Lancashire Violence Reduction Network and National
   Lead for Public Health Approaches on Policing, Preston
United Kingdom

Hazel Stuteley, OBE
Chair
C2 National Network of Connected Communities,
   University of Exeter, Exeter
United Kingdom

Felicity Thomas, PhD
Associate Professor in Culture and Health Inequalities
Wellcome Centre for Cultures and Environments of
   Health
Director of the WHO Collaborating Centre for
   Culture and Health
University of Exeter, Exeter
United Kingdom

Steve Vincent, MSc, BA (Hons), PGDMS, MiFE
Strategic Leader with experience in Strategic Planning
Operations, Command & Control
Resilience & Safety
West Midlands
United Kingdom

Phil Walters, BA (Hons), Dip PSW, CQSW
Strategic Lead
Creative Minds and Mental Health Museum
Specialist Services
South West Yorkshire NHS Foundation Trust,
   Wakefield
West Yorkshire
United Kingdom

Katrina Wyatt, BSc, PhD
Professor of Relational Health
Medical School
Health and Community Sciences, University of
   Exeter, Exeter
United Kingdom

Salma Yasmeen, MA Communication Studies, PGD Counselling, RMN, PCSC
CEO, Sheffield Health and Social Care NHS
   Foundation Trust, Sheffield
United Kingdom
Formerly Director of Strategy & Change
Strategy Directorate
South West Yorkshire Partnership Foundation Trust,
   Wakefield
United Kingdom

Acknowledgements

When I was learning about asset-based community development, I was taught by my mentor to be what is called a 'serial connector'. This means that I get to know a lot of people at all levels of society. I triangulate what I learn from everyone, and then I see who can help who with what. And then I connect them, with meaning and purpose.

In the process of editing this book, I did the same thing, except that this time, I connected all the contributors to the readers of this book in, hopefully, a meaningful way.

Many of the contributors I know personally, but that doesn't always serve you when you are seeking a range of views. You need diversity. So, others I had to track down, using my networks, asking for recommendations. I hope that you will agree with me that those who wrote chapters offer an insightful range of views on social prescribing.

So, thank you to all my contributors and especially to the seldom-heard voices that had never written for publication and whom I had to persuade. It was worth it.

A final thanks to the team at Elsevier: Robert Edwards, Abdus Salam Mazumder and Rahul Basak (from Aptara).

Prologue: Two Personal Experiences of Social Prescribing

Social Prescribing and Our Family

DAVID ASHTON, PRACTICE HEALTH CHAMPION

Born just after the war, my early days in school were blighted by asthma. When I went to secondary school, it sticks in my mind that apart from me there was one other person who suffered from asthma out of 600 pupils. But today it is an everyday illness. For children, it was a terrifying disease to have.

I loved the outdoors and walking. I would set out after breakfast and stay out all day. I was also a great bird watcher, so many a time I was late home for tea. I am telling you this now so that you get to know what kind of person I was back then.

My working life was mostly outdoors in the gardens at Lyme Park. Unfortunately, I started smoking in the early 1960s. It was the done thing to do—it was advertised on television and it was cool to smoke. As I reached the age of 55, I was diagnosed with chronic obstructive pulmonary disease (COPD), but it was something that didn't affect me at that time. I still ran every day and worked at the hospital as a domestic manager running up and down the corridors with no effect. I was still fit, so I didn't take COPD seriously and still smoked.

When I got in my 60s, my wife Julie was diagnosed with breast cancer. When we received the news, it was like a brick had hit me. I couldn't breathe and ended up on a trolley in the emergency department. It was as though COPD had been waiting to attack me. I was told that it can take years to affect you, as it is a progressive illness. Also, it can't get better, but you can slow it down by stopping smoking and exercising. Julie's cancer is clear, thank goodness, but I still have my COPD. It's not just about me or Julie, it's about how the both of us cope together. I had to retire from work, and over time I sank into depression. I became a couch potato, never going out. I did stop smoking, thank goodness. I became very unfit and my COPD was getting worse.

My GP surgery, Alvanley Family Practice in Stockport, has a Facebook page to let the patients know what was going on at the surgery, and Julie and I always commented on it. The practice business manager, Kay Keane, got a bug about alternatives to medicine: social prescribing. So she asked Altogether Better, an NHS organisation with experience of this, to help her. There were 20 people registered at the surgery who were asked if they were interested in helping set up social prescribing alongside the surgery. She asked us because we were interested in what was going on at the surgery. We all got together. Each of us had different skills. There were musicians, clerical workers, accountants and gardeners. We called ourselves 'Practice Champions'. We would meet every week to come up with ideas to bring the community together.

I was a time-served gardener, so Julie and I were asked to find an allotment and get it up and running. It took us 2 years and it was a challenge. We rang up the local allotment organizer, and they said that they had one, but it hadn't been touched for 40 years. The neighbours had been using it as a tip. There were tall trees and brambles 4 feet high. A local firm of civil engineers gave us their apprentice to clear the site under the supervision of the site manager as part of his training, and the apprentice dug up everything for us and it cost us nothing. It was a bit of a to-do because the lorry couldn't park nearby, and the loads had to be ferried to the lorry by dumper truck. It was a big job, I'll tell you. And me and my wife were overseeing it all. We were elated. We applied by ourselves for £2,000 from Tesco, and we bid for some local funding too, and that paid for a huge new cabin complete with a veranda, a garden shed and gardening equipment. It certainly kept us moving. We didn't expect that we would get this huge Norwegian cabin with a donated pool table, all the flagging and parking bays and a polytunnel. The cabin is now used by the community—for people with anxiety and depression to go and help themselves to recover.

We have a Wednesday Wonder Walking Group—a 1-mile walk that was started by the business manager and then was taken over by Practice Champions. I joined the Wednesday Wonder Walking Group. It was fabulous: there were about 20 people, and we only went as fast as the slowest person. I was the slowest person; halfway round we came to a hill and my heart sank. There was no way I could walk up that hill, it was too much for me. The group stopped and I was talking to the surgery business manager, who came along at the start with us, and she talked me into walking up that hill. I went very slowly, having to stop and get my breath back. I walked a bit further and then had to stop to take my inhalers. I stopped six times in all, but I got to the top and was delighted—all the group who had waited for me at the top clapped and cheered. I was so proud—I never thought I would be able to do it. I went on that walk week after week and eventually could walk up that hill in one go.

When I was younger and working at Lyme Park, my favourite place was up a big hill watching the planes landing at Manchester Airport. Even though I could walk up the hill on the Wednesday Wonder, I would never walk up the hill at Lyme Park, as it was a lot higher. I would dream about going up for old times' sake, but I never dreamed it would come true.

We went to Lyme Park, and Julie suggested giving it a go. Together we started up the hill. I had to sit down part way up. We were 5 miles from the road, so the choice was—do I turn round or carry on? My wife does not give up, and we carried on to the top. I made it. I was so proud—I would never have dared to think I could do this 12 months ago. I stayed there with Julie and watched the planes coming in. It was wonderful.

The community singing started when one of the Practice Champions, who plays the electric organ, suggested it. A guitarist joined him, and we all met up after the walk to sing in a local community cafe. We started inviting more people, and now we have a monthly singalong in that cafe. It takes over the whole cafe every month! It helps you to control your breathing, and for others, it offers them company.

We had a lady and she used to contact the surgery every day with this and that. Then somebody picked her up and brought her to the cafe. Eventually she phoned the surgery and apologised that she hadn't been in touch!

I was very lucky to have such forward-thinking GPs who realised that not every solution comes in tablet or medicine form. We all need different ways to keep our minds and bodies fit as well. Two of the GPs and the business manager clicked together, and they were always keen to get something going. By this, I mean they helped us, the patients, to get activities going, and eventually the whole community enjoys them.

After the champions had set several activities up, the GPs said at our regular monthly meetings that the number of frequent attenders had dropped and the GPs and nurses had more time. Neighbouring GPs said that they didn't know how our GPs found time for the Practice Champions because they themselves were too busy seeing patients. Now they have eaten their words.

It was 5 years ago that 20 of us patients had that first meeting that really changed my life. We became constituted as an unincorporated association in 2017, and we have treasurers and such to keep us in line. It shows me that anything is possible if you want it. Without our GP practice and my wife Julie, I would not have achieved it. Thank you to you all.

My Personal Experience of Social Prescribing

BY SIMON CRAMP

For me, as someone with experience of living with a learning disability, it all started with a 2006 policy 'Our health, our care, our say'. And that's where social prescribing started. And it came in a couple of years later.

The book is well resourced and well researched. Heather is very thorough and knows her stuff, but my personal experience is not great.

Social prescribing, I think, is a waste of money. It is a typical government programme: great idea but lacking in funding, long delayed and people on the ground can't work with the person. The idea, in a cost-of-living crisis in the UK and because of COVID, world events and other stuff, is great. But, like with the NHS, social prescribing is a post code lottery.

Even the NHS Long Term Plan, published in 2019, which I was part of, still lacks funding adequately. It's about making a simple system that works. People used to get referred if they had, say, a heart condition and needed exercise—there was a taster course. But with social prescribing, I got nothing. I could not walk, and my GP said, 'give it a go and tell me what you think about social prescribing'. One word: crap. In practice, lacking resources and poorly managed in some parts of the country.

Those with a learning disability don't get a fair hearing: mine is a wider problem within the NHS. In my area, there are poor staff who don't make an adjustment. You seem to have to remind people that they need to take time. Often you have telephone appointments: no, not for me—or video call—not happening. I have dyspraxia and it affects a person's coordination, and I have heart problems and arthritis and diabetes. I live in a first-floor flat, arounds hills, on benefits.

The government wanted or claims to be fair, it is not. So those that are poor get very little. It's down to the political party in power at the time.

Some of the things I will question, like shared decision making. It's not what is suggested in the book, it's just not a reality. It took a long time to be referred, and people really didn't get my situation at all—what I wanted did not matter.

So, I hope that you read all of this book, because things need to change, and the book will give you ideas.

REFERENCE

NHS England, 2006. 'Our health, our care, our say: a new direction for community services'. Available from https://www.gov.uk/government/publications/our-health-our-care-our-say-a-new-direction-for-community-services (Accessed 1 May 2024).

Setting the Scene

Chapter 1

Introduction

Heather Henry

When clinicians acknowledge that the health problems they are untangling have their roots in the social circumstances of people's lives, they start to think that the solution lies there too. This realisation has heralded the birth of social prescribing, which is variously described but essentially involves connecting people to non-clinical resources within their own communities, via a link worker, based on what matters to them and their family. Ask someone in the street, however, and they will be hard pressed to recognise the phrase or tell you what it means.

Social prescribing challenges the dominant medical model of health and begins to offer a small but significant change in direction in the UK National Health Service (NHS) system. Is this the start of a paradigm shift or is it a passing fad?

Controversy

Social prescribing is now included in health policy, general practitioner (GP) contracts and the work of integrated care systems (ICS). Although various commentators and think tanks have dissected and critiqued the approach both positively and negatively, these differing views have not so far been published together in the form of a book. This is an attempt to do something about it, by providing a 360-degree look at the concept of social prescribing. The book aims to present a balanced approach to the current debates and critiques around social prescribing.

When introducing a major change such as a social model of health, readers will want to consider the political, economic and social contexts at both local and national levels, and this book attempts to cover as much as may be relevant.

In the following pages, a wide range of contributors examine some of the world views, arguments and ways of interpreting and delivering such an approach. Some are nationally known whereas others are seldom-heard voices. Each deserves to be heard.

The concept, the premise, the evidence, the public perception, the systemisation, the commissioning, the funding and even the name 'prescribing' are all hot topics. These debates will be played out within these pages. It is for you, the reader, to interpret and decide on the way forward, for your own communities of practice.

Social Prescribing for What?

Wellbeing and health are sometimes confused or conflated, so it is important to discuss this, because social prescribing relates to both the amelioration of illness and an overall feeling that life is good, or otherwise. The World Health Organization Constitution (WHO, online), developed in 1948, defines health as 'a state of complete physical, mental and social well-being and not merely the absence of disease or infirmity'. By contrast, the What Works Wellbeing Centre (online) defines an individual's wellbeing as 'feeling good and functioning well'. It also defines national wellbeing as 'how we're doing' as individuals, communities and as a nation, and how sustainable that is for the future. It goes on to explain that there are many components that make up wellbeing, and one of these is a person's health. In this context, health is made up of four domains, including healthy life expectancy, disability, health satisfaction and levels of depression and anxiety. So, is health the same as wellbeing or is it a component of it? Should we focus on individual health and wellbeing or that of families, communities and our nation too?

The Bigger Picture

To figure out where social prescribing fits in terms of the health and wellbeing of our nation, we firstly need to consider what we are up against. The picture is bleak, with the disparity in life expectancy between rich and poor widening. Healthy life expectancy has stalled (Marmot, 2020).

Economics, power and class are woven through the explanations for inequality and offer different lenses through which social prescribing can be viewed. For example, the coronavirus pandemic highlighted how those in poverty were forced to work on the front line and live in overcrowded homes. As a result, the nation began to understand the widening gaps in health and wellbeing between the haves and have nots. Commentators such as McGarvey (2022) describe in detail how detached politicians are from the reality of working people's lives and how this is reflected in national policy that can exacerbate inequalities. In response, the mantra has become 'build back fairer' (Marmot et al., 2020) rather than 'build back better' (HM Treasury, 2021) by finally getting to grips with the social determinants of health and not just addressing the gaps in health and social care provision.

Public Perception

How do we balance the idea of social solutions with the public perception that their health is down to their individual health choices and that NHS services are the main thing that will make them better? How do we explain that health is not an individual matter but is also about how we take collective action and help one another? Amid criticism that the political culture had de-emphasised the common good (Marmot et al., 2020), COVID-19 has taught us much about community autonomy to self-determine what it needs, requiring a shift in power from national to local (Lent and Studdart, 2021).

The pandemic has helped with the public realisation that to be well, health *care* is not enough, and what we really need is decent housing, decent education, decent jobs, decent income, social contact, meaning and hope in our lives. Now that the pandemic has subsided, system leaders are learning to communicate differently about what makes us well (L'Hôte et al., 2022): de-emphasising a biomedical health care model (10–20% of what makes us well) and highlighting the importance of the social circumstances of our lives (80–90% of what makes us well; Hood et al., 2016).

There's an even more fundamental question too: Why is it important for governments to prioritise improving the health and wellbeing of the nation? Economics plays a big part in this, with influencers explaining that a lack of health is a constraint on economic growth and that a better measure of a country's progress is wellbeing rather than gross domestic product (O'Donnell, 2014). They argue that trickle-down economics doesn't improve the income of the poorest (Hope and Limburg, 2020) and that we should balance this with 'wellbeing economics' (Wellbeing Economy Alliance, online). The underlying principles here are about having economies that serve the people by addressing underlying problems to enable people to flourish.

On top of that, public health experts are saying that those in power are helpless to stop the juggernaut private sector businesses driving the commercial determinants of health (World Health Organization, 2021)—the pushing of ultraprocessed food, factories emitting pollutants and gambling organisations advertising alongside televised sports matches.

Paradigms, Perspectives and Practice

So how have people interpreted social prescribing so far? How important is it, within the context above? How should we frame and 'sell' social prescribing to the public as something that makes us well?

Section 1 of the book starts by setting the scene: the history of social prescribing, its development and the evidence base behind it. We explore how the National Academy of Social Prescribing is now driving and shaping the agenda and how this fits with addressing health inequality.

Section 2 focuses on paradigms: different ways of looking at social approaches to what makes us well, both within communities and as a nation. This includes concepts around power, control, relationships, economics, recognising strengths and assets, managing complexity and enabling self-organisation.

A range of contributors then offer differing perspectives on social prescribing in Section 3. We start with the predominant paradigm of personalised care and contrast this with views from a well-known critic, who explains his objections. We discuss how it is developing for children and young people, and we peek into the ethnography of general practice. From there we investigate social prescribing from the perspectives of NHS trusts; voluntary, community and social enterprise (VCSE); and higher education leaders.

Finally, Section 4 describes how social prescribing is being interpreted in practice, not just in health and care, but across partners connected to the wider determinants of health. We start with the experience of a social prescribing link worker in London and contrast this with how the City of London mayor's office is responding. We start to understand how the practice of community nursing, allied health professionals, emergency services and housing are responding, and we see how a former fishing town in northwest England is interpreting social prescribing in its own way, to support its renaissance.

Limitations

A book of this kind cannot cover every single aspect of social prescribing. It does not, for example, give an international perspective, although a couple of contributors allude to this. Editorial discretion has been used to curate what I hope is a range of interesting and thought-provoking voices from fields that perhaps you might not have thought to include in a book of this kind, such as the police. Over time, future editions will be able to document the evolution of social prescribing. For now, it is a snapshot of a moment where the health and care system has recognised that to be well, we need more than medicine.

REFERENCES

HM Treasury, 2021. Build back better: our plan for growth. https://assets.publishing.service.gov.uk/media/6048fd05d3bf7f1d16e263fd/PfG_Final_Web_Accessible_Version.pdf.

Hood, C.M., Gennuso, K.P., Swain, G.R., et al., 2016. County health rankings: relationships between determinant factors and health outcomes. Am. J. Prev. Med. 50 (2), 129–135.

Hope, D., Limburg, J., 2020. The economic consequences of major tax cuts for the rich. Working paper 55. London School of Economics.

L'Hôte, E., Castellina, M., Volmert, A. et al., 2022. A matter of life and death: explaining the wider determinants of health in the UK. Frameworks. Available from: https://www.health.org.uk/sites/default/files/upload/publications/2022/A%20matter%20of%20life%20and%20death_March%202022.pdf.

Lent, A., Studdart, S., 2021. The community paradigm: why public services need radical change and how it can be achieved. New Local. Available from: https://www.newlocal.org.uk/wp-content/uploads/2019/03/The-Community-Paradigm_New-Local-2.pdf (Accessed 23 December 2022).

Marmot, M., 2020. Health equity in England: the marmot review 10 years on. London: Institute of Health Equity.

Marmot, M., Allen, J., Goldblatt, P., et al., 2020. Build back fairer: the COVID-19 marmot review. The pandemic, socioeconomic and health inequalities in England. Institute of Health Equity, London.

McGarvey, D., 2022. The social distance between us: how remote politics wrecked Britain. Ebury Press, London.

O'Donnell, A., 2014. Wellbeing a sign of country's progress says ex-cabinet secretary. Huffington post. Available from: https://www.huffingtonpost.co.uk/2014/03/21/wellbeing-gdp-report-odonnell_n_5005570.html (Accessed 23 December 2022).

Wellbeing Economy Alliance. https://weall.org/.

What Works Wellbeing (online). What is wellbeing. Available from: https://whatworkswellbeing.org/about-wellbeing/what-is-wellbeing/ (Accessed 23 December 2022).

World Health Organization, 2021. Commercial determinants of health. Available from: https://www.who.int/news-room/fact-sheets/detail/commercial-determinants-of-health (Accessed 23 December 2022).

World Health Organization (online). Constitution. Available from: https://www.who.int/about/governance/constitution (Accessed 23 December 2022).

Chapter 2

Social Prescribing—Where Did It Come From and Where Is It Going?

Michael Dixon

Introduction

The concept of social prescribing is simple, and that may well be its strength. It is that our physical and social environment can have a huge impact on our health and healing—a potential that has been neglected by overmedicalisation and a culture that expects 'a pill for every ill'.

We are the air that we breathe, the food that we eat, the activities that we do and the social connections that we make. These are equally important in both health and healing. Seventy-five percent of cardiac disease is preventable, as is 25% of cancer. Our current medicine is completely failing to tackle the huge problems in society, for instance, the 40% of 11-year-old children in London who are overweight or obese, or the 25% of girls between ages 14 and 16 who are self-harming. Medicine must now extend its perspective and role from the biomedical to the psychosocial if it is to have the impact that it needs to have in the future. The National Health Service (NHS) is ideally placed to achieve this, and that may make it seem odd that social prescribing has only recently become national policy. Perhaps the vested interests of business, professionals and the NHS machine itself may have been factors, but the rapid national and now international spread of social prescribing may be evidence that we should have been doing this all along.

A PERSONAL PERSPECTIVE

In my 30s as a young general practitioner (GP) in Devon, my personal belief—that we GPs had a responsibility for the health and happiness of our local community as well as treating the individual patient in front of us—was regarded as eccentric. Colleagues would call me 'The Vicar' and say that I was treading on territory that was not relevant to the work of GPs, nor within its scope. Such ideals were simply not achievable. Now as an NHS GP in my 70s, it is a rewarding surprise to see these ideas becoming mainstream.

The Peckham Experiment

While the ideas behind social prescribing are as old as the hills, it is a relative newcomer as a national movement. Its roots can be traced back to the 'Peckham Experiment' (The Peckham Society, online), which was the brainchild of two GPs, Dr George Scott Williamson and Dr Innes Pearce, who ran a family practice in Peckham, London. The first centre operated between 1926 and 1929, with a purpose-built building replacing this in 1936 that provided a swimming pool, fitness centre, café and dance hall for their patients, with significant effects on their health and ability to resist disease. Families were encouraged to join for the sum of 1 shilling a week (£5 in today's money). Members themselves decided what activities they wanted to do and then organised them, rather than the staff. Ironically, the centre closed due to lack of funding in 1948—the year that the NHS was born. Maybe if the concept of preventing illness was understood back then, by understanding and addressing the social circumstances of people's lives rather than just by helping them when they were sick, it might have survived.

Bromley by Bow Centre

By 1984, the iconic Bromley by Bow NHS practice emerged when a church minister, Andrew Mawson, opened the church doors to the community (Bromley by Bow Centre, online). Andrew was soon joined by GP Dr Sam Everington, and the surgery now offers up to 100 social prescribing opportunities, from language and arts classes to gardening groups.

Perceiving the Role of General Practice Differently

At the beginning of the 21st century, a few GP practices were looking outside of the box in a similar way, but progress was still fragmented. Professor Chris Drinkwater, a GP in Newcastle, discovered the power of a men's fishing club to improve the mental health and employment status of its members. Another GP in Burnley, Dr James Fleming, had asked himself why he was giving antidepressants to patients who could not get jobs and set about supporting them with occupational experience instead in his 'Green Dreams' project. In my own NHS practice in Cullompton, Devon, we had 'knit and natter' groups for the isolated elderly and a range of self-help groups in our café; 'walk and talk' groups for young mothers and toddlers and patients that were stressed, depressed or overweight; as well as a wide range of gardening and health opportunities organised by the patients themselves.

In 2007, the then Secretary of State for Health, Alan Johnson, visited my practice and was surprised to hear about the wide range of problems facing GPs and their patients—such as overweight, back and neck pain, chronic fatigue, frequent infections, irritable bowel syndrome and premenstrual tension—for which modern medicine too frequently did not have effective answers. He commissioned our GP practice to produce information on these various conditions with a focus on what patients could do for themselves. Working with Bromley by Bow and taking evidence from the Universities of Exeter and Westminster (in London), our project leader, Simon Mills, a medical herbalist, produced a set of 12 guidelines for the self-treatment of a range of medical conditions (Self Care Toolkit, online). With the project completed, we then had to ask ourselves how this information could be used as effectively as possible. Leaflets and videos were the usual route, but we realised that there also needed to be a person who could initiate required changes that would both enable and motivate patients to take advantage of this information. So we recruited Ruth Tucker, with whom we had established an exercise on prescription programme in the town, to become our first 'Social Prescriber', who could be contacted by GPs in our practice via what we called a 'Desk Top Prescription'.

Social prescription was born!

The Language of 'Social Prescription'

The simplicity and clarity of the words 'Social Prescription' may have been partly responsible for subsequent events. The medical world liked the word 'prescription', while the volunteer/voluntary sector liked the 'social' bit. Conversely, many of the medics would protest at the 'social' bit entering their biomedical world with equal protests coming from the volunteer/voluntary sector that 'Social Prescription' was medicalising a good idea. By accident rather than design, it seems that we had stumbled upon something that would equally enthuse and alienate but at least capture people's imagination. Perhaps we had got it right.

THE CHALLENGE OF GAINING EVIDENCE

Our project generated widespread interest, but a number of medical professionals and managers told us that we would have to take things further and provide biomedical proof that social prescribing actually improved health and wellbeing if we were proposing it for wider use.

Things might have ended there but for two people. The first was Peter Stephens, CEO of 'Dial a Flight', who was interested in what we were doing and provided us with a substantial sum but clear instruction—'Prove your case and ensure that the idea spreads elsewhere within the NHS'. The other was Marie Polley, Senior Researcher at Westminster University. She oversaw the project in my surgery to provide social prescriptions for 142 prediabetic or diabetic patients, who were referred to Ruth as a social prescription for a period of 9 months. Our results showed that within those 9 months, a third had converted to no longer being either diabetic or prediabetic and that sustainable improvement was seen in the weight of the majority of those patients, especially if they had improved their 'patient activation index' (see Gilburt, 2014), showing that they were now in greater control of their own wellbeing and health.

Social Prescribing as a Social Movement

Our final findings (unpublished) were reported in March 2015. With the research completed it was on the train back to London with Marie that we asked ourselves the question, 'What next?' As we passed Reading station on the way from Cullompton to Paddington, we had that lightbulb moment: 'We must make this a popular national movement'.

So we wrote to around 15 clinicians, managers and researchers, who were already working on similar projects, asking if they would be interested in joining a self-elected steering group for developing and furthering social prescription. At our first meeting in the autumn of that year, we then decided to have a seminar/mini conference the following January for which Marie, much to her credit, was able to get a grant from the Wellcome Foundation. We didn't expect much interest but were surprised that 150 people applied to come to this first meeting—some of whom had to be turned away as there was only capacity for 100 at the Westminster University room that we had reserved. This was the event when social prescribing literally ignited. The energy and passion at that meeting led to a plan for a launch of social prescribing as a national movement in the House of Commons in March 2016, chaired by Stephen Dorrell, previously the Secretary of State for Health.

Representatives from NHS England came to the packed meeting and told me that they had heard about these developments and were thinking of doing some work on social prescribing themselves. They observed that our self-elected group had already got started—already with over a thousand members—and asked if we might link forces to develop social prescribing. NHS England would provide some limited funding to support the National Social Prescribing Network chaired by myself and Marie Polley and help fund regional conferences to broaden awareness. I became the NHS England National Clinical Champion for Social Prescription (I was to be the first and the last!), and at our regional conferences an increasing number of GP practices, commissioning groups and the odd health authority started taking a serious interest in social prescribing and began to provide funding for it. NHS England provided moral and practical support: Bev Taylor became the social prescribing lead at NHS England; Ian Dodge, the National Director for Primary Care, Community Services, and Strategy, maintained the profile of social prescribing at NHS England; and increasingly James Sanderson, the new head of personalised services at NHS England, injected extra energy into the movement. Inevitably there was some creative friction, but the combination of disruptive innovators working alongside national strategists led to a fruitful working relationship.

The Social Prescribing Network

The year 2017 saw the movement develop rapidly with the Social Prescribing Network now having 3000 members and uptake increasing every day. Yet there was a problem. Social prescribing had now become a postcode lottery. Its provision depended entirely upon having enthusiastic GP practices or clinical commissioning groups and/or local authorities that were prepared to fund it. An initiative that had been directly designed to address inequalities in patients who had the least—especially where health was concerned—was now creating geographical inequalities itself. This presented a challenge but also an opportunity because it then enabled us to campaign for national rollout.

To everyone's surprise at our National Social Prescribing Network national conference at the King's Fund the following year in November 2018, the then Secretary of State, Matt Hancock, declared that not only was social prescribing to become national policy, with a national rollout of social prescribing link workers, but he was also going to establish a National Academy of Social Prescribing that would help it to flourish. Today, many Primary Care Networks (a group of GP practices) have between two and three social prescribing link workers, and it has become 'business as usual' for many GP practices. Those who were initially resistant rapidly changed their minds when they found that social prescribing in practice both reduces the individual workload of the GP and creates sustainable health benefits for the patient.

A movement that had begun as a handful of enthusiasts had in just 3 years became national policy and was about to be implemented nationally with central funding. This rapid development was not the brainchild of politicians or some health policy think tank, nor was it based on incontrovertible evidence that social prescribing worked. It was partly because social prescribing became rapidly recognised as obviously beneficial and partly because patients and clinicians were seeing for themselves its often-immediate effects. This led to a mass movement nationwide that was then able to storm the barricades of conventional biomedical health policy and practice and open the floodgates to a new psychosocial model of medicine and health provision. History may well see this as the moment that we revised our thinking to see that a sustainable health system needs to be community based, making best use of the physical and social resources that are already there.

A Changing Focus

Perhaps at this point we should take a step back and describe social prescribing as it is today. Initially, the focus was on the socially isolated elderly person, someone with long-term disease or one of the 20% of patients who come to see us GPs with a primarily social problem. Increasingly, social prescribing is spreading its wings with a new focus on wider groups such as children and young people, who have particularly suffered during COVID, and an increasing number of social prescribing projects in schools, prisons and with armed forces veterans.

Then there have been changes to the prescriber of social solutions, traditionally a GP, but spreading to other members of the primary care health team, professionals in secondary care and increasingly, as word gets around, patients are referring themselves.

Link Worker Development

The crucial element in social prescribing is the skill of the social prescribing link worker. Their job is to get to know the patient—their strengths or assets, hopes, culture, history, beliefs and challenges. Many have training to learn about motivating people to self-care, to understand what matters to people and to

identify the root causes of problems. They are creating the sort of connection that GPs could initiate 40 years ago, when there was more time. Link workers' effectiveness depends upon their local knowledge, interpersonal skills and passion for the job. Many have a clinical background in nursing, occupational therapy, nutrition and other clinical areas. Increasingly, the link workers are people who themselves have benefitted from social prescription.

The rapid expansion of social prescription has led the link worker community to develop their own membership organisation—The National Association of Link Workers. This has led to developing a national training programme and the exchange of ideas.

Health, Hope and Happiness

Link workers develop a trusting relationship that enables them to formulate a plan with the person that is designed to improve their life, happiness and health. The end point is to provide someone, who may be lost and at their lowest ebb, with meaning, significance and hope in their lives to lead them towards a happier and healthier life.

The success stories behind social prescribing are endless. Debs Taylor (online), one of our College of Medicine national patient champions, describes how social prescribing took her from someone very wounded and dependent upon mental health services and drugs to becoming an artist and master of her own destiny, now working to ensure that others have the same opportunities. Sean Jennings (online), another patient champion, was addicted to high doses of medically prescribed opiates for back pain and was able to stop them entirely as a result of social prescription. Professor Chris Drinkwater, a key member of our original leadership group, paid for social prescribing (before it was supported nationally) in Newcastle West using a 'Social Impact Bond' where organisations invest money and gain financial returns related to social outcomes (Bridges, online). This was paid off after 6 years through the financial return on delivery of outcomes (improved wellbeing and savings in secondary care costs). The original programme is now NHS funded and the delivery organisation (Ways to Wellness) has subsequently developed a range of other social prescribing services.

Criticisms

Nevertheless, academics still say, quite reasonably, that social prescribing does not yet have an absolutely firm evidence base, but as the Rotherham social prescribing commissioning manager once said, 'It is just plain common sense'.

The health and care system is now creating supportive partnerships with communities that understand what they need to thrive—and developing their services accordingly. This is beneficial to both. Early exploitative approaches, where the NHS described the voluntary sector as a cheap money-saving solution, have dissolved into more respect and investment. The truth to tell is that the success of social prescribing as a movement has not been built upon evidence but upon mass enthusiasm based on what people are seeing with their own eyes. The use of penicillin did not initially require evidence as we now know it because it was obvious that people were getting better. Social prescribing may, historically, fit into the same category.

Apart from comments that social prescribing had not built up a sufficient evidence base, there was also some early criticism that social prescribing was really a side show and seemed to be overshadowing the much more important task of developing 'Health Creating Communities', which would in the long term be a more important factor in enabling health services themselves to be sustainable. The concepts behind health creation are covered in Section 2. I have often described social prescribing as the 'Trojan horse' for doing exactly that—developing healthier communities. This is now visibly beginning to happen.

A Capacity Challenge

In the early days of social prescription, where it was successful, we found that it was rapidly swamping the capacity of local volunteer and voluntary services to provide help. Social prescribing has created a demand for extending local community groups and increased the supply and thus the potential for using the local physical and social environment to improve the health of everyone. For many people, this enhanced range of activities can be easily accessed through 'signposting'. But in communities that are 'easily overlooked', such as males of working age, the social prescribing link workers are as relevant as ever in helping those most in need or most invisible to get started and fulfill their potential for health and happiness. In this way, social prescribing is not just addressing the inequalities of the individual patient but also beginning to help communities develop their offer for everyone.

Inevitably, social prescribing has put increasing demands on the voluntary, community and social enterprise sector, whose funding has been hard hit by COVID. The job of 'increasing local social capital' has led voluntary, community and social enterprise support organisations to develop various ways to support local community groups. The sector has also lobbied for sustainable investment, leading to different funding models (Kimberlee et al., 2022). Local and national initiatives such as The National Academy of Social Prescribing's 'Thriving Communities' Fund have aimed to fill this funding gap. With the NHS increasingly struggling to provide sufficient resources and professionals to meet demand, leading to a subsequent negative impact on quality and access, the role of the community is becoming increasingly important in extending what is available for improving health and care. Integrated care systems hold the keys to collectively make this happen and will be the new engine room, shifting away from the traditionally secondary care–centric, disease-focused NHS. This is largely because of their combined ability to mobilise local resources as social prescribing has done. This is not a pipe dream.

Reconnecting Public Services With Their Communities

Some areas of the country are working to re-create the connections that we have lost in our increasingly alienated societies. For instance, in Frome in Somerset, there are now 1800 volunteer community connectors—taxi drivers, hairdressers, shop assistants, students etc.—who support their local social prescribing link workers and help to connect local people to the various physical and social various opportunities available. In Ilfracombe, Devon, each street has a volunteer coordinator, who ensures that everyone on that street can get the relevant volunteer/voluntary services. 'Altogether

Better' (https://www.altogetherbetter.org.uk), a spin-out social enterprise from the NHS, has helped general practices across the country to mobilise around 25,000 voluntary Patient Champions in GP practices throughout the country. These champions self-organise to create social solutions such as allotment groups, mirroring the approach of members of the Peckham Experiment.

During the COVID pandemic, we saw 750,000 volunteers come forward wanting to support the health service. With three-quarters of the population already volunteering at least once a year, there lies an immense potential to develop this whole area and create sustainable healthy communities. It just needs leadership and a process of 'normalising' volunteering so that it becomes part of life—similar to the path that social prescribing itself has trod. It also needs minimal seed funding, which will require some flexibility and original thought on the part of financially squeezed health commissioners used to the rigid processes for funding evidence-based biomedical interventions.

A Global Alliance

Social prescribing is developing rapidly right across the United Kingdom. In Scotland there is a nascent Social Prescribing Network, and social prescription is widely available, for instance via 'community connectors' in East Ayrshire. In Wales there are many clusters of social prescribing excellence, and social prescribing is currently part of a Welsh Government consultation (August 2022). Northern Ireland has also developed social prescription in many areas, including a women's prison in Belfast. The Social Prescribing Network lead there, Tony Doherty, works closely with his Republic of Ireland counterpart, David Robinson, a consultant physician, as part of a pan-Ireland initiative to progress social prescription.

As I write, 22 countries are now signed up to the Global Alliance on Social Prescribing led by the National Academy of Social Prescribing and supported by a number of organisations including the World Health Organization and the United Nations. Britain should take pride in having been the birthplace of this. In some countries, such as the Republic of Ireland, the Netherlands and Finland, they are approaching national rollout. Canada and Australia are well on their way, while Portugal and the United States are taking their first steps but accelerating in a similar way to the UK experience. New countries are joining the Alliance every month with the same enthusiasm and willingness to burn the midnight oil that enabled social prescribing to thrive in the United Kingdom. Their values and recognition of the central role of the social prescribing link worker are the same. The models differ. For instance, in the Netherlands the link worker is a professional social worker in a different role, while most are being supported by their municipalities/local authorities rather than their health service. The United Kingdom—albeit with the advantage of having an NHS—has been able to assemble and support this rapid development on the international scene.

Conclusion

Make no mistake, there are numerous bridges still to be crossed and battles to be fought. Endless problems remain, as ever, whether it be convincing GP colleagues, supporting investment in the voluntary and social enterprise sector, preventing the bureaucratisation and throttling of social prescription or navigating the ebb and flow of political change. Nor does any movement ever stand still. Nevertheless, it seems that the concepts behind social prescription are now here to stay and that the medical landscape has changed forever.

At our last National Social Prescribing Network international conference in March 2022, Sir Michael Marmot noted the horrific health inequalities in the United Kingdom, especially post COVID. He said that beyond changing national policy to reduce the difference between the wealthy and the poor, social prescription at local level was in his opinion now the most powerful instrument for addressing those health inequalities.

This development, as I have described, has been a mass movement fired by a few leaders, who have given up their time and on occasion their credibility to make things happen. Many of them are still part of the steering group of the National Social Prescribing Network. It is to them as friends, colleagues and co-conspirators that I give my eternal thanks.

REFERENCES

The Bridges. Available from: https://www.bridgesfundmanagement.com/bridges-commits-1-65m-first-active-social-impact-bond-uk-health-care-sector/.

Bromley by Bow Centre. Available from: https://www.bbbc.org.uk/ (Accessed 24 August 2022).

Debs Taylor. Available from: https://www.youtube.com/watch?v=GT35aDMbTAI.

Gilburt, H., 2014. Supporting people to manage their health: an introduction to patient activation. King's Fund, London.

Kimberlee, R., Bertotti, M., Dayson, C., Elston, J., Polley, M., Burns, L., Husk, K., [On behalf of the NASP Academic Partners Collaborative]., 2022. '(Sustainable) funding models for social prescribing'. National Academy for Social Prescribing, London.

The Peckham Society. Available from: https://www.peckhamsociety.org.uk/ (Accessed 24 August 2022).

Sean Jennings. Available from: https://www.england.nhs.uk/south/2019/06/25/seans-story/.

Self Care Toolkit. Available from: https://selfcaretoolkit.net/ (Accessed 24 August 2022).

Chapter 3

What Is Wellbeing and What Keeps Us Well?

Nancy Hey

Introduction

Improving wellbeing and reducing wellbeing inequality are key measures of a country's success, something for us all to aim for, now and for the future.

To help improve wellbeing in the United Kingdom, What Works Centre for Wellbeing accelerates research and democratises access to robust wellbeing evidence. We do this by collaborating and sharing insights with the research community and decision-makers in government, business, third-sector organisations and communities. We work closely with partners to answer key questions and identify gaps in the research to be filled.

The Centre was established in 2014 under the 2010 to 2015 Conservative and Liberal Democrat coalition government and is part of the What Works Network and The Evidence Quarter. This network improves the way the UK government and other organisations create, share and use high-quality evidence for decision-making.

As wellbeing evidence has gained prominence in the integrated health care system, this chapter provides an introduction to what works to improve wellbeing. We hope readers will be able to use these insights to build their understanding and to design practices using a wellbeing lens.

What Do We Mean by Wellbeing?

National wellbeing is 'how we're doing' as individuals, communities and as a nation, and how sustainable that is for the future. At an individual level, it concerns

With thanks to Robyn Bignall-Donnelly, Lizzy Hvide, Stewart Martin, Margherita Musella, Ingrid Abreu Scherer and Joanne Smithson.

whether we are feeling good and functioning well. Community wellbeing is 'being well together'.

In economics, wellbeing is sometimes referred to as social welfare or social value.

WHAT MAKES UP WELLBEING?

Wellbeing encompasses the environmental factors that affect us and how we function in society, and the subjective experiences we have throughout our lives.

It can be defined as having 10 broad dimensions:

1. The natural environment
2. Personal (subjective) wellbeing
3. Our relationships
4. Health
5. What we do
6. Where we live
7. Personal finance
8. The economy
9. Education and skills
10. Governance

These dimensions were identified through national debate, run by the Measuring National Wellbeing Programme at the UK Office for National Statistics (ONS) from 2010 to 2011, and benefitting from guidance by leading international experts (Oman, 2016). The dimensions of wellbeing provide a useful starting point for the exploratory 'what matters to me' conversations which are at the heart of social prescribing.

Crucially, wellbeing recognises the aspects of our lives that we determine ourselves, through our own capabilities as individuals. This subjective wellbeing is an important dimension, related to how satisfied we are with our lives, our sense that what we do in life is worthwhile (purpose), our day-to-day emotional experiences (happiness and anxiety) and our wider mental wellbeing.

If these dimensions are a way of understanding 'how we're doing', then social prescribing digs into 'what matters' to us: How do these dimensions translate into our everyday lives, and how are they balanced differently for different people at different stages of their lives?

These psychological needs are an important part of what makes us human. It matters how often, and for how long, we experience positive emotions—such as pleasure and a sense of purpose—or potentially negative emotions, like anxiety.

Wellbeing is responsive and dynamic, fluctuating across people's lives. Evidence indicates that we can adapt to some changes, such as relationship breakdown, although our wellbeing is less resilient to other negative circumstances such as longer-term unemployment.

POPULAR MODELS AND FRAMEWORKS FOR UNDERSTANDING WELLBEING

Perhaps the most well known to health care practitioners is the **Five Ways to Wellbeing (2018)**, developed by the New Economics Foundation. These are simple, evidence-based actions that individuals can do in their everyday lives: connect, be active, take notice, keep learning, give. Since their publication, they have been commonly used as an engagement tool in school curriculums, the NHS, the voluntary sector and by local authorities.

A way of understanding wellbeing is how well people are able to flourish—whether they feel positive emotions, can function well in society, can respond to challenges and find meaning in their lives—even as things change. Recent definitions of flourishing combine hedonic (pleasurable) and eudaimonia (living well) elements to create a more comprehensive and holistic approach, implying feeling satisfied with life and having the ability to live to the fullest (Chaves, 2021).

This approach is referred to as **PERMA** (Positive emotion, Engagement, Relationships, Meaning and Accomplishment [Seligman, 2012]) and is most commonly found in the field of positive psychology.

At its best, social prescribing looks at people's hopes and aspirations—as well as challenges—to build a sustainable plan for flourishing. In that context, PERMA can help social prescribers to explore drivers to gain deeper insight and offer a more nuanced and effective referral. For example, in the past there may have been a tendency for general practitioners (GPs) to refer directly to gyms for physical fitness, which was not always a sustainable intervention. Now, link workers dig into the barriers to starting physical activity (engagement); suggest activities that are stimulating, like nature walks (positive emotion); and connect people to volunteer 'buddies' who can help them get started and keep going (relationships).

New Economic Foundation's model of wellbeing (Fig. 3.1) describes how someone's external conditions interact with their personal resources to allow them to function well and experience positive emotions.

An applied example of the dynamic model of wellbeing (Fig. 3.1) might be a person who loses their job. The change to their *external conditions* affects their ability to feel good and function well; their self-esteem and optimism (*personal resources)* fall due to the loss of professional identity, which is compounded by the financial strain of lost income and financial stability. They feel isolated without anyone to talk to, and their mental health worsens. When they visit their GP with depression, a link worker signposts them to a self-help group. Their *personal resources* start to build as they connect with and learn from others about how to cope. Feeling supported, they successfully apply for another job, improving their security and independence, which positively feeds back into their ability to feel good and function well.

Well-known international wellbeing frameworks include the Sustainable Development Goals, endorsed by more than 150 countries and including targets for the environment, safety and health (United Nations, 2022), and the Organisation for Economic Co-operation and Development Better Life Index (OECD, 2022). Governments and regional bodies around the world, from the European Union to New Zealand, are explicit in their goals to target and value key aspects of wellbeing using frameworks and regular measurement.

IS WELLBEING UNIVERSAL?

Wherever you are and whatever your cultural background or personal circumstances, people intuitively understand the value of happiness and wellbeing.

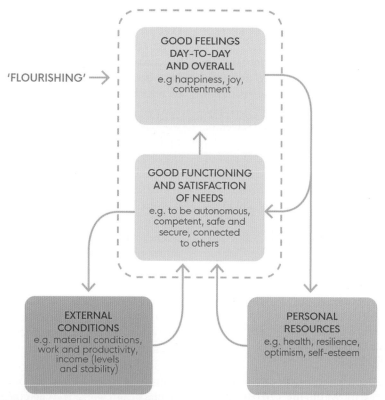

'FLOURISHING' →

GOOD FEELINGS
DAY-TO-DAY
AND OVERALL
e.g happiness, joy,
contentment

GOOD FUNCTIONING
AND SATISFACTION
OF NEEDS
e.g. to be autonomous,
competent, safe and
secure, connected
to others

EXTERNAL
CONDITIONS
e.g. material conditions,
work and productivity,
income (levels
and stability)

PERSONAL
RESOURCES
e.g. health, resilience,
optimism, self-esteem

Fig. 3.1 New Economic Foundation's dynamic model of wellbeing. From Abdallah, S., Mahony, S., Marks, N., Michaelson, J., Seafod, C., Stoll, L., and Thompson, S., 2011. *Measuring our progress: the power of well-being.*

Despite the universality of these concepts, everyone has a different starting level when it comes to wellbeing. If you imagine people on a wellbeing ladder, those who are towards the bottom may have a harder time moving up towards better wellbeing than those nearer the top. This is because the rungs of the ladder are not equal. Low wellbeing tends to be caused by serious or multiple factors which are not easy to overcome.

If we accept that some aspects of wellbeing are subjective, we can better understand the interactions and trade-offs between different experiences. We can also take into account the longer-term effects and the varying importance of the domains to different people.

We know that most of these aspects have a diminishing influence on our wellbeing the more we have. For example, £10 makes a much bigger difference to someone on minimum wage compared to someone already earning £35,000 a year. Similarly, having one more friend to rely on makes a bigger difference to those with a small social network compared to someone with many friends.

What affects wellbeing is different for everyone. So, no matter how many positive things we have in our lives, if we don't experience or feel that our lives are going well, then this is our reality. No one factor will make us completely happy if another important factor is missing. For example, a person with high financial security but no meaningful social connections may experience low wellbeing due to loneliness and lack of connection. In short, a balance is important in order to thrive.

WELLBEING INEQUALITIES AND LEVELLING UP

Some people are more likely to experience low wellbeing than others. People with the poorest personal wellbeing are most likely to have at least one of the following characteristics or circumstances:

- Self-report very bad or bad health

- Be economically inactive with long-term illness or disability
- Be middle-aged
- Be single, separated, widowed or divorced
- Be renters
- Have no or basic education

The COVID-19 pandemic has amplified inequalities across society, including wellbeing. The pressures of the pandemic on health, jobs, social connections and education have meant that some groups are now at greater risk of having low wellbeing.

To combat geographical inequality and give everyone the opportunity to flourish, the UK Government laid out 12 cross-society missions in its *Levelling Up the United Kingdom* white paper (2022). The missions reflect the key drivers for wellbeing, such as housing, skills and pride in place. They include closing gaps related to the aims of social prescribing, such as in healthy life expectancy and wellbeing, by 2030.

MEASURING WELLBEING

Wellbeing measurement is widely recognised as an evidence-informed approach to understanding how services, projects or programmes make a difference.

Used alongside traditional indicators of progress such as gross domestic product (GDP) or life expectancy, measuring wellbeing can capture what matters most to us and the places where we live.

Detailed guidance on measuring wellbeing is available on the Centre's website: measure.whatworkswellbeing.org.

What Do We Know About What Makes People Well?

The three biggest drivers of adult life satisfaction are physical and mental health, relationships and work. This can be thought of as feeling loved, feeling safe and feeling fulfilled.

Our wide-ranging rapid evidence reviews indicate that creative, social and physical health interventions improve overall wellbeing, as well as decrease loneliness (Blodgett et al., 2022). These include many of the activities that are socially prescribed, such as culture and sports programmes, group exercise, arts-based interventions, volunteering, adult learning and nature therapy, including gardening.

This positive effect may be because such activities can:

- Be fun and facilitate engagement and social connection
- Be relaxing or absorbing
- Offer an interesting learning opportunity and challenge
- Provide structure and achievement
- Cultivate a sense of agency and control

Here we offer an overview of things we know work to improve wellbeing so far, based on the evidence.

1. *Physical and mental health*

On average, the experience and perception of our mental and physical health is the biggest single factor that explains how we rate our wellbeing.

For example, outdoor activities and exercise have been found to have a positive impact on mental health (Mansfield, 2018). This includes engaging with green (nature) and blue (water) spaces, which is associated with a higher sense of purpose (What Works Centre for Wellbeing, 2021) and reduced place-based disparities in wellbeing (Abdallah et al., 2017).

The relationship between health and wellbeing is two-way, with one influencing the other. Good physical and mental health is associated with higher life satisfaction, while high wellbeing correlates with health outcomes such as improved immune system response and higher pain tolerance (Fig. 3.2).

2. *Relationships*

Getting involved in **community activities** can:

- Affect both physical and mental health
- Help people to connect to others, which can particularly help in terms of building trust and self-confidence
- Increase social cohesion by bringing different groups together
- Help people to increase their skills

The places where we live, work and spend time have an impact on our wellbeing. So do the people we know—and encounter—in these places. Activities that take place in community hubs or cultural heritage spaces may improve a sense of trust, belonging and pride in the local area (Bagnall et al., 2018).

Music, arts and **crafts** activities can create the conditions for wellbeing (Tomlinson, 2018; Daykin, 2016). They have been found to have a positive effect on mental health, as well as helping some groups to

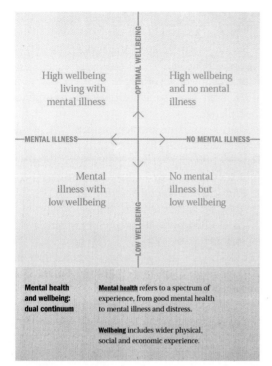

High wellbeing living with mental illness

High wellbeing and no mental illness

OPTIMAL WELLBEING

—MENTAL ILLNESS— ⟵ ⟶ —NO MENTAL ILLNESS—

Mental illness with low wellbeing

No mental illness but low wellbeing

LOW WELLBEING

Mental health and wellbeing: dual continuum

Mental health refers to a spectrum of experience, from good mental health to mental illness and distress.

Wellbeing includes wider physical, social and economic experience.

Fig. 3.2 Grid. From de Pury, J., Dicks, A., 2020. *Step change: mentally healthy universities.* Universities UK.

improve their self-esteem, share their experiences and feel a sense of purpose.

Volunteering has an impact on physical and mental health, as well as creating a sense of identity and purpose (Grotz, 2020). It can also help people to build their social relationships and encourage people to continue to volunteer in their communities.

When done well, community engagement in decision-making can directly impact on wellbeing, build social networks and improve social cohesion (Pennington et al., 2018).

The National Academy of Social Prescribing (2022a; 2022b) has created a guide for volunteer-involving organisations that identifies key steps to make the experience work for people who may come to volunteering as part of a social prescribing journey.

3. *Work and what we do*

Being employed is the third biggest factor associated with wellbeing after our mental and physical health and our personal relationships.

Being out of work is damaging for wellbeing, regardless of age, gender, location, ethnicity and level of education. The effect is as big as bereavement, and the longer the period of unemployment, the worse the effect. Support that helps people to find work through high-quality information is effective at boosting wellbeing (What Works Centre for Wellbeing, 2017a).

Beyond employment, job quality matters (What Works Centre for Wellbeing, 2017b). Our feelings of wellbeing at work are influenced by day-to-day experiences with colleagues and management, and how purposeful or meaningful we feel.

Employers have a major influence on a person's sense of wellbeing, which can have a multitude of benefits for the organisation itself. For example, research funded by the Department of Health shows that 'good management of National Health Service (NHS) staff leads to higher quality of care, more satisfied patients and lower patient mortality. Good staff management offers significant financial savings for the NHS, as its leaders respond to the challenge of sustainability in the face of increasing costs and demands' (West et al., 2011, p. 2). Working with employees and providing in-work support can help career progression and retention.

Learning at work can help people to build confidence and feel a sense of purpose and progress (What Works Centre for Wellbeing, 2017c). According to research by the Department for Business Innovation and Skills, taking a part-time course for work has been estimated to give wellbeing benefits equivalent to £1584 of income per year (Dolan and Fujiwara, 2012).

When learning is through a hobby or leisure activity, this can have a large impact on life satisfaction, especially for those living in more disadvantaged areas (What Works Centre for Wellbeing, 2018).

THE ROLE OF SOCIAL PRESCRIBING

We know that creative, social and physical health activities are likely to have a wellbeing benefit. These can be accessed in a variety of ways, so what is it about social prescribing that might be making an additional difference?

Evidence suggests that interventions need to be tailored to individuals to be effective (Victor, 2018). Social prescribing does this by using a person-centred approach—asking 'what matters to me' rather than 'what's the matter with me'—and an asset-based methodology that harnesses the person's strengths, experience and skills. Working collaboratively to co-develop an action plan can help individuals to have a sense of agency while also giving them the tailored support they need. In this way the mechanism of social prescribing itself enhances the wellbeing benefit of prescribed activities.

GROWING THE EVIDENCE BASE

The What Works Centre for Wellbeing has a variety of digital resources detailing key findings, knowledge gaps and recommendations from systematic and rapid evidence reviews from 2016 to present. This also includes an interactive, searchable knowledge bank consolidating insights from 16 systematic reviews on wellbeing and culture and sport, work and learning and community wellbeing (What Works Centre for Wellbeing, 2019).

We are continuing to investigate not just what works but the how and why.

In the case of social prescribing, approaches need to be further explored so we can pull out the 'golden threads'—the key elements or benefits underpinning activities that help to improve wellbeing—to enable us to better understand what works and deliver more robust recommendations.

Summary

Wellbeing has 10 dimensions:
1. The natural environment
2. Personal (subjective) wellbeing
3. Our relationships
4. Health
5. What we do
6. Where we live
7. Personal finance
8. The economy
9. Education and skills
10. Governance

Wellbeing:
• Varies over time
• Is both objective and subjective
• Is about feeling good and functioning well
• Is multidimensional
• Is measurable
• Has a two-way relationship with health
• Can be thought of as a ladder with unequal rungs, leading to inequalities with those experiencing low levels of wellbeing finding it harder to experience high levels of wellbeing
• Is used alongside traditional indicators of progress to understand what matters most and inform future decision-making
• Can be improved through creative, social and physical health activities

The three biggest drivers of adult life satisfaction are:
1. Physical and mental health
2. Relationships
3. Work

Models and frameworks to conceptualise wellbeing include:
• Five Ways to Wellbeing
• PERMA
• New Economic Foundation's model of wellbeing
• Sustainable Development Goals
• The OECD Better Life Index

Further What Works Wellbeing Resources

For charities, practitioners and community organisations:
• What Works Wellbeing, 2022. *Brief guide to measuring loneliness.* Available from: https://whatworkswellbeing.org/resources/brief-guide-to-measuring-loneliness/ (Accessed 9 December 2022).
• Bagnall, A., Jane South, J., Mitchell, B., Pilkington, G., Newton, R. Salvatore Di Martino, S., 2017. *Systematic scoping review of indicators of community wellbeing in the UK VERSION 1.2.* Available from: https://whatworkswellbeing.org/resources/community-wellbeing-indicators/ (Accessed 9 December 2022).

For employers:
• What Works Wellbeing, 2022. *Workplace wellbeing question bank.* Available from: https://whatworkswellbeing.org/resources/workplace-wellbeing-question-bank/ (Accessed 9 December 2022).
• What Works Wellbeing, 2022. *Guide to better workplace wellbeing.* Available from: https://whatworkswellbeing.org/guidance-for-better-workplace-wellbeing/ (Accessed 9 December 2022).

- What Works Wellbeing, 2022. *Employee wellbeing snapshot survey.* Available from: https://whatworkswellbeing.org/category/employee-snapshot-survey/ (Accessed 9 December 2022).
- What Works Wellbeing, 2022. *Wellbeing benchmarks—how is your organisation doing?* Available from: https://whatworkswellbeing.org/wp-content/uploads/2020/04/www-benchmarks1.pdf (Accessed 9 December 2022).
- What Works Wellbeing, 2020. *How cost effective is a workplace wellbeing activity?* Available from: https://whatworkswellbeing.org/resources/how-cost-effective-is-a-workplace-wellbeing-activity/ (Accessed 9 December 2022).
- What Works Wellbeing, 2022. Brief guide to measuring loneliness. Available from: https://whatworkswellbeing.org/resources/brief-guide-to-measuring-loneliness/ (Accessed 9 December 2022).

For government—national, devolved, local and wider public sector:

- Guide to wellbeing economic evaluation. Available from: https://whatworkswellbeing.org/resources/a-guide-to-wellbeing-economic-evaluation/ (Accessed 9 December 2022).
- UK Government, 2022. *The green book* Available from: https://assets.publishing.service.gov.uk/government/uploads/system/uploads/attachment_data/file/1063330/Green_Book_2022.pdf (Accessed 9 December 2022).

REFERENCES

Abdallah, S., Wheatley, H., Quick, A., 2017. Drivers of wellbeing inequality: inequalities in life satisfaction across local authorities in Great Britain.

Bagnall, A., South, J., Di Martino, S., Southby, K., Pilkington, G., Mitchell, B., Pennington, A., Corcoran, R., 2018. A systematic review of interventions to boost social relations through improvements in community infrastructure (places and spaces). Report for what works Centre for Wellbeing. Available from: https://whatworkswellbeing.org/product/places-spaces-people-and-wellbeing/ (Accessed 9 December 2022).

Blodgett, J., Kaushal, A., Harkness, F., 2022. Rapid review of wellbeing evaluation research using the Warwick-Edinburgh mental well-being scales (WEMWBS) commissioned by the what works centre for wellbeing. Available from: https://whatworkswellbeing.org/wp-content/uploads/2022/05/WEMWBS_Rapid_Review_final.pdf (Accessed 9 December 2022).

Chaves, C., 2021. Wellbeing and flourishing. In: Kern, M.L., Wehmeyer, M.L. (eds.), The Palgrave Handbook of Positive Education. Palgrave Macmillan, Cham, pp. 273–295. https://doi.org/10.1007/978-3-030-64537-3_11.

Daykin, N., 2016. Music, singing and wellbeing in healthy adults. Report for what works centre for wellbeing. Available from: https://whatworkswellbeing.org/wp-content/uploads/2020/01/1-systematic-review-healthy-adult-music-singing-wellbeing-nov-2016final.pdf (Accessed 9 December 2022).

Dolan, P., Fujiwara, D., 2012. Valuing adult learning: comparing wellbeing valuation and contingent valuation. Research paper number 85. Available from: https://assets.publishing.service.gov.uk/government/uploads/system/uploads/attachment_data/file/34598/12-1127-valuing-adult-learning-comparing-wellbeing-to-contingent.pdf (Accessed 9 December 2022).

Five Ways to Wellbeing, 2018. *Five ways to wellbeing.* Available from: http://www.fivewaystowellbeing.org/ (Accessed 9 December 2022).

Grotz, J., 2020. *Volunteering – wellbeing – volunteering: a virtuous cycle?* Available from: https://whatworkswellbeing.org/category/volunteering-and-wellbeing/ (Accessed 9 December 2022).

Mansfield, L., 2018. A systematic review of outdoor recreation (in green space and blue space) for families to promote subjective wellbeing. Report for what works Centre for Wellbeing. Available from: https://whatworkswellbeing.org/product/family-and-outdoor-recreation/ (Accessed 9 December 2022).

National Academy for Social Prescribing, 2022a. *NASP evidence note: social prescribing and mental health.* Available from: https://socialprescribingacademy.org.uk/our-work/accelerating-innovation/volunteering-for-wellbeing-guide/ (Accessed 9 December 2022).

National Academy for Social Prescribing, 2022b. *Volunteering for wellbeing guide: how to link to social prescribing.* Available from: https://socialprescribingacademy.org.uk/our-work/accelerating-innovation/volunteering-for-wellbeing-guide/ (Accessed 9 December 2022).

OECD (Organisation for Economic Co-operation and Development), 2020. *Better life index.* Available from: http://www.oecdbetterlifeindex.org/#/11111111111 (Accessed 9 December 2022).

Office for National Statistics, 2022. *Measures of national wellbeing dashboard.* Available from: https://www.ons.gov.uk/peoplepopulationandcommunity/wellbeing/articles/measuresofnationalwellbeingdashboardqualityoflifeintheuk/2022-08-12 (Accessed 9 December 2022).

Oman, S., 2016. Measuring national wellbeing: what matters to you? What matters to whom? In: White, S.C., Blackmore, C. (eds.), Cultures of Wellbeing. Palgrave Macmillan, London, pp. 66–94. https://doi.org/10.1057/9781137536457_3.

Pennington, A., Watkins, M., Bagnall, A., South, J., Corcoran, R., 2018. A systematic review of evidence on the impacts of joint decision-making on community wellbeing. Report for what works Centre for Wellbeing. Available from: https://whatworkswellbeing.org/product/joint-decision-making-briefing/ (Accessed 9 December 2022).

Seligman, M.E.P., 2012. Flourish: a visionary new understanding of happiness and well-being, Atria.

Tomlinson, A., 2018. Visual arts and health. Report for what works Centre for Wellbeing. Available from: https://whatworkswellbeing.org/wp-content/uploads/2020/01/Full-report-art-mental-health-wellbeing-Jan2018_0146725200.pdf (Accessed 9 December 2022).

UK Government, 2022. Levelling up the United Kingdom. Available from: https://www.gov.uk/government/publications/levelling-up-the-united-kingdom (Accessed 9 December 2022).

United Nations, 2022. The sustainable development agenda. Available from: https://www.un.org/sustainabledevelopment/development-agenda/ (Accessed 9 December 2022).

Victor, C., 2018. An overview of reviews: the effectiveness of interventions to address loneliness at all stages of the life-course. Report for what works Centre for Wellbeing. Available from: https://whatworkswellbeing.org/resources/tackling-loneliness-review-of-reviews/ (Accessed 9 December 2022).

West, M., Dawson, J., Admasachew, L., Topakas, A., 2011. NHS staff management and health service quality. Available from: https://assets.publishing.service.gov.uk/government/uploads/system/uploads/attachment_data/file/215455/dh_129656.pdf (Accessed 9 December 2022).

What Works Centre for Wellbeing, 2017a. *Unemployment, (re) employment and wellbeing*. Available from: https://whatworkswellbeing.org/product/unemployment-reemployment-and-wellbeing/ (Accessed 9 December 2022).

What Works Centre for Wellbeing, 2017b. *Job quality and wellbeing*. Available from: https://whatworkswellbeing.org/product/job-quality-and-wellbeing/ (Accessed 9 December 2022).

What Works Centre for Wellbeing, 2017c. *Learning at work and wellbeing*. Available from: https://whatworkswellbeing.org/resources/learning-at-work-and-wellbeing/ (Accessed 9 December 2022).

What Works Centre for Wellbeing, 2018. *Adult learning and life satisfaction*. Available from: https://whatworkswellbeing.org/product/adult-learning-life-satisfaction/ (Accessed 9 December 2022).

What Works Centre for Wellbeing, 2019. Evidence knowledge bank. Available from: https://whatworkswellbeing.org/resources/evidence-knowledge-bank-draft/ (Accessed 9 December 2022).

What Works Centre for Wellbeing, 2021. What matters for our sense of purpose? Available from: https://whatworkswellbeing.org/resources/sense-of-purpose-covid/ (Accessed 9 December 2022).

Chapter 4

History of Social Prescribing

James Sanderson

Introduction

Modern medicine is arguably one of humanity's greatest achievements—the discovery of antibiotics, the development of vaccines, the ability to X-ray the human body, the multiple advancements in surgery and complex treatments for major diseases, to name just a few major leaps.

The positive advancements we have seen in health care over the past 100 years have contributed to people enjoying longer lives in developing countries across the globe. In the United Kingdom, we have seen life expectancy increase by over 15 years since the creation of the NHS in 1948—a remarkable jump over a relatively short period of time.

However, we know that longer lives do not necessarily equate to healthier lives, and during this same period we have also seen a rise in multimorbidity and a level of complexity in health that can limit the effectiveness of a single-treatment pathway.

This has created new pressures both for people and health care systems. The consequence of longer survival means that the population of the world is ageing—we have just passed the 8 billion threshold of people living together on our planet, and we are seeing the pressures that this brings to our infrastructure, our resources and our climate.

We know modern medicine is amazing. However, we are increasingly seeing the drawbacks too—antimicrobial resistance puts our ability to fight infections at risk, there are increasing consequences of addiction to opiates, and polypharmacy is placing new pressures on health systems. To illustrate just one of the challenges, it has been found that one in five people over the age of 65 who are in hospital in the United Kingdom are there not because of the conditions they are living with, but because of the drugs they have been prescribed (Department of Health and Social Care, online).

We also know from countless studies that the effects of social determinants of health are having a big impact on people's health outcomes, which, unless we tackle them, will only bring wider gaps and inequalities between the richest and poorest in society.

Societal issues frequently manifest in presentations to health professionals; in the United Kingdom, at least one in five GP appointments are for issues that do not have a medical origin (Citizens Advice, online). The pressures of modern living, loneliness, social isolation, debt, housing and relationships are all common issues resulting in a visit to general practice.

So, whilst medicine is amazing, medicalising social problems is not the answer, nor does medicine hold all the keys to supporting people throughout their lives. And alongside the power of medicine, we know that nonmedical interventions can greatly enhance health outcomes.

That's where social prescribing comes in.

History

Social prescribing responds to these challenges by adopting a holistic and asset-based approach to health and focusing on what matters to an individual. Then, based on individual circumstances and needs, a plan is developed that supports and delivers psychosocial interventions to improve health outcomes. It helps build relationships, unlock individual strengths, increase choice and control, and support connections within the communities where people live.

In England, social prescribing has been around in various forms for many years. Some point to the origins being in 1928 as part of what was known as the Peckham Experiment, which ran until 1950 and provided local families with a range of activities in a purpose-built centre for a nominal fee. Doctors monitored and observed the families and found that they would thrive when given the freedom to make choices about their activities; that they would choose activities which would help their development; and that, given resources in a community, people would be active in their community and help it to grow. They concluded that health is more than simply an absence of disease and identified the critical role of environment in promoting good health. The centre closed after the founding of the modern NHS, as, despite its success, it did not fit with the new systems being put in place.

Forward-thinking GPs have practiced modern forms of social prescribing for perhaps 30-plus years, but these examples were somewhat fragmented and limited. Momentum gathered in 2015 when NHS England supported the creation of the Social Prescribing Network (www.socialprescribingnetwork.com) to bring together like-minded people who saw the opportunities of a new approach to health. At this same time, work had commenced on creating new approaches to involving people in their care and support. There was growing recognition that as a health system, we needed to rethink medicine and embrace the opportunities for the delivery of more personalised care.

The Universal Model of Personalised Care

Personalised care in England, as defined within the 2019 publication *Universal Personalised Care*, means giving people 'choice and control over the way their care is planned and delivered, based on what matters to them and building on the assets that they bring to their own care' (NHS England, 2019). Whilst not a new approach, the Comprehensive Model for Personalised Care establishes a new pathway that considers patients' lives in a holistic way and puts them at the heart of the care they received, rather than simply focusing on one particular condition or disease pathway.

Human beings are complex, and it is difficult to separate the issues that we face in our daily lives from each other. For example, someone living with cancer and experiencing issues with their mental health does not live with cancer one day and have mental health issues the next. Nor do we always respond to things in the same way or desire the same outcomes from people who have experienced the same challenges in life. A one-size-fits-all approach to health care simply does not meet either the complexities of modern health challenges or the expectations of people living modern lives.

The National Academy for Social Prescribing 'ecosystem' (Fig. 4.1) and the NHS comprehensive personalised care model demonstrate both the process of social prescribing and the population impact. The comprehensive personalised care model defines six evidence-based and interlinked components, including social prescribing (Table 4.1) needed for health, that would support people at the whole population level, those living with one or more long-term conditions, and those with highly complex needs (NHS England, 2019). Similar approaches have been adopted in Wales, Scotland and Northern Ireland.

Shared Decision-Making

Shared decision-making fundamentally changes the clinical conversation and the relationships between clinician and patient—it moves far away from the age-old adage of 'Doctor knows best' in order to enable the knowledge and expertise of a patient to be used alongside the clinical and professional expertise of the doctor, enabling decision-making based on a full appraisal of the circumstances and opportunities. Whilst clinicians can be experts in conditions and diseases, people are the only experts in themselves, in the goals they want to pursue and in the care or support they need to enable them to achieve those goals.

Choice of Provider and Services

Choice might seem like a simple concept, but the availability of information upon which to make a fully informed decision is often a complex process. Legislation supports several choice options, for example, deciding on which hospital to visit for

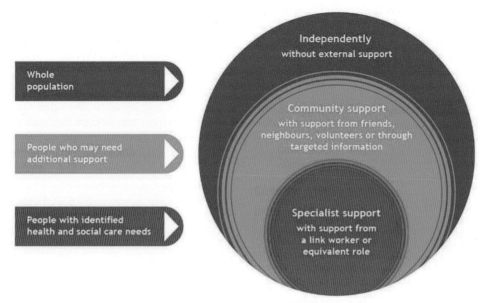

Fig. 4.1 Social prescribing—ecosystem. From the National Academy for Social Prescribing (2022) nasp_annualreview_2122.pdf. socialprescribingacademy.org.uk.

TABLE 4.1   Six Key Components of Comprehensive Personalised Care
1. Shared decision-making
2. Choice
3. Personalised care and support planning
4. Social prescribing and community-based support
5. Personal health budgets and integrated personal budgets
6. Supported self-management.

From Comprehensive Personalised Care Model. (n.d.). Available at: https://www.england.nhs.uk/wp-content/uploads/2019/02/comprehensive-model-of-personalised-care.pdf (Accessed 9 February 2023).

elective treatment, alongside everyday choices, such as whether to take a particular medication, or major decisions about invasive treatments that can have a significant impact on outcomes.

Personalised Care and Support Planning

For people living with complex long-term conditions and particularly those with multimorbidity, having a personalised care and support plan may be effective in enhancing their outcomes, and also reducing their reliance on health care services (Coulter et al., 2015). A plan that looks holistically at someone's circumstances and documents their care and treatment wishes enables them to be in greater control of their health and enables health care professionals as well as non-statutory service providers to support them in a more meaningful way.

These three approaches—shared decision-making, choice and personalised care and support planning—established the context for a new approach to patient care and created the circumstances for the deployment of new approaches to creating health.

The comprehensive model then concentrates on three innovative interventions to respond to the plan developed via this introductory process.

Personal Health Budgets

Personal health budgets, or PHBs, enable people to organise and purchase their care and support in a way that meets their individual needs. Their origins came from campaigns led by disability rights groups in the 1970s and 1980s that called for choice and control over their lives.

The NHS subsequently followed with the introduction of PHBs, firstly as a right to request, then as a right to have for people receiving support under the continuing health care scheme. Since the introduction and small-scale trials, personal health budgets have been expanded to support multiple groups of people, including those requiring a wheelchair and those receiving support for their mental health. There are now over 120,000 people in receipt of a PHB, and evidence demonstrates them to be cost effective, saving on average 17% on the direct cost of home care packages, whilst enabling people to take more active control over their lives (NHS England, online-b).

Supported Self-Management

The second intervention is a broad-based approach known as self-management support. This builds on the fact that people living with long-term conditions who have greater knowledge, skills and confidence to manage their health and wellbeing are more likely to experience improved outcomes. Helping people to build skills, knowledge and confidence can reduce GP visits and hospital admissions. This can be achieved by:

1. access to formal self-management education programmes—either face to face or digital;
2. health coaching;
3. peer support.

Self-management programmes usually focus on providing education and support for people with single long-term conditions. For people with diabetes, COPD or heart problems, there is strong evidence that they improve outcomes (Bodenheimer et al., 2002), so they have become part of the standard care package.

There is a spectrum of self-management programmes available in England, and they tend to range from those that are primarily educational and aim to teach people specific skills (e.g., pulmonary rehabilitation programmes) to those that aim to mobilise the group dynamic in order to effect change (e.g., group CBT programmes in mental health).

Health coaching focuses on providing support for people to set individual goals for what they want to achieve in their lives. These goals might not necessarily be directly health related, but nevertheless they tend to improve health-related outcomes by helping people to build a sense of agency that generalises to a sense of agency over their health condition.

A final component of self-management is peer support. Our sense of connection with people experiencing similar challenges can directly influence how we feel about the impact on ourselves. Connecting people with peers to enable them to learn from others who have shared experience and developing a sense of community has been a key pursuit of the comprehensive model, recently leading to a major new initiative to connect people living with type 1 diabetes.

Social Prescribing

This is the final part of the model of comprehensive personalised care, introduced into health policy via the comprehensive model and the long-term plan for the NHS (2019). This brought the formerly fragmented parts into a single model that works more harmoniously together. Core to the successful deployment of each of the components is a 'what matters to you' conversation.

Concept and Terminology Debate

Social prescribing is simply an asset-based mechanism which supports people to connect with their community and engage in meaningful activities in pursuit of improved health and wellbeing outcomes.

The term *social prescribing* has been hotly debated over the years with some, who generally have alternative models to sell, asserting that it is paternalistic and an embodiment of 'Doctor knows best', due to the suggestion that activities are prescribed based on clinical view rather than that of an individual. However, this is far from the case, and the name simply originates from the need to differentiate between biomedical interventions and those that are psychosocial in nature. The other aspect that some fail to recognise is that many people, due to a lack of skills, knowledge and confidence, need support, and support from a trusted professional to help them achieve a connection or enable them to be assured that a particular intervention is good for their health. Too much time has been spent debating these concepts, with the creation, on occasion, of an unnecessary conflict between what in essence are similar models focused on delivering positive outcomes for people.

The Link Worker Role

One of the most significant shifts in the implementation of social prescribing came with the introduction of the link worker role by the NHS. Link workers, community connectors or a myriad of other terms have been used for some time to describe those people who support others to make connection into the community. The link worker role had existed before 2019, but by placing this role within the contract for General Practice in England (NHS England, online-a), the NHS had something of a first: placing the pursuit of psychosocial support alongside medical interventions and demonstrating the importance of this—not just as a nice-to-have venture alongside health care, but as an integral part of a health care system.

As part of the government's commitment to 26,000 new roles in primary care, including pharmacists, first contact physiotherapists, health coaches and care navigators, link workers became a new profession in the NHS which has since grown to see over 3000 people recruited to the role.

Whilst many people in society have the means to connect to communities themselves or take up a particular activity to support their health, some lack the means—be it personal knowledge, connection or finances—to be able to achieve their goals. Whilst some communities are excellent in supporting their neighbours, even in the most connected communities some people unfortunately go unnoticed, which is why approaches to community development alone can't fix the multiple issues facing people.

This is why the link worker role is so important. The NHS regularly ranks as the country's most trusted institution, and GPs are one of the most trusted members of society. It is therefore obvious that when people face difficulties in life and lack either their own resources or are unable to access those of the community around them, they reach out to General Practice.

Prior to the introduction of the link worker role, GPs had relatively few tools to support people living with primary psychosocial challenges: a referral to a specialist service, a prescription for a medicine or words of reassurance. Many have said that good GPs have always practised a form of social prescribing— the knowledge of a local group or a service that can be passed on in the consultation, the discussion about

ways to stay well through exercise—but what the link worker brings is something very different and powerful. They bring time and conversation.

Link workers take the time to get to know a patient and talk to them about their particular health concerns and what their goals are. They use the power of shared decision-making, offering choice and work with the individual to develop a comprehensive personalised care and support plan, working through the first three steps of the Comprehensive Model.

The 'Ecosystem' of Social Prescribing

Social prescribing activity generally happens across four 'zones' with a myriad of examples within each zone of asset-based community programmes:

1. Arts and Culture—Everything from singing for the brain groups, to community choirs, to dance for health programmes which support balance and falls prevention, to art classes which alleviate loneliness and social isolation
2. Sport and Exercise—Programmes tailored to individual ability, from walking football and chair aerobics to parkrun and specialist cycling clubs
3. Natural Environment—Green social prescribing has seen a huge expansion over recent years with local nature reserves and parks enabling activities from bush skills, to open water swimming, to forest bathing and conservation work
4. Knowledge and Learning—A big category with everything from housing and financial advice and relationship support to courses to learn about specific medical conditions and general learning and life skills advancement programmes

These social prescribing zones exist within an ecosystem of social prescribing where people are generally connected at three levels to the same activities.

Some people can connect themselves—through realisation of the types of activities that might improve in their lives. This tends to be true for those who have the individual agency or means—either socially or financially—to access the right activity for themselves. But just because vibrant community activity can exist in many areas doesn't mean that it is accessed by those who might really benefit from it, and there is a risk that models only concentrating on the development of community can miss reaching people.

TABLE 4.2	**Five-Point Plan for Social Prescribing**

- **Make some noise—raising the profile of social prescribing**
To expand social prescribing, we need to get the message out there—that connecting people for wellbeing is vital for people and communities.
- **Find resources—develop innovative funding partnerships**
We recognise the challenges faced by social prescribing link workers, the local voluntary, community, social enterprise and arts sector and will seek to improve resources to realise their social prescribing goals.
- **Build relationships—broker and build relationships across all sectors**
Social prescribing relies on strong, mature relationships at national and local levels across multiple sectors.
- **Improve the evidence—shape and share the evidence base**
There is already an evidence base for social prescribing, but it is not comprehensive. We need to build a consensus about what we know and don't know, improve accessibility and visibility of evidence.
- **Spread what works—promote learning on social prescribing**
We will share what is good, what has been learnt and draw from multiple sources to ensure continued development of social prescribing.

From National Academy for Social Prescribing (2020 online-d). A social revolution in wellbeing: our strategic plan 2020-23. Available from https://socialprescribingacademy.org.uk/about-us/our-vision/ (Accessed 1 February 2023).

That is where the next level of the ecosystem comes in: the opportunity of support for connection and signposting via trained individuals offering light-touch support.

There are great examples of this happening across the country, for example in Frome, where people ranging from taxi drivers to supermarket assistants and hairdressers have been trained to become community connectors who can help people to find a route to support (Firman, 2019).

The final part of the ecosystem is where the link worker model comes in, to ensure that those people requiring dedicated and multifaceted help can be supported effectively in order to experience the same sort of life chances as others in their communities.

When people connect to social prescribing, they tend to do so through three levels of involvement—experience, participation and intervention. If we take music as an example, experience will come from going to watch a live concert or simply putting on your favourite playlist—we know that music is proven to have the power to support our mental health and wellbeing, and so using music to support us through life is a positive pursuit. Beyond simply listening, participation in a community choir or orchestra can hold additional benefits, especially due to the opportunity of community connection and friendship that can be created via the activity. Finally, using music as an intervention for a particular health need is also rapidly gaining attention—for example, the work of the English National Opera through their programme 'Breathe'. Here, professional singers support people impacted by COVID by using singing and breathing exercises to improve their lung health.

The National Academy for Social Prescribing

The momentum for social prescribing gathered pace with the launch of the National Academy for Social Prescribing (NASP). NASP was built through co-production with a wide number of individuals and organisations who developed a 3-year strategy. The result was a five-point plan (Table 4.2) which was articulated in the organisation's first strategy.

NASP launched a series of initiatives within a flagship programme: Thriving Communities (online-c), developed in partnership with NHS England, Sport England, Natural England, The Money and Pensions Advisory Service, Arts Council England and Historic England—organisations spanning the four zones for social prescribing.

Thriving Communities offered not only a grant programme but also a network for voluntary sector organisations, enabling them to collaborate across the zones to form coalitions to develop innovative social prescribing programmes.

Alongside Thriving Communities, NASP worked with the Royal Voluntary Service to launch the Accelerating Innovation Programme (online-a) focusing on innovation at a national level, which gathered over

100 national organisations to create a learning and support programme. Additionally, an academic partners' programme brought together seven academic institutions to develop the evidence base (National Academy for Social Prescribing online-b) via a series of detailed evidence summaries across key sectors.

NASP has also supported the continued expansion of the Social Prescribing Student Champion Scheme, alongside the Social Prescribing Network, the College of Medicine, and NHS England (online). This was established by medical students in 2016 to engage the next generation of health care professionals to promote social prescribing. The scheme is now a multicentre national project led by young health care professionals and health care students representing all UK medical schools. The scheme played a crucial role in successfully embedding the principles of social prescribing and personalised care in the official curriculum of the majority of universities and medical schools across the United Kingdom.

Since its establishment, it has recruited thousands of medical and health-related students to spread awareness of social prescribing through peer teaching and focusing on aspects of personalised care. Student champions have delivered over 1250 peer teaching sessions at local universities and a total of four national conferences.

The scheme has also supported international partners across the world in developing similar student programmes with successful examples taking place at the national level in Australia, Canada, the United States, Japan, Portugal, Singapore and several other countries. A 'Social Prescribing International Student Movement Framework' (2021a, online) was published as a call to action for clinicians, students and academics to challenge a pathogenic health paradigm.

NASP and the World Health Innovation Summit (WHIS) collaborated to develop the Global Social Prescribing Alliance (GSPA, www.gspalliance. com), which develops alliances with partners around the world dedicated to developing social prescribing in their country or region. Following this, the World Health Organisation (WHO) and the United Nations Global Sustainable Index Institute (UNGSII) became partners in the GSPA, followed by 25 country representatives.

GSPA worked with global partners to publish a Playbook for Social Prescribing (online, 2021) which documents the key steps for the establishment of social prescribing in a country or region.

The Global Social Prescribing Alliance International Playbook (2021a; 2021b) builds on the momentum and vision set out by global leaders in September 2015 at the UN General Assembly when the Sustainable Development Goals were announced in New York. It showcases best practices for social prescribing and highlights shared learning that can support health systems around the world to navigate and deliver Good Health and Wellbeing during and after the pandemic.

It lists the seven steps to developing good social prescribing (Table 4.3).

The Future of Social Prescribing

In the future, we will hopefully see continued expansion of the link worker model across the country and indeed the wide ecosystem within which it exists. To deal with the challenges faced by modern society and to support people in improving their health and wellbeing to live their best life, social prescribing needs to continue to adapt and evolve. But what is clear is that this evolution needs to continue along the lines within which social prescribing was originally formed—as a social movement, not owned by one particular organisation, but as an

TABLE 4.3 Seven Steps to Developing Good Social Prescribing
1. Bring everyone together to build social prescribing locally
2. Community development and support for local community groups
3. Develop the role of the social prescribing link worker or community connector
4. Create shared plans with the person
5. Training and workforce development
6. Ensure clinical engagement
7. Measure impact

From Global Social Prescribing Alliance International Playbook (2021). Available from https://www.gspalliance.com/gspa-playbook.

organic and non-profit-making venture that truly unites people who share the goal of improving lives.

Conclusion

Across the United Kingdom, the NHS has made significant progress to deliver services built around the principles of personalised care. In England, the comprehensive model for personalised care defines six evidence-based and interlinked components, including social prescribing.

Link workers connected to primary care and others support people needing psychosocial support, giving time and a listening ear.

Social prescribing exists within a wide ecosystem that enables community connection at three levels: independently, community support and specialist support. People can then access support within four zones of activity (arts and culture, sport and exercise, nature and learning and knowledge), and this support can be through three different levels of engagement (experience, participation and intervention).

NASP continues to support the development of social prescribing in the United Kingdom, and The Global Social Prescribing Alliance continues to make connections across the world.

REFERENCES

Bodenheimer, T., Lorig, K., Holman, H., et al., 2002. Patient self-management of chronic disease in primary care. Journal of the American Medical Association 288 (19), 2469–2475.

Citizens Advice *A very general practice* (n.d.). Available at: https://www.citizensadvice.org.uk/Global/CitizensAdvice/Public%20services%20publications/CitizensAdvice_AVeryGeneralPractice_May2015.pdf (Accessed 7 February 2023).

College of Medicine (Online). National Social Prescribing Student Champion Scheme. Available from https://collegeofmedicine.org.uk/national-social-prescribing-student-champion-scheme-the-social-prescribing-network-the-college-of-medicine-and-nhs-england/ (Accessed 1 February 2023).

Coulter, A., Entwhistle, V., Eccles, A., Ryan, S., Shepperd, S., Perera, R., 2015. Effects of personalised care planning for people with long-term conditions. *Cochrane Library*. https://www.cochrane.org/CD010523/COMMUN_effects-of-personalised-care-planning-for-people-with-long-term-conditions#:~:text=Personalised%20care%20planning%20aims%20to%20provide%20support%20from,become%20more%20able%20to%20manage%20their%20own%20health (Accessed 9 February 2023).

Department of Health and Social Care (n.d.). *National overprescribing review report.* [online] Available at: https://www.gov.uk/government/publications/national-overprescribing-review-report (Accessed 6 February 2023).

Firman, S., 2019. Case Study: The Frome Model of Enhanced Primary Care. Shift Design. Available from. https://shiftdesign.org/case-study-compassionate-frome/ (Accessed 1 February 2023).

Global Social Prescribing Alliance (2021a, online). Social Prescribing International Student Movement Framework. Available from https://www.gspalliance.com/student-movement-framework (Accessed 1 February 2023).

Global Social Prescribing Alliance (2021b). Global Social Prescribing Alliance International Playbook. Available from https://www.gspalliance.com/gspa-playbook (Accessed 1 February 2023).

National Academy for Social Prescribing (online-a). Accelerating Innovation Programme. Available from https://socialprescribingacademy.org.uk/our-work/our-workaccelerating-innovation/ (Accessed 1 February 2023).

National Academy for Social Prescribing (online-b). Evidence on Social Prescribing. Available from https://socialprescribingacademy.org.uk/evidence-on-social-prescribing/ (Accessed 1 February 2023).

National Academy for Social Prescribing (online-c). 'Thriving Communities' Available from https://socialprescribingacademy.org.uk/our-work/thriving-communities/ (Accessed 1 February 2023).

National Academy for Social Prescribing (online-d). A social revolution in wellbeing: our strategic plan 2020-23. Available from https://socialprescribingacademy.org.uk/media/rxtc2zbh/nasp_strat-plan-summary.pdf (Accessed 15 February 2023).

NHS England (online-a). GP Contract. Available from https://www.england.nhs.uk/gp/investment/gp-contract/ (Accessed 1 February 2023).

NHS England (online-b). Evidence and case studies. Available from https://www.england.nhs.uk/personalisedcare/evidence-and-case-studies/ (Accessed 1 February 2023).

NHS England, 2019. Universal Personalised Care: Implementing the Comprehensive Model. [online] England.nhs.uk. Available at:. https://www.england.nhs.uk/publication/universal-personalised-care-implementing-the-comprehensive-model/ (Accessed 7 February 2023).

Chapter 5

The Link to Health Equity

Interview between Professor Sir Michael Marmot and Heather Henry

HH

Well hi, Michael, thank you so much for agreeing to this interview about the link between health equity and social prescribing.

I think my first question to you is: What's your overall opinion of social prescribing?

MM

Let me put social prescribing in context. For a very long time and in some parts of the world, when people think about inequalities in health, they think about inequalities in access to health care. So there's been a real disjunction, and particularly in the US, because the US has such an inequitable health system. Let me define what I mean. Those inequalities that are judged to be avoidable by reasonable means and are not avoidable are unfair and hence inequitable. So we've kind of switched from using health inequalities to inequities. So, in the United States in particular, because there are gross inequities in access to the health care system, when they think about health inequities, they think about health care inequities. And it's still the case here, but to a lesser extent. My whole approach has been the social determinants of health. It's the conditions in which people are born, grow, live, work and age and inequities in power, money and resources that drive inequities in health.

Then the question is what's the role of the health care system. Obviously if people get sick, they need health care, and we don't want inequities in access to health care to compound inequities in health that arise from unequal conditions in daily life, so health care is vital. Social prescribing in a way is somewhere in

between. In other words, when people seek care, the practitioner—usually a doctor, could be a nurse or other health care practitioner—could pay attention to the conditions in which people are born, grow, live, work and age do what they can within their span of control to address those conditions. And that's where social prescribing comes in.

There are two ways, I think, to look at it. One is, that's great, it's terrific that health care practitioners should be addressing the conditions that make people sick. The other way of looking at it is it's not enough. If people are getting sick because of government policy, for practitioners to prescribe something on an individual basis—a bit more exercise, a bit more food, a bit more nutritious food, older people going to a dance class—they're good things, I don't want to decry them, but you could say that they're not getting at the real drivers of health inequalities.

Let me continue the argument myself: the fact that you can't do everything doesn't mean that you should do nothing. So the argument for social prescribing is, Okay, we are not addressing the fundamental drivers of health inequities, but we are trying to make a difference to the conditions of people's lives—what's wrong with that?' So my answer to my argumentative self is, 'That's pretty good'. So the fact that social prescribing doesn't do everything doesn't mean that we should say therefore it's useless. It's not; it's potentially very useful.

HH

And when it comes to thinking about integrated care then—this is the context within which social prescribing is being developed—do you see potential? So, for example, your own report on Build Back Fairer in Greater Manchester (Marmot et al., 2021), and you talk about the things that need to be done there in order to build back fairer—is there a link between that and working in an integrated way on social prescribing?

MM

Potentially, very much. The work we've done in Greater Manchester, Cheshire and Merseyside, we're doing elsewhere. The East London foundation trust wants to be the first Marmot ICS. It doesn't let national government off the hook. We do need national policies that are in the direction of creating a fairer distribution of the social determinants of health. That said, national policies are what they are, and the question is what can be done at a place-based level, and we were commissioned by the ICS in Cheshire and Merseyside and working with the ICS (as it developed into) in Greater Manchester and Lancashire and Cumbria—in east London as well—to put forward proposals for how the ICS could address the social determinants of health. And we get a very enthusiastic uptake in both Greater Manchester and Cheshire and Merseyside. And that's encouraging because it needs people at a local level saying yes, we do need national policy change. I mean, if more children are in poverty because of government policy, that makes the challenge in places at local level much more difficult. Then the question is: How can you break the link between increasing levels of child poverty and worse outcomes for children? Can local services make a difference? And our hypothesis is yes, they can, and that ICSs have a crucial role to play in delivering that.

HH

I'm guessing that you're going to say that devolution will help with this then?

MM

I'm very interested in the high priests of devolution, but I haven't joined the church. I think that empowerment of communities is absolutely vital. If devolution helps that, then great. And the second argument is that in my experience, local authority level people involved—both the civil servants involved and the political people involved—have a much keener understanding of how the conditions in which people live and work impact on their health and wellbeing. In Westminster we have this pathetic charade of candidates to lead the Conservative Party and each one says, 'I'm a tax cutter', 'No I'm a better tax cutter', 'No I'm going to cut even more taxes', 'I want to cut taxes. I want to cut taxes'. I haven't heard one of them yet say no, I'm interested in greater equity in health and wellbeing of the population. Listening to their language it doesn't seem to have entered their calculus that that's got anything to do with them becoming Prime Minister. What's health and wellbeing of the population got to do with being Prime Minister? What you've got to do is show that you're a tax cutter. What? How degraded can our political debate be? I don't hear that at local level—Conservatives, Greens, Lib Dems, Labour—they're not identical, you can distinguish them, but I don't hear people say it's all about cutting taxes or getting rid of waste and forget the content of people's lives. So at local level, politicians and employed civil servants—local government officials—are I think much more sensitive to the reality of people's lives. So, if devolution helps, that's great. If devolution means being starved of funds and letting national government off the hook, that's not such a good solution.

HH

So, what do you think of the government's levelling up agenda?

MM

Well, I wrote a commentary on it for the *British Medical Journal* [Marmot, 2022] on the [Levelling Up] white paper [2022] and I said … 4 objectives … 12 missions … this is terrific. And I thought I would have been pleased to have written this. Great. Then the sneaking suspicion that this might be better than I could have written—that was humbling. So that was the analysis part.

Then we get to okay, what are we going to do? In the white paper the writers point out that when Germany levelled up, when the former Democratic Republic of Germany, East Germany, joined the Federal

Republic but they were economically and socially behind, Germany spent €2 trillion over 25 years. That by my calculation is about £70 billion each year. In the Levelling Up White Paper (HM Government, 2022) the budget for 4 years was £4.8 billion—that's £1.2 billion a year. What? We need £70 billion and we're going to spend £1.2 billion? This is two-orders-of-magnitude too small.

Ah, I thought. This is just a start of the 10. I think the chancellor has made three budgets since then. I don't think he even mentioned levelling up. There was no money for levelling up … nothing … not a single programme for levelling up. Well, now the Prime Minister has gone, and we don't know what the next Prime Minister will do. It wasn't serious. So, the first part of the white paper, I thought if you meet these 4 objectives on these 12 missions, you will reduce health and equalities by my analysis, so I was full of admiration for it. It's the 'what are we going to do in the light of this analysis', and it was empty. Nothing serious.

HH

Now, I'm a member of the voluntary community and social enterprise sector. The difficulty for us when we think about social prescribing is that it's short-term funding. It's grant funding, it's 1-year contracts … rolling and things like that. How do we properly resource communities to deliver social prescribing? Is that a local role, a national role or both?

MM

The answer is yes. It's local, it's national, it's both. Let's come back to levelling up. IPPR North (Webb et al., 2022) calculated that in the 2021 Levelling Up budget there was £32 per person per year for communities in the north. I had documented in my 2020 report (others have too) (Marmot et al., 2020) the decline in local authority spend per person. The decline was greater the more deprived the area, and IPPR North said the annual decline in funding over the last 10 years was £413 per person per year. So, take away £413 per person per year, give back £32, and then you've got levelling up. This is insulting, it is derisory, it's not serious. I mean that's part of the policy incoherence. The Prime Minister was brought down because he was dishonourable and

untrustworthy, but there was a policy incoherence. And if you're serious about levelling up, you can't take £400 plus away and give £32 pounds back and think you're going to level up. So, funding for local government has to come from the centre and it has to come locally, but you can't keep raising local track taxes if you're stripped of funding from the centre. And there's got to be stable funding for the voluntary community and social enterprise sector for local government, for the ICSs. They will need stable funding.

HH

And in terms of local authorities and how they actually work … you know I'm a big fan of the Wigan Deal down the road here from me … they had one of the biggest cuts, if not the biggest budget cut, in the country about 15 years ago. They decided to take that different tack and go into partnership with the community … You go around the country and do a lot talking to local authorities—do you advise them in any way in terms of how they might need to change the way that they invest their money, a bit like Wigan council did? And what do you see? Do you see differences, what works?

MM

We worked with them. So, we would like to think we're not just visiting experts who come in with a recipe and say do this; we work with them, we review the evidence. We've done a lot of work, so we don't come in naïvely. We've done a lot of work reviewing the evidence on what's likely to make a difference. But we then engage the different players locally—local government, both political and employees, ICSs, the voluntary and community sector, the police, fire and rescue, education—and now we're trying to get businesses involved as well … to get a partnership. And yes, we end up through these deliberations with a set of recommendations about how money should be spent. Now, there's political considerations, there's statutory duties, there's all kinds … So what we recommend is not the only set of recommendations or set of approaches, but it's a way of saying how to orient what councils do.

In the case of Coventry, the first Marmot city, they took the six domains of recommendations from my 2010 report, and they planned the development of

Coventry around them. And they even claimed on one of my visits to Coventry that when they applied successfully to be the City of Culture, it was because they were a Marmot city, and I said, 'Come on, I bet you say that to all the boys!' And they said, no really … because we could show that we were the kind of city that was focused on people's health and wellbeing through the life course which we got from your report, and we were worthy nominees to be a City of Culture.

HH

It seems to me that the work of you and your team is much like a system convener: you know, getting people together and encouraging that system's leadership. A strong thread through that is relationship building and communication with a very wide range of players there. I'm also thinking about housing, fire and rescue and police within this book. But some of the criticisms of social prescribing is that it's still a little bit of a medical model—it's still a little bit doing unto people rather than enabling them. And in some cases, some commentators have suggested that it's very exploitative of the VCSE sector. What's your view on that?

MM

My view is what I said at the beginning about social prescribing. I don't see my role when we work with local communities … city regions like Greater Manchester … as promoting social prescribing, I see my role as I was trying to encourage action on the social determinants of health. And getting people in primary care active there is a good thing. So, I see social prescribing as a good thing. As I said, it is not everything that we need … I'm not saying what you need is social prescribing … no, social prescribing is one of the steps that can be taken. I'd much rather see primary care practitioners doing social prescribing the not doing it. So yes, it's a medical model, yes, you could say it's just a sticking plaster … it's not addressing the fundamental drivers … you could say all of those things. In some sense it's true. But as I said at the beginning, I'd much rather see them doing it than not doing it; social prescribing doesn't solve everything, but it's a good step, a good direction.

HH

So primary care contractors, general practitioners—you know, it's written into their contracts—that's a positive step then for primary care?

MM

Very much. Doctors and nurses are highly respected by the public, that's what the evidence shows. Politicians are highly disrespected, that's what the evidence shows. So if people who are highly respected by the public … are trying to address aspects of people's lives that are important for their health, it's a good thing. I mean, yeah it's not perfect, you could say it's a medical model, it's this, it's that … it's a good thing. It's trying to, in my view, do two things. One is get individuals to change in a way that might be beneficial to their health. But the second is it's a step in terms of changing the climate of understanding of what the drivers of ill health are.

In the past (and I think this is changing) if you asked the general public about health, they'd say, 'Oh, when my grandma was in hospital, the nurses were wonderful' or 'Do you know how difficult it is to get a GP appointment?' That's what they think health is. Then you ask them about problems they face in their lives: 'I can't afford the rent where I live', 'There are gangs all around, I don't want my children to play outside and get caught up in gangs', 'The schools are inadequate', 'No opportunity for kids to run around the park' and on and on. Well, those are the social determinants of health. They're the concerns in people's lives—and people in primary care can play an important educative role in helping people recognise that the things that bother them in their lives are the social determinants of health—are important influences on their health. It's not having wonderful nurses look after granny when she's in hospital or getting to see your GP. Wonderful nurses are a contribution to our civilization, and getting to see your GP is very important, but so is recognition of how those things in your life—early childhood education, employment, having enough money to live on, housing, environment, community—all of them are key to your health as well. And the very act of social prescribing is in a way an educative act by helping people understand.

HH

And how far are health care professionals in primary and community on their journey of moving towards that understanding of the social determinants of health and particularly that idea of proportionate universalism? Because, you know, I see sometimes a lot of the attention goes towards older adults when in fact you're saying that you get the biggest bang for your buck early on in the life course. How do you see that journey?

MM

Well, I'm always hopeful. I could be quite critical about politicians, but I always take a positive view. I wrote my first paper on health inequalities in 1978, so I've been doing this a while. And I've never in all my time seen so much interest in health inequalities—recognition of the social determinants of health—as we have now. When I produced my 2020 report 'Health Equity in England: The Marmot Review 10 Years On', the Royal College of Physicians convened others of the medical royal colleges and wrote an open letter to the Prime Minister urging him to act on my recommendations. And following that, the medical royal colleges then started to attract other health care organisations. Initially there were about 70 organisations in this so-called Inequalities in Health Alliance. I was doing the Christmas lecture at the Royal College of Physicians in December 2020. I looked at these 70-odd organisations (that had joined), and most of them were either royal or British, you know, British Lung Foundation, British Heart Foundation, Royal College of Nursing and so on. There are now more than 200 organisations that have joined this Inequalities in Health Alliance!

Now, you might be critical, but the fact is that the leaders of the health professions—the medical royal colleges, these medical charities and other organisations—have joined up with the Inequalities in Health Alliance, which is not just about equity of access to health care but about broader issues on the social determinants of health. For much of it, and rightly so, it's about what can we do within our specialty—whether it's primary care, obstetrics and gynaecology, psychiatry, physicians, paediatrics and child health—what can we do within our specialty and how can we get involved in the wider issues. So the climate's changing for the better, I'd say.

HH

That's cheered me up hugely, I'm so glad you said that.

Lastly, what about prevention? You talk passionately, of course, about prevention. How can prevention be part of social prescribing?

MM

Well, social prescribing really is about prevention. My nervousness with prevention is the way it's interpreted within medicine. You do something to a patient—you tell them give up smoking. You tell them watch your food, don't get obese. But that's a very limited effectiveness. It's not a bad thing to do, but it's limited effectiveness. Public health, yes of course, is about prevention, but the social determinants of health, it's not just what a doctor does with a patient, it's about creating the conditions for people to lead healthy lives. So if social prescribing means recommending that an older person join a dance club, sing in a choir, helping people get access to a food bank or some way to subsidise their home heating, that's great and potentially along the lines of prevention. But also the structural drivers need addressing.

HH

Any last thoughts on the future then of social prescribing—what might you predict or what might you want?

MM

I'm no good about predicting the future. I have enough difficulty explaining the past, so I'm not going to predict what the future might look like. But the encouragement that I've taken from the various medical royal colleges and practitioners is really important, I would say. It looks like more and more medical practitioners are understanding how important addressing the condition of people's lives are and asking what they can do, whether it's in the context of an integrated care system or whether it's what an individual practitioner can do with a patient, working in partnership with others. Certainly, it's been moving in a very positive direction. Let's hope that continues.

REFERENCES

HM Government, 2022. White paper: levelling up the United Kingdom. Available from: https://www.gov.uk/government/publications/levelling-up-the-united-kingdom (Accessed 29 December 2022).

Inequalities in Health Alliance. Available from: https://www.rcplondon.ac.uk/projects/inequalities-health-alliance (Accessed 29 December 2022).

Marmot, M., Allen, J., Boyce, T., et al., 2020. Health equity in England: the marmot review 10 years on. Institute of Health Equity, London.

Marmot, M., Allen, J., Boyce, T., et al., 2021. Building back fairer in greater Manchester: health equity and dignified lives. Institute of Health Equity, London.

Marmot, M., 2022. The government's levelling up plan: a missed opportunity. Bri. Med. J. 376, o356.

Webb, J., Johns, M., Roscoe, E., et al., 2022. State of the North 2021/22; powering northern excellence. IPPR. Available from: http://www.ippr.org/research/publications/state-of-the-north-2021-22-powering-northern-excellence (Accessed 29 December 2022).

Chapter 6

Does Social Prescribing 'Work'?

Marie Polley

Introduction

When I set up the Social Prescribing Network in 2015, we launched a report of our first national conference at the Palace of Westminster, with support from all the major political parties. The report contained ideas and priorities for taking social prescribing forwards (Social Prescribing Network, 2016). Our speaker who hosted us commented that social prescribing is common sense—the idea that we listen to a person in need and then help them to get the appropriate support. And on the face of it, I agree with him.

The need for evidence-informed innovation in social prescribing, however, is paramount to getting a rich understanding of how and when social prescribing works and for whom. High-quality research requires well-designed studies using appropriate and relevant methods of collecting research data. One of the most frequent questions I have been asked is: What is the evidence that social prescribing works? Maybe we could rephrase this question and ask: How do you know that common sense works? Social prescribing as a model of care across all the different sectors is a new way of working for many professionals, so we also need to ask: Who does social prescribing work for? Are there contexts in which social prescribing is particularly beneficial? Are there groups of people or situations where social prescribing is not appropriate?

Social Prescribing as an Architecture, Not an Intervention

Social prescribing is defined in many ways, and to explore this briefly is fundamental to how one

approaches determining if social prescribing works. In our first report (Social Prescribing Network, 2016), we co-produced a definition of social prescribing with all the conference delegates which involved a patient being connected to a link worker by a health care professional. The patient was then supported to co-produce solutions to their unmet needs, often via voluntary community and social enterprise groups. Social prescribing has evolved around the world (Morse et al., 2022), and a recent Delphi study was carried out to provide a universal definition of social prescribing, reflecting how social prescribing has evolved in the UK and globally (Muhl et al., 2022). The definition broadly reflects a person's unmet needs being supported by a person in a connector role, helping them to find a solution, often in the community. It moves away from the use of the word 'patient', instead preferring the word 'person', since some people are referred to social prescribing by professionals outside of the health care profession and therefore are not patients.

I personally speak about social prescribing as an architecture that enables a person to move more efficiently between the different parts of our society, for example, health service, social care and other services that support how a person's housing, finances, legal or employment issues are resolved and organisations available in the local community.

You may wonder why it is so important to have a sense of architecture or structure and not use the more common word 'intervention'. An intervention can set up a picture of a more linear model that you do something to a person, and it has an effect.

Cause-and-effect thinking works well for medication, that is, there is a direct attribution to the medication of the change it causes in the person. This type of intervention lends itself well to research trials that compare the effect of a single medicine in people who take it to the effect of giving a placebo to people who think they are taking the real medicine but are only having a 'look alike'. The trials here are called randomised controlled trials, and they are the standard by which the biomedical world determines how well a medicine works.

When you think about the architecture of social prescribing, however, there are multiple factors which will affect how well social prescribing works for a person. Furthermore, social prescribing is a personalised service. Each person who speaks with a social prescribing link worker has concerns and needs specific to them. These may have been partially identified by the professional who refers them to the social prescribing link worker, but the concerns will be more fully identified when they spend time with a link worker. The link worker then helps a person to be more ready to receive appropriate support and connects them to the support. And the combination of support will also be designed for that person specifically.

One can more easily research the effectiveness of social prescribing and demonstrate that the change in wellbeing of a person is *associated* with the social prescribing service they visited. The association leaves room to say other factors could also have contributed to the impact on a person. Only when you can create a control group to compare the effects of people who do and don't have social prescribing can you start to attribute change rather than associate it.

Evidence That the Prescribed Activities Work

There is already a huge amount of evidence of benefit when a person engages in creative activities or physical activity, receives social welfare support or becomes a volunteer. For example, a review by the World Health Organization concluded that engagement in the arts can benefit child development, support neurodevelopmental and neurological conditions, encourage health-promoting behaviours, assist with management of chronic conditions, support care for people in hospital with acute conditions, prevent ill health through enhancing mental health, support formal and informal caregiving, reduce risk of cognitive decline and frailty and support end-of-life care (Fancourt and Finn, 2019). Volunteering is associated with lower levels of mental distress and greater levels of health-related quality of life (Mak et al., 2022), as well as improved life satisfaction and quality of life (Matthews and Nazroo, 2021). Gardening and horticulture are linked with improved mental wellbeing, increased physical activity and a reduction in social isolation (Howarth et al., 2020). Becoming more physically active can decrease the risk of getting chronic conditions, improve existing conditions and support mood levels (Costa Santos et al., 2022; Kerr and Booth, 2022). Health Justice partnerships (collaborations between health care and legal services which support patients with social welfare issues such as welfare benefits) can benefit disadvantaged groups in society (Beardon et al., 2021). Furthermore, recent evidence shows that the effect of depression medication is negatively mediated by housing or employment issues (Buckman et al., 2022).

Social prescribing as a model is intended to create additional or alternative routes to supporting health and wellbeing, instead of just prescribing medications, and therefore draws on existing evidence of how nonmedical approaches can benefit wellbeing.

The Impact of Social Prescribing on a Person

The Medical Research Council guidance on evaluating new and complex interventions provides a road map of types of data to be determined before designing an RCT (Skivington et al., 2021). This involves qualitative data, case studies, proof-of-concept research and identification of appropriate outcomes to measures and the effect size where pre–post change of outcomes occurs. The majority of data collected about social prescribing since 2016 therefore fall into this category, with the exception of a few controlled trials.

Data can be collected using interviews, focus groups and case studies to identify the range of outcomes a person experiences in a social prescribing service. Other benefits of the social prescribing service can be identified by collecting qualitative data from other stakeholders to see if there is benefit to the referrers, the link workers, the commissioners, and the organisations providing the social prescribing activities. These data can, for example, also be used to create a theory-of-change model for that specific social prescribing scheme and identify mechanisms of action.

Trends in population health differ in different parts of the UK, so social prescribing schemes in different geographical settings are often focused on supporting specific and different groups of people. As an example, the qualitative meta-analysis by Liebmann et al. (2022) documents the populations studied in the 19 papers analysed; these included people with multiple complex needs, psychosocial and economic needs, people living with multiple chronic conditions, people experiencing loneliness or social isolation, people with low to moderate mental health issues, and people who were carers. The ages ranged from 16 to 95 years with a variety of age groupings within this range. The needs being addressed through social prescribing often change as people get older—this was seen in an evaluation by Polley et al. (2021), where people over 65 years old needed support with independent living, caring responsibilities, finance and housing. People between 18 and 64 years old were more likely to need support with lifestyle changes. This all makes direct comparisons of quantitative data between different social prescribing schemes difficult and inappropriate in many ways.

A mapping project carried out by Polley et al. (2020) identified social prescribing outcomes reported in peer-reviewed published literature, grey literature and through interviews with a range of non–health-based stakeholders. The findings showed that only some aspects of social prescribing schemes were being monitored and reported. The final analysis identified 99 potential outcomes relevant to social prescribing schemes, only 40% of which were being quantified. Moreover, 37 outcomes were directly associated with the determinants of health, but only 20% of these outcomes were being reported in the social prescribing literature. It was also noted that there was a bias towards health-based outcomes (Polley et al., 2020; Polley and Fixsen, 2021). It stands to reason, therefore, that to effectively capture the impact of social prescribing schemes, one needs to understand the support needs and the associated outcomes of the cohort of people being referred into that social prescribing scheme. Additionally, it is critical to choose a validated measurement tool that captures these outcomes to determine if social prescribing works and for which groups of society. This tool or tools used to measure change are likely to be different across schemes, as you wouldn't measure loneliness specifically using the same tool to monitor how active a person is at managing their chronic health condition, for example.

Using Social Prescribing Link Workers to Identify Support Needs

Let's take a step back from outcomes and examine the value that social prescribing link workers bring to this architecture. It is easy to presume as a researcher, a clinician, a commissioner or other professional that we know what problems or concerns a person wants support with and how a person will benefit from social prescribing. We must not presume, however, to know another person's thoughts and must hear from them directly.

Many social prescribing schemes use a link worker who acts as a bridge between the person with their unmet needs and the different sources of support available. The professional who refers a person to a link worker often does so because they don't have capacity to explore all the issues affecting a person. Whilst the reason for referral is recorded, once a person has spent up to an hour with a link worker, their priority may be established as different from the initial referral.

A good example of this was reported in Polley et al. (2021). Table 6.1 has been adapted from this work to show the proportion of referral reasons recorded by professionals who referred a person to a social prescribing link worker. This is compared with the proportion of types of support then prescribed by the social prescribing link worker, after they had spent time with a person.

There are many points to make about these data. It is based on over 6000 people and therefore provides a reliable picture of what is happening. If you compare why people were referred, the majority were for lifestyle risk factors and emotional/mental health issues (77% of referrals), showing the medical bias previously referred to in this chapter. Once a person spent time talking to a link worker, a further two categories of support were identified which were not initially present on referral data. One was related to learning and development, for example, getting support for education or training opportunities (6%). The second area was actually

TABLE 6.1   Proportion of Reasons for Referring to a Social Prescribing Link Worker Compared With the Proportion of Types of Support Then Prescribed

Referral Reason	Reason for Referral to Social Prescribing Link Worker (n = 6050)	Areas of Support Prescribed After Discussion With Social Prescribing Link Worker (n = 34,606)
Lifestyle and modifiable risk factors (weight, physical activity etc)	55%	33%
Emotional/mental wellbeing	22%	11%
Social contact	8%	19%
Independent living	4%	6%
Carer support	3%	6%
Finance and housing	2%	10%
COVID specific	2%	1%
Unmet needs with existing clinical condition	0%	9%
Learning and development support	0%	6%

From Polley, M., Seers, H., Johnson, R., 2021. Tandridge district council wellbeing prescription service final evaluation report. https://www.researchgate.net/publication/353038388_TANDRIDGE_DISTRICT_COUNCIL_WELLBEING_PRESCRIPTION_SERVICE_FINAL_EVALUATION_REPORT_APRIL_2021.

identifying unmet needs with clinical conditions (9%). This could be related to ongoing pain, issues with medications or the need to see a primary or secondary care professional about their existing condition. This is interesting given that many referring professionals in this scenario were mainly medical professionals.

It is also notable that whilst modifiable and lifestyle factors were the primary referral reason (55%), only a third of the support was for this (33%). Instead, more support was needed for housing, finance, social support, carer burden, as well as the two previously unidentified issues. A similar situation related to emotional and mental health. Overall, this highlights the importance of a link worker having time to spend with a person and understand their situation—which is often complex. One could argue that these data demonstrate how a link worker is identifying the root causes of a person's poor wellbeing.

The final point to draw the reader's attention to is that there were, on average, six forms of support per person referred. People with complex situations often need a range of support that runs concurrently, as exemplified by the quote below.

I have a client who is terminal [terminally ill]. She could no longer work but didn't know where to get financial support. She has used loan sharks and is feeling threatened. House is damp and unsuitable, and her son has just been released from prison and needs to get out of the neighbourhood but doesn't know how to do this and fulfil probation requirements.

*(**Link Worker**) (**Polley et al., 2020**)*

The value of a link worker here is that they can support the coordination of the different types of support and remove that burden from the patient who in this situation often has a low level of self-efficacy.

These data demonstrate that investing in the time a link worker spends with a person is having a successful outcome—it is showing that the issues a person has are being identified, and therefore a person is getting the support they need in a coordinated and non-judgemental way. It shows that this part of the social prescribing architecture is working.

The importance of the link worker has been picked up in several research studies (e.g., Husk et al., 2020; Pescheny et al., 2018; Polley et al., 2019, 2021; Wildman et al., 2019). Data have shown that being able to talk with a social prescribing link worker and develop a strong, supportive and sustained relationship was key to a person then feeling able to explain the things that are going on, as shown in the quotes below.

Meeting someone [a link worker] and being able to talk things through and feeling supported has given me confidence.

(Polley et al., 2019)

The advisor has been a sensitive and helpful advisor, who's given me enough latitude to open up about what are quite private matters.

(Polley et al., 2019)

Changes in Outcomes for People Before and After Social Prescribing

Considering the high level of variation between different social prescribing schemes, much of the known benefits of social prescribing have been identified through qualitative research or research that has measured changes before and after a person goes through a social prescribing scheme. Many of the themes that have been captured in social prescribing research were identified in a qualitative meta-synthesis review by Liebmann et al. (2022) as well as in other research studies. These themes reveal commonalities in how social prescribing works and help us to understand how social prescribing can have a positive effect on people's wellbeing.

In addition to highlighting the beneficial role of social prescribing link workers in identifying unmet needs, the relationship with the link worker was seen to increase levels of confidence to try out new social activities. Both of these aspects were seen to support a person's mental health as well as reduce their levels of social isolation and loneliness (Dayson and Bennett, 2015; Polley et al., 2019).

Thomson et al. (2018) noted that through carrying out new activities via the community groups and organisations, people have the opportunity to learn new skills and feel more empowered to meet and talk to people and share their experiences. Todd et al. (2017) found that the locations the activities were held in also acted as a positive enabler to improved wellbeing, and sharing of experiences with people in a similar position also made people feel less lonely.

Outcomes such as improvements in mental health, social wellbeing, the number of people in a person's social network as well as levels of confidence and empowerment are frequently reported as being positively impacted by social prescribing schemes (Bertotti et al., 2020; Bertotti and Temirov, 2020; Dayson et al., 2020; Dayson and Batty, 2020; Dayson and Damm, 2020; Woodall et al., 2018). The range of potential outcomes is broad, and many people can have improvements in several areas of their lives. These improvements may occur soon after seeing a link worker and being connected to the right support, or there may be a gradual improvement, or one that comes 1 to 2 years later, as exemplified by the quotes below.

Talking to [Wellbeing Advisor] really helped me. She made me feel like I am not fighting this alone. She referred me to several services, and I am now getting help. I think I have turned a corner now.

(Service User) (Polley et al., 2021)

People who were in crisis three years ago are now interested in volunteering, for example, a very long journey, but yeah…

(Link Worker) (Polley et al., 2020)

Some of these improvements in outcomes act as catalysts or stepping stones for a person to become more active, start volunteering or get back to work, for instance. This increased activity and socialising further improve their wellbeing. When working with people who have complex situations and multimorbidity, it is important to be realistic about what outcomes are expected to improve and the time frame in which this will happen, as well as the fact that there are often multiple outcomes that change.

Another example of improvements is in physiological outcomes for people. The evaluations of two different social prescribing services in the West and Southeast England showed improvements in weight, blood pressure and cholesterol levels (Polley et al., 2019, 2021). The number of people analysed in these two evaluations was low, therefore limiting the generalisability of the data. Another evaluation of a social prescribing programme in Northern England, supporting people with type 2 diabetes, analysed data from 8086 people. The social prescribing group (n = 4752) was compared with a control group of patients who weren't able to access the service but lived in the same area (n = 3334). The study concluded that the people who received social prescribing support had statistically significant improvement in their blood sugar levels compared to the control group. Given the number of people involved in this study, these results signal that a social prescribing approach could help to reduce the public health burden of type 2 diabetes (Wildman and Wildman, 2021).

Economics and Service Usage Implications

Whilst the actual premise of this chapter is 'does social prescribing work?', it is important to address the slightly different question of cost effectiveness of social prescribing, as this is often seen—rightly or wrongly— as a way of determining if social prescribing works. In 2017, a team of us first started to look at the potential impact of social prescribing on health service usage. We analysed 14 sources of data and found a variable level of reduction of health service usage, including emerging evidence of reductions in visits to GPs, A&E and unplanned secondary care (Polley et al., 2017). It was enough to be able to conclude that social prescribing appears to have a protective effect on health service usage and that social prescribing services could achieve greater value for money if they were better targeted to the population that completes and responds to social prescribing. There were many caveats to this early work, including the need for more research data to confirm the findings.

In the social prescribing service evaluation from West England (Polley et al., 2019), we used a retrospective case-matched approach to developing a control group of patients in the same GP practices who fit the same referral criteria and didn't have social prescribing. These data showed a reduction in 0.74 GP visits per patient, which was statistically significant. This was only based on 190 people in total but again showed a modest reduction in visits to the GP.

Another, more recent study, also based on a small sample size, reported an economic analysis of frequent attenders to GP services who were using social prescribing. The results identified a direct cost saving of £78.37 per participant over the 5 months of social prescribing in frequent attenders to GP practices. As with conclusions from Polley et al. (2017), the authors suggest targeting referrals to social prescribing to achieve maximum cost benefit (Lynch and Jones, 2022).

Further strong data have come from the Ways to Wellness social prescribing service. The service aimed to support people between 40 and 74 years old with specific long-term conditions. The service was run in the west of Newcastle upon Tyne where deprivation is higher than the average for England and many people had multiple, complex medical, practical and social needs. As well as demonstrating an improvement in different wellbeing domains, there was a 27% lower secondary care cost in the Ways to Wellness patients, compared to a control group of patients in the same area who didn't use the social prescribing service. The reduction in use of hospital services equated to an annual cost reduction of £1.56 million in 2019–2020 (Case et al., 2021).

Much of the economic analysis to date has looked at the value of social prescribing to the health service. Social prescribing as demonstrated throughout this chapter identifies and supports issues that have an impact in many other aspects of society. For instance, there is an impact of social prescribing (yet to be determined) on the criminal justice system, local authority services, the Department of Work and Pensions and the Department of Education. Neither has much research been undertaken to value the ripple effect of social prescribing. For example, if an adult takes up a creative activity, their child is more likely to engage in a creative activity, and this has been shown to be protective to mental health (Mak and Fancourt, 2021). This broader economic analysis is still to be carried out, although Dayson and Batty (2020) have written on this area if you want to read further.

Conclusion

When sticking to the question 'does social prescribing work?', this chapter has demonstrated many ways in which the positive impacts of social prescribing schemes have been captured. These impacts are primarily to a person's wellbeing but can range from supporting determinants of health through to specific long-term conditions. Many researchers are now seeking to understand which groups of people benefit the most from social prescribing schemes and in what circumstances. It is likely that these suppositions will be tested out over the next decade using carefully designed controlled trial situations.

Simply put, if social prescribing is about compassionately identifying unmet social, welfare and health needs and supporting these through a range of non-medical interventions, then yes, on balance, I do think social prescribing works.

REFERENCES

Beardon, S., Woodhead, C., Cooper, S., Ingram, E., Genn, H., Raine, R., 2021. International evidence on the impact of health-justice partnerships: A systematic scoping review. Public Health Rev. 42. https://www.ncbi.nlm.nih.gov/pmc/articles/PMC8113986/pdf/phrs-42-1603976.pdf.

Bertotti, M., Frostick, C., Temirov, O., 2020. An evaluation of Social Prescribing in the London Borough of Redbridge: Final evaluation report. Available from: https://repository.uel.ac.uk/item/887zw (Accessed 26 February 2024).

Bertotti, M., Temirov, M.O., 2020. Outcome and economic evaluation of city and Hackney Social Prescribing scheme.

Buckman, J.E.J., Saunders, R., Stott, J., Cohen, Z.D., Arundell, L.L., Eley, T.C., Hollon, S.D., Kendrick, T., Ambler, G., Watkins, E., Gilbody, S., Kessler, D., Wiles, N., Richards, D., Brabyn, S., Littlewood, E., Derubeis, R.J., Lewis, G., Pilling, S., 2022. Socioeconomic indicators of treatment prognosis for adults with depression: A systematic review and individual patient data meta-analysis. JAMA Psychiatry 79 (5), 406–416. https://doi.org/10.1001/jamapsychiatry.2022.0100.

Case, T., Drinkwater, C., Moffatt, S., Bromhead, S., 2021. Ways to Wellness: The First Six Years Approach, Findings and Learning the First Six Years: Approach, Findings and Learning.

Costa Santos, A., Willlumsen, J., Meheus, F., Ilbawi, A., Bull, F.C., Willumsen, J., Ilbaw, A., 2022. The cost of inaction on physical inactivity to healthcare systems. https://ssrn.com/abstract=4248284.

Dayson, C., Batty, E., 2020. Social prescribing and the value of small providers evidence from the evaluation of the rotherham social prescribing service. Available from: https://www.shu.ac.uk/centre-regional-economic-social-research/publications/social-prescribing-and-the-value-of-small-providers-evidence (Accessed 26 February 2024).

Dayson, C., Bennett, E., 2015. Evaluation of the rotherham mental health social prescribing service. Available from: https://www.shu.ac.uk/centre-regional-economic-social-research/publications/evaluation-of-the-rotherham-mental-health-social-prescribing-service-2015-16-2016-17 (Accessed 26 February 2024).

Dayson, C., Damm, C., 2020. Evaluation of the rotherham social prescribing service for long term conditions. https://www.shu.ac.uk/centre-regional-economic-social-research/publications/evaluation-of-the-rotherham-social-prescribing-service-for-long-term-conditions (Accessed 26 February 2024).

Dayson, C., Painter, J., Bennett, E., 2020. Social prescribing for patients of secondary mental health services: Emotional, psychological and social well-being outcomes. J. Public Ment. Health. 19 (4), 271–279. https://doi.org/10.1108/JPMH-10-2019-0088.

Fancourt, D., Finn, S., 2019. What is the evidence on the role of the arts in improving health and well-being? A scoping review. (WHO). World Health Organization Regional Office for Europe https://iris.who.int/bitstream/handle/10665/329834/9789289054553-eng.pdf.

Howarth, M., Brettle, A., Hardman, M., Maden, M., 2020. What is the evidence for the impact of gardens and gardening on health and well-being: A scoping review and evidence-based logic model to guide healthcare strategy decision making on the use of gardening approaches as a social prescription. BMJ Open 10 (7). https://doi.org/10.1136/bmjopen-2020-036923.

Husk, K., Blockley, K., Lovell, R., Bethel, A., Lang, I., Byng, R., Garside, R., 2020. What approaches to social prescribing work, for whom, and in what circumstances? A realist review. Health Soc. Care Community 28 (2), 309–324. https://doi.org/10.1111/hsc.12839.

Kerr, N.R., Booth, F.W., 2022. Contributions of physical inactivity and sedentary behavior to metabolic and endocrine diseases. Trends Endocrinol. Metab 33 (12), 817–827. https://doi.org/10.1016/j.tem.2022.09.002.

Liebmann, M., Pitman, A., Hsueh, Y.C., Bertotti, M., Pearce, E., 2022. Do people perceive benefits in the use of social prescribing to address loneliness and/or social isolation? A qualitative meta-synthesis of the literature. BMC Health Serv. Res. 22 (1), 1264. https://doi.org/10.1186/s12913-022-08656-1.

Lynch, M., Jones, C.R., 2022. Social prescribing for frequent attenders in primary care: An economic analysis. Front Public Health. doi:10.3389/fpubh.2022.902199.

Mak, H.W., Coulter, R., Fancourt, D., 2022. Relationships between Volunteering, Neighbourhood Deprivation and Mental Wellbeing across Four British Birth Cohorts: Evidence from 10 Years of the UK Household Longitudinal Study. Int. J. Environ. Res. Public Health 19 (3). https://doi.org/10.3390/ijerph19031531.

Mak, H.W., Fancourt, D., 2021. Do socio-demographic factors predict children's engagement in arts and culture? Comparisons of in-school and out-of-school participation in the Taking Part Survey. PLoS One 16 (2), e0246936. https://doi.org/10.1371/journal.pone.0246936.

Matthews, K., Nazroo, J., 2021. The impact of Volunteering and its Characteristics on Well-being after state pension age: Longitudinal evidence from the English longitudinal study of ageing. J. Gerontol. B Psychol. Sci. Soc. Sci. 76 (3), 632–641. https://doi.org/10.1093/geronb/gbaa146.

Morse, D.F., Sandhu, S., Mulligan, K., Tierney, S., Polley, M., Chiva Giurca, B., Slade, S., Dias, S., Mahtani, K.R., Wells, L., Wang, H., Zhao, B., de Figueiredo, C.E.M., Meijs, J.J., Nam, H.K., Lee, K.H., Wallace, C., Elliott, M., Mendive, J.M.,..., Husk, K., 2022. Global developments in social prescribing. BMJ Global Health 7 (5), e008524. https://doi.org/10.1136/bmjgh-2022-008524.

Muhl, C., Mulligan, K., Bayoumi, I., Ashcroft, R., Godfrey, C., 2023. Establishing internationally accepted conceptual and operational definitions of social prescribing through expert consensus: a Delphi Study Protocol. Int. J. Integr. Care 23 (1): 3, 1–9. https://doi.org/10.5334/ijic.6984.

Pescheny, J., Randhawa, G., Pappas, Y., 2018. Patient uptake and adherence to social prescribing: A qualitative study. BJGP Open 2 (3). https://doi.org/10.3399/bjgpopen18X101598.

Polley, M., Bertotti, M., Kimberlee, R., Pilkington, K., Refsum, C., 2017. A review of the evidence assessing impact of social prescribing on healthcare demand and cost implications. Available from: https://www.researchgate.net/publication/318861473.

Polley, M., Fixsen, A., 2021. Capturing the whole effect of social prescribing—meaningful outcomes and theoretical positions. Eur. J. Integr. Med. 48. https://doi.org/10.1016/j.eujim.2021.102006.

Polley, M., Seers, H., Fixsen, A., 2019. Evaluation report of the social prescribing demonstrator site in Shropshire-final report. https://westminsterresearch.westminster.ac.uk/item/qx18z/evaluation-report-of-the-social-prescribing-demonstrator-site-in-shropshire-final-report.

Polley, M., Seers, H., Johnson, R., 2021. Tandridge district council wellbeing prescription service final evaluation report. https://www.researchgate.net/publication/353038388_TANDRIDGE_DISTRICT_COUNCIL_WELLBEING_PRESCRIPTION_SERVICE_FINAL_EVALUATION_REPORT_APRIL_2021.

Polley, M., Whiteside, J., Elnaschie, S., Fixsen, A., 2020. What does successful social prescribing look like? Mapping meaningful outcomes. https://www.researchgate.net/publication/340115811.

Skivington, K., Matthews, L., Simpson, S.A., Craig, P., Baird, J., Blazeby, J.M., Boyd, K.A., Craig, N., French, D.P., McIntosh, E., Petticrew, M., Rycroft-Malone, J., White, M., Moore, L., 2021. A new framework for developing and evaluating complex interventions: Update of Medical Research Council guidance. BMJ 374, n2061. https://doi.org/10.1136/bmj.n2061.

Social Prescribing Network. 2016. Report of the Annual Social Prescribing Network Conference https://www.researchgate.net/publication/359393191_REPORT_OF_THE_ANNUAL_SOCIAL_PRESCRIBING_NETWORK_CONFERENCE/citation/download.

Thomson, L.J., Lockyer, B., Camic, P.M., Chatterjee, H.J., 2018. Effects of a museum-based social prescription intervention on quantitative measures of psychological wellbeing in older adults. Perspect. Public Health 138 (1) 28–38. doi:10.1177/1757913917737563.

Todd, C., Camic, P.M., Lockyer, B., Thomson, L.J.M., Chatterjee, H.J., 2017. Museum-based programs for socially isolated older adults: Understanding what works. Health Place 48, 47–55. https://doi.org/10.1016/j.healthplace.2017.08.005.

Wildman, J.M., Moffatt, S., Steer, M., Laing, K., Penn, L., O'Brien, N., 2019. Service-users' perspectives of link worker social prescribing: A qualitative follow-up study. BMC Public Health 19 (1), 98. https://doi.org/10.1186/s12889-018-6349-x.

Wildman, J., Wildman, J.M., 2021. Evaluation of a Community Health Worker Social Prescribing Program among UK patients with Type 2 diabetes. JAMA Netw. Open 4 (9), e2126236. https://doi.org/10.1001/jamanetworkopen.2021.26236.

Woodall, J., Trigwell, J., Bunyan, A.M., Raine, G., Eaton, V., Davis, J., Hancock, L., Cunningham, M., Wilkinson, S., 2018. Understanding the effectiveness and mechanisms of a social prescribing service: A mixed method analysis. BMC Health Serv. Res. 18 (1). https://doi.org/10.1186/s12913-018-3437-7.

Chapter 7

Summary Section 1 Setting the Scene

David Buck and Laura Lamming

Social prescribing has come a long way in a short amount of time. As Michael Dixon's chapter shows, that does not mean it is new or novel in itself—but what is new is how it has been accepted and embraced by large parts of the health policy and practice world and its acceptance as part of the toolkit of primary care and beyond.

As recently as 2016, when we were writing about social prescribing, also known as community referral, in the specific context of 'the evidence' on gardens and health, it still seemed on the fringes (Buck, 2016). By the time we were researching the Additional Roles Reimbursement Scheme (Baird et al., 2022) under which many social prescribing link workers are funded through the GP contract, the enthusiasm for social prescribing across areas of the primary care workforce was clear. However, it is worth noting that even at that time, there still appeared to be challenges and confusion around these roles, reinforcing the message in the preceding chapters of this book that there is still work to be done.

Indeed, social prescribing is now at a similar place as many other ideas that have made their way into health policy and practice. We have passed the first stage, characterised by a long struggle to get traction through the leadership, persistence and vision of relatively few critical leaders and the creation of strong and diverse networks. We have got to a recognised but still developing approach with an institution, the National Academy for Social Prescribing, and a professional body, the National Association of Link Workers, to support the future of social prescribing both in the UK and globally. This has been accompanied by NHS institutions adopting social prescribing as part of the intervention framework of primary care, as James Sanderson lays out. Academic studies have started to 'catch up', applying their own frameworks of evidence and taxonomy to social prescribing as a subject of study even as the debate about where social prescribing fits between 'wellbeing' and health continues, as the chapters by Marie Polley and Nancy Hey set out. Finally, an edited volume, this one, has been commissioned to summarise the canon, and to look forward to what could happen next.

The King's Fund has played a very small part in this, not bringing any particularly creative thinking directly, but perhaps performing a role as a socialiser and normaliser, helping to bring social prescribing to a mainstream audience in the health and care system, putting on a number of events and publishing explanatory articles on social prescribing (Buck and Ewbank, 2020) and wider community approaches to health (Buck et al., 2021) and periodic reading lists (see resources section) for a wider audience. From that standpoint, some reflections are set out below.

The health and care system has been changing; social prescribing's acceptance is a part of that—as is the shift to personalised care, integrated care systems and a serious focus on population health. This is all stated policy, legislated for, and underpins the future direction of travel. The supertanker of health and care has been slowly but genuinely changing course. The experience of COVID-19 has sharpened many leaders' understanding of inequalities and what drives them, and the role that community played in the response. But the health and care system has emerged under severe pressure following the pandemic; rising waiting lists and workforce pressures are top of the agenda for politicians in a way they have not been since the late 1990s and early 2000s. Responding to these acute pressures therefore risks crowding out effort and attention on social prescribing and the wider context in which it sits. This must be resisted.

It is tempting to resist it by jumping to justify social prescribing primarily by arguing that it will reduce waiting lists or workforce pressures or save the NHS money. But, in our view, this risks subverting the underlying purpose and power of social prescribing as demonstrated throughout this book. It is not a scalpel—an instrument to be wielded to 'save the NHS'—but a way of connecting people to activities to provide comfort, wellbeing and health. Several chapters have set out this argument from different perspectives: Marmot puts it in the context of the medical profession connecting to the social determinants of health. He sees it as contributing to wider wellbeing through evidence-based activities. We know those activities and the social connections they forge and strengthen are connected to long-term improvement in all sorts of quality-of-life–related outcomes (Munford et al., 2020). This is what social prescribing is for; if a byproduct of it is a reduction in medical demand, or some form of cost saving to the NHS, that is all to the good—but it is not the purpose.

That does not mean we should not be interested in finding out more about its effects, particularly who 'it works' for and why; by knowing more, social prescribing can be better designed, used and targeted where necessary. But we should not expect it to work for everyone; it is not a cure-all, and we should not overclaim its benefits. The findings set out earlier in this section are fascinating, and it is encouraging that there is increasing nuance with the question less 'whether it works' and more what does it mean 'to work' and 'for who'. The insights on how important the link worker is and their role in mediating social prescribing and its effects are particularly powerful. The recent workforce development framework (NHS England, 2023) for these roles is encouraging, as it demonstrates recognition of the value of the roles and individuals themselves beyond the activities or services which they may be sign-posting people to.

Turning to the future, we hope that social prescribing both develops itself and draws more focus and attention to related models of communities and health. Professor Jane South of Leeds Beckett University and colleagues did many people a service with her work for Public Health England, setting out the family of community-orientated interventions (2015) that helped to demystify a complex landscape of related approaches. Our King's Fund explanation of communities and Health (Buck, Wenzel and Beech, 2021) is in a similar vein, including social prescribing as part of a wider set of community approaches, with some more focused on communities in service design and delivery and others on community empowerment and the creation of health directly (see Fig. 7.1).

That brings us to the final point, one that has been made many times but can never be made enough. Social prescribing is only possible because of the complex and dense social fabric that exists in our societies, where there is something, someone and somewhere to prescribe to. We know that places with poor social fabric, fewer community groups and ties and low levels of social infrastructure do worse on social and health outcomes than you would expect even given levels of deprivation. The pioneering work of Local Trust (2019) demonstrates that relatively small but certain levels of resources—but long-term, and not tied to

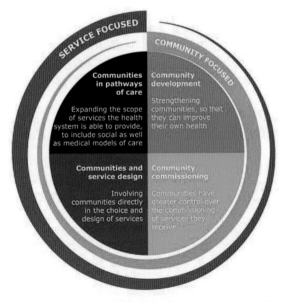

Fig. 7.1 Service- and community-focused approaches to communities and health. Courtesy The King's Fund. 2023. Social prescribing reading list. https://www.kingsfund.org.uk/publications/communities-and-health (Accessed 20 March 2023.)

specific short-term outcomes—can make a huge difference to communities, stimulating the growth of that social fabric and the conditions for social prescribing to work. We look forward to a future where social prescribing is embedded as part of much deeper work so that we have no need for the term *left-behind neighbourhoods*.

Resources

The King's Fund. 2023. Social prescribing reading list. https://koha.kingsfund.org.uk/cgi-bin/koha/opac-shelves.pl?op=view&shelfnumber=133 (Accessed 20 March 2023).

REFERENCES

Baird, B., Lamming, L., Bhatt, R., et al., 2022. Integrating Additional Roles into Primary Care Networks. King's Fund, London. https://www.kingsfund.org.uk/publications/integrating-additional-roles-into-primary-care-networks (Accessed 17 March 2023).

Buck, D., 2016. Gardens and Health: Implications for Policy and Practice. King's Fund, London. https://www.kingsfund.org.uk/publications/gardens-and-health (Accessed 17 March 2023).

Buck, D., Ewbank, L., 2020. What Is Social Prescribing? King's Fund, London. https://www.kingsfund.org.uk/publications/social-prescribing (Accessed 20 March 2023).

Buck, D., Wenzel, L., Beech, J., 2021. Communities and Health. King's Fund, London. https://www.kingsfund.org.uk/publications/communities-and-health (Accessed 21 March 2023).

Buck, D., Wenzel, L., Beech, J., 2021. Communities and Health. King's Fund, London. https://www.kingsfund.org.uk/publications/communities-and-health (Accessed 21 March 2023).

Local Trust., 2019. 'Left behind' neighbourhoods. https://localtrust.org.uk/policy/left-behind-neighbourhoods/ (Accessed 21 March 2023).

Munford, L., Panagioti, M., Bower, P., et al., 2020. Community asset participation and social medicine increases qualities of life. Soc. Sci. Med. 259. https://www.sciencedirect.com/science/article/pii/S0277953620303683 (Accessed 21 March 2023).

NHS England, 2023. Workforce development framework: social prescribing link workers. https://www.england.nhs.uk/long-read/workforce-development-framework-social-prescribing-link-workers/#summary (Accessed 21 March 2023).

Public Health England, 2015. Health and wellbeing: a guide to community-centred approaches. https://www.gov.uk/government/publications/health-and-wellbeing-a-guide-to-community-centred-approaches (Accessed 21 March 2023).

Paradigms

Chapter 8

Personalised Care

Kim Ryley

Introduction

From the legacy of our genes to the particular life experiences that condition our thinking and behaviour, we are all unique. We all differ too in the complex and delicate web of interactions between our mind and our body that determine our personal sense of wellbeing. Yet, there is much in the operation of our fragmented and over-specialised health and care services that seem often to forget or overlook this. As a result, despite the best intentions of caregivers, the empathy and compassion that are the key to all effective treatment are put at risk.

The Current Paradigm Underpinning Social Prescribing

The current NHS paradigm that incorporates social prescribing is part of the Comprehensive Model of Personalised Care (NHS England, 2019; see Chapter 4). This consists of six key components:

1. Shared decision-making
2. Choice
3. Personalised care and support planning
4. Social prescribing and community-based support
5. Supported self-management
6. Personal health budgets and integrated personal budgets

These are designed to overcome failings of fragmented, depersonalised care. Fundamentally, it replaces the question 'what's the matter with you?' with a deeper enquiry of 'what matters to you?' In doing so, it sees the person receiving care as a key asset in the team of experts needed to ensure their good health and quality of life and seeks actively to support and empower them to have greater agency in the process of ensuring their maximum possible wellbeing in the context of their individual lives.

A Revolution

The widescale implementation of this model is nothing short of a revolution that replaces the current provider-driven, 'industrialised', bio-medical model of health care that we have created in this country. Instead, we have a kinder and more compassionate approach that treats the physical, psychological and social needs of those requiring support in holistic and life-affirming ways. Achieving this depends on ready access to local, flexible, high-quality community-based solutions.

The Personalised Care Framework is not a 'pick and mix' approach. Rather, its elements need to be delivered together, in full, to get maximum benefit. Intrinsically, it is co-designed and co-produced, utilising the lived experience of those they intend to benefit. As such, the framework needs to be supported by several key enablers, including leadership to support culture change, to overcome tensions and contradictions within our current health care systems and to reshape them with the active participation of those at the frontline.

Systems Leadership

However, on the ground, the adoption of Personalised Care at the frontline remains piecemeal and uncertain, despite the growing evidence of emerging good practice. There is not yet a widespread, shared understanding of the need for and benefits of personalised care, nor a strong desire more widely to explore new approaches which challenge current outdated systems and orthodoxies. This is now the main challenge for all those who are passionate advocates of a more compassionate and effective approach to meeting future health and care needs.

We need to raise awareness by better communicating our successes and create a 'buzz' and excitement amongst health and care professionals at all levels. We need to focus on sharing case studies of innovative new practice, to make a switch in the way things are done, despite vested interests in maintaining the status quo. Effective influencing on this scale will require more than persuasion to change frontline practices and guidelines; it means winning the hearts and minds of all those involved in creating and maintaining a better quality of life for all those in need of support.

Fundamentally, this means that health and care practitioners need to be helped to believe that personalised care offers tangible benefits for them, as well as for those receiving treatment and care. A bad system will beat a good person every time, but good people working collectively can change the system, if motivated and incentivised to do so.

We know that strong system leadership is the most important factor influencing culture and practice. This is needed to embed new organisational cultures that positively change the current power imbalance between caregivers and care-receivers. This depends on the comprehensive engagement and reskilling of current workforces, new service-commissioning arrangements, and the building of new relationships with local voluntary and community-based providers. The NHS, in particular, is learning a new 'language' of partnership. It is recognising that social prescribing has the power to change lives by enabling innovative, frontline approaches, shared decision-making, self-organisation and supported personal management of one's own health care.

Such a proactive and flexible approach can be seen in the example of the London Borough of Sutton's initiatives to tackle health inequalities across the Borough, through changing roles and relationships by design locally. Its successes are the product of innovations such as local outreach teams, the use of health coaches and effective social prescribers who bring the whole system together and make it more accessible to all local residents. Another great example of tackling health inequalities through local partnership working

and outreach is the Healthy Hyde PCN's integrated team of 34 multidisciplinary staff. These provide a holistic approach to meeting individual needs, using shared local knowledge, against a backdrop of a severely overstretched primary care service (Harvey, 2021).

A Coalition for Change

For over 10 years, the 50 diverse organisations that make up the Coalition for Personalised Care (C4PC) have pursued their shared mission of ensuring that true personalised care is the norm in all health and care settings. The Coalition has had some significant achievements in this revolutionary approach, not least in changing health and care policy at national level. Personalised care is now a key part of the NHS Long Term Plan and is supported by a dedicated team of expert staff who can help practitioners (and patients) to understand its benefits and demonstrate what good practice looks like. Similarly, a wholesale shift to personalised care approaches and practice permeates the changes recommended in the recent stocktake review of primary care provision (Fuller, 2022). The report says this, reflecting the expansion of personalisation to population:

Integrated neighbourhood 'teams of teams' need to evolve from Primary Care Networks (PCNs) and be rooted in a sense of shared ownership for improving the health and wellbeing of the population. They should promote a culture of collaboration and pride, create the time and space within these teams to problem solve together, and build relationships and trust between primary care and other system partners and communities.

(Fuller, 2022)

Workforce Development

Breaking down uncertainty and possible anxieties about how such changes might affect job security, pay levels and career progression for health and care staff are a new priority for the Coalition. A key way into this will be to demonstrate that training to re-skill around personalised care approaches can actually protect against such worries, as demand for such expertise increases, while also providing greater job satisfaction. Working more closely to create a framework for greater empowerment and self-management is challenging. It means engaging with a wide range of other agencies, community-based service providers and receivers of care as equal partners. It requires greater humility by the professionals involved to realise that, rather than threaten traditional practices, it enables a more rewarding professional working life.

The Coalition's partner organisations include the Institute for Personalised Care and the NHSE Personalised Care Group. They are already making impressive progress with innovative programmes of learning and development to equip thousands of key workers with the future skills they will need to thrive in the new health and care systems.

The wider benefit of personalised care is that it can (and should) be applied also to the way health and care staff are treated. Given current and foreseeable pressures on them, together with pandemic burnout, trauma, high turnover and vacancy rates, it is essential that NHS and Social Care bosses understand the equal need for organisational culture change to a more compassionate model.

Trust and Relationships

System change to support personalised care is all about trust and relationships. For example, our research into vaccine hesitancy during the COVID pandemic showed clearly that, to be effective, not least in ensuring health equity for all, personalised care requires the active participation of a wide range of community-based organisations across the spectrum of statutory, voluntary, social enterprise and private sector organisations. Citizens trust those closest to them, who understand them, live in their community and are accessible. Such collaboration involves 'turning the NHS inside out', where system leaders act as convenors to develop sustainable local networks of health and care provision working collaboratively on the wider determinants of health and wellbeing, such as good-quality affordable housing for all and secure employment with an adequate living wage.

Bringing the Assets Together

The Coalition's partner organisations recognise that the NHS will need help and advice on how to invest wisely in new forms of commissioned local provision, and how to create frameworks which are sustainable in the long term. This change will bring in new expertise and a wider workforce to help tackle future health and care challenges effectively. That is why the Coalition has expanded recently and includes key partners such as the National Association of Link Workers, major charities with a health and care focus, and key community-based organisations.

We are also reviewing our links with the social care sector, whose crucial role in guaranteeing good, personalised care is now widely recognised and valued. Years of funding restrictions have greatly reduced the universal support role of such services, as they have been required increasingly to ration such access. The need for extensive reform to create fresh energy, enhanced pay and status for its workforce and a new focus in the sector is supported enthusiastically by the Coalition.

Innovation

There is an irony in that a move to personalised care (whether for caregivers or those receiving care) has never been more needed, but current and post-pandemic pressures, such as workforce shortages and a rising cost of living, make such a shift more difficult. Effective ways are required to prioritise innovation in personalised care where needed, whilst also giving priority to tackling the significant backlog of those awaiting overdue treatment or diagnosis. Indeed, personalised care and community-based solutions—for example, 'hospital at home'—are already being used imaginatively to help those on waiting lists maintain a better quality of life prior to treatment and even to find alternative care arrangements that are preferable to hospital-based solutions.

Power Shifting

This shift requires a bolder rethink of what, as a society, we expect our health and care systems to do, and how they can be better integrated to provide a comprehensive, more holistic, flexible 'customised' response. This means a shift in power towards those experiencing disadvantage and those with complex needs. New models of good practice need to prioritise reducing future demand for services through better prevention of need and by avoiding the current 'revolving doors' of repeat demands, so that people maintain their well-being for longer periods.

For example, although the sound principles of personalised care are applicable to everyone in need and in all settings and circumstances, they are particularly effective for the rapidly growing number of people, like me, who suffer multiple long-term conditions and who can place the most pressure on services that may not be best designed to meet complex needs. These new pressures are not just the result of increased longevity, as research by the Richmond Group of Charities (2022) has shown that factors such as ethnic background and deprivation can increase the number and complexity of those needing particular, long-term care and support at an early age, while also exacerbating current health inequalities.

Such 'multi-morbidity' (as it is often unhelpfully known) is a conundrum for health and caregivers, as, by definition, those who experience it cannot be 'cured' but need regular and extensive monitoring, support and treatment to maintain their wellbeing as much as is possible. As the receivers of such support, our focus is on how we can best sustain our quality of life without the need for constant 'external' (and frequently uncoordinated) interventions. As people with lived experience of our particular conditions and needs, we are often eager and willing to do more to self-manage our own treatment and care. We also need ready access to carefully target expert support, ideally from an integrated team who understand the complexities of our interacting conditions and treatments and our particular preferences about how we want to be helped to maintain independence, agency and an acceptable quality of life.

Technology

To illustrate this more personally, as someone with three potentially life-threatening medical conditions, who has generally had good care and treatment, it has been an interesting journey for me to acquire the knowledge and confidence necessary to be able sometimes to successfully challenge the apparent inability or unwillingness of some parts of the health and care system to respond to my particular overall needs and preferences efficiently and effectively. For example, initially it took me many months of negotiation to be allowed to self-test to monitor my rare blood disorder (thereby avoiding frequent disruption to my work because of the need to attend hospital or clinic for this), and such self-management of my condition depended on me purchasing my own testing equipment. The freedom and reassurance this has given me showed this to be one of the best investments I have ever made. My next challenge is to see if I can be allowed to adjust the dosage of my medication when testing shows this to be necessary, given that such efficient self-management arrangements have long been in place for diabetics.

A recent breakthrough in diabetic treatment shows how new technology will give many people even greater control over their own treatment. This is part of a welcome major growth in the use of new technology to help both remote monitoring and treatment, within a wider NHS@Home (www.england.nhs.uk/nhs-at-home) initiative that shifts the need for this to be done solely on medical or care premises. Properly designed, such technology can greatly extend personalised care options, but it also risks a greater health inequality if appropriate access and personal support in its use are not freely available to all.

Mental Health

Nowhere are the benefits of personalised care more necessary than in the treatment and support of mental health, where worrying exponential growth in demand (particularly from children and young adults) makes access very difficult for most. There are a growing number of innovative new approaches to meet this need, such as Barnet's Wellbeing Service (www.barnetwellbeing.org.uk) which aims to support local residents to self-manage their emotional wellbeing, remain independent and reduce their reliance on emergency services. This is a partnership of community-based and statutory services, managed by a local charitable organisation, and has a strong input from voices of lived experience. With an emphasis on prevention and early intervention, its formalised social prescribing process ensures access to locally delivered, integrated, whole system solutions through a single point of access. The service promotes awareness of and de-stigmatises mental health issues, as well as maps out clearer pathways of care for the future users. Based on the World Health Organization recommendations (2021) on person-centred and rights-based community services, nearly 200 local people a month now receive support that also provides better and cheaper outcomes.

Conclusion

There is a growing consensus nationally that much of our current health care system is no longer fit for purpose because it cannot provide effective, joined-up solutions to health demands that are increasingly caused by growing social and economic inequalities in the UK. As a result, there is increasing discontent amongst both care users and medical/care professionals. Staff satisfaction and morale are at an all-time low, and there is a growing sense of a system now experiencing 'permacrisis'. Given the sense of urgency for an ambitious and radical overhaul of both service design and delivery, the post-pandemic era must be seen as an essential turning point in the way things are done.

This shift needs to locate care at the heart of our communities, where local needs are better understood and where local solutions are more readily accessed at neighbourhood level. Necessarily, this requires a re-prioritisation by system leaders from over-specialised, hospital-centric approaches to alternatives delivered by integrated, co-located, multidisciplinary teams, with greater capacity and flexibility, as well as an ethos of genuine partnership between themselves and the communities they serve. More flexible, 'bridge-builder' support roles will be needed to tackle health disparities and inequalities. Helping everyone to stay well longer means also putting a new emphasis on prevention, whole population health creation and investing in community initiatives that grow social capital and build greater resilience, to reduce future demand on statutory health care services.

Personalised care is not a 'magic silver bullet', but it offers a compelling vision of viable alternative approaches, with proven benefits. To be successful, change needs to be locally 'owned' and driven, within a framework of supportive national policies which devolve power and resources to the point of need. Workforce development and redesign can lead to a more autonomous frontline staff, free from top–down micro-management, generating more innovative solutions to improve outcomes. Strong connections with local communities and trust from local people will be the key to restoring the badly battered public confidence in the ability of our health care services to protect and enhance our wellbeing and quality of life. Personalised care offers the revolutionary inclusion of social prescribing into a historical biomedical, sickness model and gives us hope that the future will be better.

REFERENCES

Fuller, C., 2022. Next steps for integrating primary care: Fuller stocktake report. NHS England and NHS Improvement. https://www.england.nhs.uk/publication/next-steps-for-integrating-primary-care-fuller-stocktake-report/ (Accessed 3 March 2023).

Harvey, J., 2021. Written evidence submitted by Dr Jane Harvey. UK Parliament. https://committees.parliament.uk/writtenevidence/41641/pdf/ (Accessed 22 March 2023).

NHS England, 2019. Universal personalised care: implementing the comprehensive model. https://www.england.nhs.uk/wp-content/uploads/2019/01/universal-personalised-care.pdf (Accessed 1 March 2023).

The Richmond Group of Charities, 2022. No time to lose: Changing the trajectory for people living with long-term health conditions. https://richmondgroupofcharities.org.uk/sites/default/files/final_rg_mltc_report_a4_0.pdf (Accessed 3 March 2023).

World Health Organization, 2021. Guidance on community mental health services: Promoting person-centred and rights-based approaches. https://www.who.int/publications/i/item/9789240025707 (Accessed 3 March 2023).

Chapter 9

Going Upstream: Community Power and the Community Paradigm

Chris Dabbs

*'We cannot just pull people out of the river.
We need to go upstream and stop them falling in.'*

Introduction

The think tank New Local has been setting out a case for a fundamental shift in how public services work (Lent and Studdert, 2019). The 'community paradigm' means an equitable relationship between communities and public servants, designing and delivering things together, by focussing on the underlying causes of inequality, such as intergenerational trauma. Communities would have both more control and more responsibility.

This 'community paradigm' is based on three broad principles:

- Empowering communities – shifting decision-making power from institutions to communities
- Resourcing communities – communities having genuine power over and responsibility for decisions on public funding
- Creating a culture of community collaboration – collaboration between communities and public service organisations, rather than behaviour based on hierarchies and transactions

Paradigms Over Time

Public services exist within the prevailing culture of their time.

From the 16th to the early 20th century, there was a largely 'civic paradigm'. There was an evolving patchwork of independent bodies delivering limited public services. These were funded by voluntary contributions and, increasingly, some tax.

By the 1940s, there was predominantly a 'state paradigm'. This was characterised by a hierarchy, featuring professionally dominated siloes. People were seen and treated largely as passive 'service users'.

During the 1980s, there was a shift to a 'market paradigm'. This emphasised efficiency and cost, with relationships described in transactional terms. People were seen and treated largely as 'customers' or 'consumers', although without any economic power.

Although social, economic and environmental circumstances have changed, these two paradigms, the 'state' and the 'market', still hold heavy sway over public services. As responses to challenges of the distant past, they are often inappropriate to meet either rising demands or people's appetite for greater control over their own lives, including through the use of technology.

This situation also tends to reinforce a declining faith in representative democracy and central government. Many people increasingly feel either alienation from a remote political class and/or powerlessness up against corporate interests.

New Local argues that 'more power and resources should be given to communities rather than be held by central government or public services'. This 'community paradigm' reflects a belief that 'people and communities themselves have the best insight into their own situation', and that public services therefore need to work with this insight to be effective and sustainable.

Such a shift would involve communities supporting each other and creating long-term solutions, with public services focussed on prevention and early intervention, rather than reaction to acute situations and crises.

Social Prescribing

Officially, 'social prescribing' is described as 'an approach that connects people to activities, groups, and services in their community to meet the practical, social and emotional needs that affect their health and well-being' (NHS England, online). It tends to focus on people with health problems or complex social needs.

The standard model involves people being referred to a 'social prescribing link worker'. The worker discusses what matters to the person and works with them to produce a personalised care and support plan. The aim is to support the person to take control of their health and wellbeing.

This approach has been criticised by some, such as Cormac Russell (2017). He argues that the term 'social prescribing' can be counter-productive and disabling. Social prescribing in the UK often focusses on referrals to programmes and services within the voluntary sector, rather than encouraging people to be valued for their gifts and to become interdependent members of their communities. In short, there is too much emphasis on referrals to organisations and not enough on the associational life of communities themselves.

The very language of 'referrals', 'prescribing' and 'care and support plans' clearly base 'social prescribing' within a traditional medical mindset and context in which some people are held in higher value and hold much more power than others. This tends towards seeing and describing people as individual 'clients' or 'service users' and risks transactional relationships with professionals.

For the person, the risk is being linked to programmes and services, rather than actively exchanging their skills, knowledge and experience with others within a complex social context. There is scope, as articulated by the Camerados movement (online), to focus on being 'a bit more human' through purpose and friends. This includes having fun with others, being asked for help and being alongside people (rather than trying to 'fix' them).

This is not to say that 'social prescribing' activity is without value. Clearly, linking people to meaningful activities is better than leaving them languishing. It does, however, question the framing and approach of many 'social prescribing' services and programmes.

What Really Matters to People?

During 2021, a series of in-depth conversations were held with a range of adults in Salford, Greater Manchester, who had been on the 'shielding' list since March 2020 as a result of the COVID-19 situation. They reflected a diversity of ages, genders, races, sexual orientations, backgrounds, faiths and reasons for 'shielding'.

People were asked about what they enjoyed doing and what they most valued in their lives. Many people said that, to manage their experience of having long-term health conditions, they 'take things day by day' (Unlimited Potential, 2021).

Six themes emerged from people's stories and experiences:

- **Being respected**—people talked about the importance of being believed and understood by other people, as well as fair access. Some people spoke of not wanting other people to perceive them as 'ill', in order to avoid prejudice.
- **Health**—people talked about access to green spaces, exercise, being in spaces that felt clean and safe, day-to-day management of their health, and access to the health care system.
- **Understanding yourself**—people spoke about mental health training and therapy, as well as expressive creative outlets, such as writing poetry or expressing their personality in their style.
- **Purpose and being valued**—people talked about the importance of their work, learning new things, participating in social support groups or their faith community. They spoke as much about helping others as they did about being helped.
- **Quality relationships**—people talked about their friendships, romantic relationships, pets and their family.

- **Enjoyment**—people talked about things that were simply fun or distracting, such as television and movies, music, puzzles, shopping, travelling, art and crafts.

These priorities reflect not only themes that are important for all people but also those of more specific importance to people living with long-term health conditions and/or in complex social situations. There is particular scope to address them through community and using community power, complemented by appropriate support by and engagement with public and voluntary sectors.

How Might Things Be Different?

Both within communities and as a nation, we need different ways to look at social approaches to what makes us well. This includes exploring power, control, relationships and economics, recognising strengths and assets, managing complexity and enabling self-organisation.

There could be a different approach that reflects the 'community paradigm', which would be more effective than traditional 'social prescribing'.

Such an approach would actively address the determinants of health and wellbeing, rather than the symptoms. It would involve system leadership over the long term, integrating in 'one system' with both other social approaches and public services. It would also engage with other arenas, such as local employers.

Practically, rather than link workers, there would be a network of community-connecting champions (or 'participation advocates'). They would elaborate and strengthen connections within communities, as well as enable people to address the determinants of their own health and wellbeing through participation.

Rather than being led by either statutory or voluntary organisations, this would require governance that is more citizen/peer-led, being more efficient and streamlined while still enabling cooperative and partnership working.

Sustainability of this approach requires not only long-term funding from the public sector but also multiple income streams. Rather than a focus on funding to pay for services, it would shift towards investment in communities and their assets.

What Would Be Different for Communities?

Participation advocates would enable citizen-led discovery, connecting and mobilisation to embed community power within communities. Citizens—especially those people whose voices are quieter or often unheard (being 'easy to ignore' in the present system)—could then feel more valued and listened to.

The offer would be more a community offer than a service offer. It would support peer networks to enable people to connect and get involved in community life. It would reach all communities, especially those that experience the greatest inequalities (whether by class, geography or identity).

This approach is more likely to be widely recognised and trusted, with greater recognition of community-based ways to address issues, on par with the medical model for genuinely clinical issues.

Case Study: The Elephants Trail

The Elephants Trail in Greater Manchester creates spaces in which people who have experienced multiple disadvantages come together to develop collective solutions to issues. They first build relationships and explore power, wealth, inequality and the most difficult issues. Then, using techniques such as deep democracy and legislative theatre, they 'lean' into situations and make decisions together.

Either within their communities or, where necessary, partnering with local agencies, the teams work together for practical change on issues that directly affect the lives of people with the hardest lives. The aim is to create long-term solutions in which people believe and trust.

Along the way, the teams learn how to work together effectively. Some people have described their Elephants Trail experience as 'life changing' and 'the best thing that has ever happened to me'.

What Would Be Different for Individuals?

As of now, conversations with professionals and others should start with 'what matters to you?' rather than 'what is the matter with you?'

People would, however, primarily be seen in terms of their strengths (rather than their needs and deficits) and described by professionals as 'people I support' or equivalent, rather than as 'clients', 'service users', 'patients', etc.

Rather than a single gateway (such as a primary care practice), the approach would enable a broad range of entry points, especially for those who are isolated or marginalised (such as neighbours, family, friends, employers, local businesses and delivery services).

Increasingly, people would seek social rather than clinical or service solutions, including a balanced blend of direct and digital engagement. People would learn how to support and help themselves, often in a family or social approach (rather than an individual one). This would be encouraged through greater opportunities to link with like-minded people from diverse backgrounds.

This approach would also provide the conditions for more appropriate activities and social engagement for specific people, such as people with learning disabilities, people with dementia, D/deaf people and people from minority cultural or religious backgrounds. For example, a group of people with learning disabilities could create their own group to enable them to do physical activity together, rather than only staying in a day centre.

As a result, people would experience success as participating, interdependent members of their community, recognised and valued for their gifts, skills and passions, which they exchange with others. In some cases, people will feel liberated from what has limited or repressed them.

Key Principles

There are six key principles on which to base this new approach:

- Everyone has strengths that are needed to produce solutions.
- All types of power must be shared, and unequal power addressed.
- Good relationships are crucial. They need time, respect and trust.
- Diversity of people is important for high-quality thinking.
- There are different types of knowledges. Lived experience is valuable.

- It is important to test new ideas. There is no failure, just learning.

(co-produced with local people through the Elephants Trail, see www.elephantstrail.org.uk)

System Change ('The What')

We have learned through many diverse projects with local people and communities that such a system change towards this new approach requires action both by communities and at a system level.

Communities have the agency to do three key things themselves:

- Organise: gather and share local strengths (knowledge, skills, awareness); come together to take action on things that matter to communities; set up groups, organisations and enterprises.
- Take collaborative action: create trusted responses and social/emotional support that the usual services cannot meet; mutual aid—practical support, sharing resources, etc. (including in crises); community-run activities that improve wellbeing; build wealth, including through social/mutual ownership of assets.
- Spread with others: reach out and build trust with people 'not on the radar' or who do not want to engage with services and organisations; work alongside young people; spread the approach through spaces in other localities.

At the same time, four key things need to be done at a system level:

- Focus on prevention, rather than reaction: break the cycles that lead to disadvantage, poverty and trauma; help and support people long before they get into trouble and hit rock bottom; support people to develop life/social skills and political and economic literacy.
- Increase power held by communities: provide flexibility and shift/share control, resources and budgets to communities so that they can do more for themselves. (Power is not finite, so this does not necessarily mean a reduction in power held by professionals/agencies.)
- Build social/mutual ownership of wealth by communities: redistribute wealth socially to change people's economic status so that local

investment is realised and communities generate income within and outside 'the system'; shift procurement and funding towards communities, away from extractive outsiders who 'helicopter'/'parachute' in and out to produce 'outputs'; more high-quality jobs for local people.

- Work mutually alongside communities: reach out, see in person the reality on the ground for diverse people, beyond the data and the 'gatekeepers'; develop a culture of genuine co-production with local people; have real transparency and accountability at all levels about whether or not things are changing, and whether or not people feel more control and influence.

Co-Production With Local People and Communities ('The How')

To realise the vision in practice requires genuine co-production with local people and communities, crucially involving an equitable sharing of power and wealth.

Exploration with local people and communities has concluded that this means four key areas of activity:

- Value and invest in people and communities. This means to: appreciate the value and *strengths* already in communities (skills, *knowledges* and experience)—turn disadvantage into an advantage (lived experience); encourage *diversity* of backgrounds, life experiences and mindsets for high-quality thinking; invest time, energy and resources, and recognise that this needs to be different for people facing severe and multiple disadvantages; engage people throughout the process to develop ownership; ensure practical benefits for participants (such as personal development, life opportunities and payment for specific tasks/roles).
- Focus on a clear purpose—change. This means to: start with a very clear core purpose (system change, not fitting within the system or a 'sticking plaster' approach); reach consensus on direction, focus and priorities; work together and collaborate for practical change; be honest about *power*, how the system works and how to 'play the game'; *power* is critical—increase the power held by local people and communities so

they have more agency to do things together for themselves, and can lead on their own issues, without having to wait for others.

- Create a supportive environment and trusting relationships. This means to: create a gentle, caring, thoughtful environment/space in which people feel safe and trusted, and can be authentic and understood; from the start, enable the *diversity* of people to get to know each other, and nurture and value trusting *relationships* between them; early on, establish ground rules, including how conflicts or inappropriate behaviour will be addressed; encourage and support honest speaking, deep listening and structured team building; create and facilitate spaces for people to grow, develop and act together; connect, engage directly and build *relationships* with professionals and agencies for mutual understanding, co-production and collaboration.
- Support and share action learning. This means to: accept the complexity and let it run; exchange ideas in a democratic environment; prioritise *relationships* and principles (not performance indicators and outputs) to enable *testing*, experimentation and capture of learning (rather than 'success' or 'failure'); enable local people to contribute their narratives and *knowledges* on their own terms while learning how to present effectively to 'the system'.

Conclusion

Modern social, economic and environmental circumstances require an equitable relationship between communities and public servants, designing and delivering things together, with a focus on prevention. This means the creation of environments in which new solutions can be nurtured, and the conditions for those solutions to spread.

Things can evolve to address what really matters to people, and the determinants of their health and wellbeing. This requires investment in communities and their assets, strengthening and multiplying the connections within communities. This encourages community life, involving more diverse people in greater numbers. As a result, social solutions for many issues become as or more attractive than service solutions.

This requires system change at both community and system levels, with an open and honest reflection on, and redistribution of, collective power and wealth. This can be achieved only through true co-production between the 'system' and local people and communities.

There is a wide range of such activity at neighbourhood and local levels, but these are rarely nurtured or spread and so tend to remain small and isolated examples. Inspiring as these may be, we need a more systemic approach for a broad impact, both in unity with local communities and together with the 'system'.

In this way, people will not only feel that they can make or help to shape the decisions that affect their lives but actually do it!

REFERENCES

Camerados. Available from: https://camerados.org/what-is-camerados/ (Accessed March 2023).

Lent, A., Studdert, J., 2019. The community paradigm. Why public services need radical change and how it can be achieved, London: New Local. Available from: https://www.newlocal.org.uk/publications/the-community-paradigm/ (Accessed 27 February 2024).

NHS England, online. What is Social Prescribing? Available from: https://www.england.nhs.uk/personalisedcare/social-prescribing/ (Accessed 6 March 2023).

Russell, C., 2017. Social prescribing, a panacea or another top-down programme? Available from: https://www.nurturedevelopment.org/blog/abcd-approach/social-prescribing-panacea-another-top-programme-part-1/ (Accessed 6 March 2023).

Unlimited Potential, 2021. Day by day. Priorities of people with long-term health conditions. Available from: https://www.unlimitedpotential.org.uk/enterprise/innovation-projects/day-day (Accessed 6 March 2023).

Chapter 10

Interview With Lord Gus O'Donnell

Heather Henry

HH

What on earth prompts a former cabinet secretary to three prime ministers and an influential economist to become such an outspoken advocate for wellbeing?

GO'D

Very good question. Basically, I moved from academia—I was teaching economics—into government … most of my time working within the civil service, in the treasury and also abroad as well. And one of the things that I thought was missing in all of my time, there was governments being really clear about what it was that they wanted to achieve—what was their success measure—and what were they trying to do for the country, the nation, the people? And it just struck me that all my life I'd really, as an economist, bought into the idea that we are trying to (and here the economists have their own jargon) maximise people's utility or improve what they call a social welfare function, which is basically the sum of everybody's utility. By that we're basically saying we want people to have high-quality lives, satisfied lives that are worthwhile. And to me that was clearly the ultimate goal of what government should be.

Now, along the way you have interim measures which see whether you're improving people's wellbeing, but to me that was what it fundamentally should be about. And of course when you start to think about that, as an economist you want to measure everything. 'If you treasure it, measure it'. And the question was then, well, how do we measure wellbeing? And we could go on for hours about that, but

one of the important aspects of wellbeing—not the only one by any means but the important one—is people's perception of their own wellbeing, what's known in the trade as subjective wellbeing.

And one of my last acts as cabinet secretary with the coalition government and particularly with David Cameron as Prime Minister was to start this process of asking people questions: about how satisfied our people were with their lives, how worthwhile they thought they were, and questions about happiness and anxiety. And we've now got data on that going back to about 2012. And it was incredibly useful for us during the COVID period to track what was happening to people's wellbeing. And it's also incredibly useful to look at variations across age, across different parts of the country, across different states … you know, the level of people's wellbeing when they're unemployed versus employed … the relationship with income … all sorts of things. To actually understand what are the drivers of wellbeing.

And once you get that, it's like coming back to governments and saying, 'So, isn't this what you're really trying to achieve?' And we've seen it most recently with the new Prime Minister saying, 'It's all about growth'; well, growth in what? If it was growth in the quality of people's lives, that would be brilliant. But I'm afraid rather lazily people may translate it as growth in gross national product. Or something like that, which would be quite a big mistake.

HH

Because you've talked about changing the gross national product measure into basically wellbeing, have you had much traction on that?

GO'D

It's slightly more complicated than that in the sense that we have gross national product, gross domestic product, which economists have used as a measure of activity, what's going on in the economy. And it's been going for decades now. But the people that put it together said, 'For God sake, don't use this as a success measure'. But I'm afraid that message has got lost along the way. And people think of when we say 'oh, growth's gone up 2% this year,' well that's unambiguously good. It means that there's been 2% more activity. It depends on whether the activity's good or not.

We've just noticed in the health field that actually GDP fell recently because we weren't testing and vaccinating so many people, and that's because we'd succeeded in the work on COVID. So you have to realise actually that more activity here is because of a bad thing. More activity here doesn't mean that people's lives are better, it means that they're worse. Wouldn't it be great if we didn't have to vaccinate anyone or test anyone because COVID hadn't happened? But because we had to, that's been a positive push. Obviously, COVID's had many, many more negative effects on the economy as well. So I think the question is … GDP … I don't want to say we want to drop it, but we do need a better measure of what constitutes success for society, and I'm saying that GDP really measures what income we've got, how much we're producing—which is very relevant and important—but actually if as a society everybody is getting more miserable, even if we were getting richer, would you really be happy with that?

What I think should be our goal is to give people very satisfying, worthwhile lives … that they feel proud of themselves and feel happy. That's kind of ultimately what it's about.

HH

And has the government and treasury listened to you when you talk about these measures of success?

GO'D

The fact that David Cameron started things off—I think that it was really important. In terms of where we've got to, I think the civil service as a whole has now got the tools to measure these things. They've put out a manual called the HM Government (2022a) to show people how to measure these things and to allow for them.

Have we succeeded at a political level? I think that's pretty much work in progress. I think this is much more understood at the community level, at local levels. Is it understood nationally? Do I hear politicians talking about how to improve wellbeing? No. Politicians will always want to use their own language. So, they may not use the word 'wellbeing'. They may use quality of life, standard of living—things like that. But it's work in progress, and I wish we'd got a lot further. Some countries like New Zealand, Iceland, the devolved nations—Wales and Scotland—have shown some interest. There are examples around the world and places where it's starting to get more traction. For many years we've had world happiness reports (https://worldhappiness.report/) which look at the determinants of wellbeing and have suggested policies. So, it's growing, but it's growing more bottom up than top down.

HH

I've got to agree with you because I see in the third sector, in the communities that I work with, in the commissioners that I work with—they now understand and accept that there are methods for measuring social value and wellbeing and encourage us as providers of wellbeing services to accept them. I use the Office for National Statistics 4 wellbeing questions (happiness, anxiety, a worthwhile, satisfying life; ONS4, online)—were you involved in those?

GO'D

Yes. Very much at the start. We should give a shout-out to David Halpern who set up the Behavioural Insights Unit (https://www.bi.team/). David and I talked about this a lot. I knew that the way that we would get this taken seriously … to get the evidence together … to convince particularly those hard-nosed folk in the treasury, you need really good evidence. We weren't even able to say what's been happening to wellbeing in the country—we didn't have an agreed definition.

So, the ONS4 questions … they had roadshows … they went round the country and asked people about it. And in the end those are the four we've got, and now they have the status of official national statistics, which is very important. So, they generate good, reliable, consistent data. The OECD (Organisation for Economic Co-operation and Development, online) does this, so many, many more countries are now measuring very similar things.

When you got that data, you begin to have a more serious conversation about it, otherwise people say, 'Well this is all very fluffy, what does it mean, we haven't got any evidence?' So all these things we can now say that actually we have. There's the Oxford Centre (https://wellbeing.hmc.ox.ac.uk/) that Jan de Neve has set up; there's the What Works Centre for Wellbeing (https://whatworkswellbeing.org/); I chair a charity called Pro Bono Economics (https://www.pro-bonoeconomics.com/). We are emphasising improving wellbeing and reducing inequalities in wellbeing. I think it's taking off, and when you go to communities, you think about levelling up.

Andy Haldane, who went into government, who's a founder of Pro Bono Economics, was the chief economist at the Bank of England and worked on the Levelling Up white paper for this government (HM Government, 2022b). In there you'll see that improving wellbeing is part of the missions and successes. So, it's getting there. I wish we had some more courageous politicians who would go out and start saying, 'Okay guys, so you want to increase wellbeing? Well, what should we do?' And starting to say, 'I'm pursuing this package of improving the amount of money that we're spending on mental health—or looking at mental health issues in the young', and moving away from just measuring success in schools by exam results, by looking at the wellbeing of the kids—that would be great for me. As yet, I think the politicians are a little bit behind the people.

HH

Now, you mentioned the Behavioural Insights Team or the so-called 'nudge unit' that help people make better choices. Is behavioural science relevant to social prescribing, and if so, in what way?

GO'D

Massively. I was brought up as an economist and taught economics. It's known as 'the dismal science'. But it certainly had a dismal view of human nature, which is that the only way that you could describe people in an economic model is as basically as 'positronic robots'— I think Isaac Asimov had it about right (Asimov and Silverberg, 1992). We work out fine calculations about what's going to maximise our utility over the course of our lifetimes, subject to the money will have. And we make these perfectly rational decisions. We never make mistakes. We're never short-sighted. If we've got a world of people like that, there's not much role for government, to be honest, and everything sorts itself out very nicely.

Surprise, surprise, the world is full of people like you and me who make mistakes! We can be short-sighted and we can get things wrong, we can sometimes be quite selfish and sometimes altruistic. We need to build government policy around the real world, around what real people do and what matters to real people. And I think that's where we've gone wrong. So, trying to cope with things like addiction, where a rational model would say, 'Once people know that smoking is bad, they'll stop'—well, actually they don't. So building it around real human nature has been really important.

I'd say, all policy analysts need to understand a lot more about what drives human behaviour, and that's every area, be it how to persuade people to pay their taxes or anything else—there's a lot of behavioural insights gone into that and it's been quite successful. How do we persuade people to stop smoking? Social prescribing comes in there. How do we persuade people in the current circumstances to economise on energy? For one thing, it's expensive, but we can try to explain to people, as David Halpern was recently doing on BBC Radio 4—is it really necessary to have a shower every day?

But in all of that we need to be incredibly careful about one of the lessons of behavioural public policy, which is that it really really matters who the messenger is. If the messenger is seen as an all-powerful state, we get a nanny state … the government is telling you you can't have a shower every day, then people will rebel against it. We need to think about actually providing people with information and understanding of the issues, so they make their own choices. Have faith in people making better choices but also help them and incentivise them to make the choices that are not only good for them but good for society as a whole.

HH

So I can see a lot of hope there in terms of the development of social prescribing link workers or community connectors who, certainly in this part of the world, in Greater Manchester, they are local people who understand other local people and local community. And so I think that's really helpful, and also within health and social care there's a lot around motivational interviewing, so me as a nurse that used to sit in general practice and used to tell people what they should and shouldn't do for their lifestyle and moving much more to that conversation about what matters to people, what they're interested in and following that link into understanding their wellbeing rather than going straight for the blood pressure or the heart disease. It makes a lot of sense to us as practitioners.

GO'D

Absolutely, and I would say that your whole point about getting this closer to the people, doing it at local and community level—because nationally and centrally the kind of messages that might work in a rich Surrey suburb might be very different from those that work in a deprived area. And the pressures that people face would be very different in those areas. So, spending more time walking and playing golf may be more appropriate in one area and be completely wrong for somewhere else. We need to be quite local in this. Which is why I say one of the good things that is happening at the moment in wellbeing is that it is being understood locally at community level. It is in a sense devolving power to them, to say, 'Look, we recognise what we want to do we want to improve, let's say, parenting skills but we're not sure how to do it'. The last thing they need is a government edict. In Manchester you've got a brilliant initiative called the Bee Well initiative (https://www.manchester.ac.uk/discover/social-responsibility/civic/beewell/) which is looking at surveying kid's wellbeing and looking at those areas

where there are particularly low levels and trying to work out what's the source of that and what can be done about it. I think that's a brilliant initiative. But it had to happen at local level because nationally we're still obsessed with measuring success by exam results.

HH

You seem to have a lot of interest in children and young people compared to adults and older adults.

GO'D

You can take the man out of the treasury but you can't take the treasury out of the man, they say. If you do things early, then you get it right. You will know from a health point of view that those first few weeks of life are massively important in terms of the development of babies, and in general the sooner you can get at problems to either correct them or prevent them, the better.

From a treasury point of view, quite often you're dealing with the cost of failure, which is really high. So failure from a treasury point of view is someone who, rather than contributing positively to society, has been unemployed, then they've committed crime, they're now in prison … it's costing you a lot of money, both in benefits and in looking after them in prison. Whereas if you have that earlier initiative, let's say at school—those 'sliding doors' moments where someone's been tilted by a great teacher, or someone who's motivated them to push their lives in a different direction—and then they become a success, they're earning money, they're volunteering, they're working for charities and they're paying lots of tax. They're not costing the state a lot. Everybody wins. To me, that's an example of success. So, the earlier we do these interventions, the better, because otherwise we're just dealing with the costs of our previous failures.

HH

And alongside that around earlier intervention you also talk quite a lot about why are we still spending on failure and shouldn't we be spending more on health promotion. And now I'm thinking: In an era of long waiting lists post COVID, what should health and care leaders be doing with their budgets, or is it a treasury issue? Is it a matter of poking the treasury and saying, 'Well, I know that we've got to catch up with all the long waiting times, and things like that, but also if we don't do that work on improving wellbeing, keeping people as well as they can, rather than catching up on their operations, we're gonna fail surely?' We're going to be spending on failure rather than spending on wellbeing! But I'm just wondering how much you think local leaders can help with this, in the new integrations and the relationships that we're developing, beyond health and social care, housing, policing?

GO'D

There are two dimensions to this. There's the macro—the big end from treasury about how much we should spend on health overall. With our ageing society we're going to have to spend more on health. And then comes the question on how we allocate that money then. For me it would be trying to bias it towards exactly the things that you've been talking about: the integrated care systems, the whole system on prevention. But you do then hit the problem of politics. You just need to look at the kind of things that politicians say and the promises they make on health care. It's 'so many thousand more nurses, doctors or hospitals', it's not actually 'what we're going to do is improve quality of life or life expectancy'—it's these intermediate inputs. To me a successful health system would be one where we are having fewer hospitals, fewer people in hospitals because we're actually preventing them going in—there's less need for these things because we've reallocated some of the money towards the prevention end, the front end, the integrated care that's keeping people out of these problems, rather than just letting that happen and saying, 'OK, well, we've got loads of people with diabetes or issues with increasing obesity, let's spend a lot of money on dealing with their diseases'. I want to prevent them in the first place, I don't want them getting there.

My esteemed colleague Nigel Crisp wrote a very good book, *Health Is Made at Home, Hospitals Are for Repairs* (2020). And I think that's it really—we should regard everybody going into hospitals as a bit of a failure—we should have kept them out.

One thing I would also add is a book by John List (2022), an economist, called *The Voltage Effect*, and it is all about how you scale up. Believe me, he's worked a lot with the private sector with Uber and with Lyft in the United States. And there are some really important lessons in there about how to go from something that looks really successful locally to try to range it out nationally, because it's really hard.

HH

Now I want you to turn to the capacity of voluntary community and social enterprises, because social prescribing basically relies on that capacity, and you've done some work on attempting to measure the economic output of charities. What did you discover in that work?

GO'D

We're coming to the end of a 2-year [project] called The Law Family Commission on Civil Society (The Law Family Commission and Pro Bono Economics, 2023) which looks at the broader social sector. But yes, if you just looked at the charity sector (slightly narrower than the whole civil society), [it] is worth in monetary terms about £22 billion, according to the national accounts—that's 1% of GDP. We reckon that the social value that it adds is about 10 times that £22 billion; so there are about 1 million people working in the sector—about 180,000 charities! So, I think this is a massively underresearched and undervalued part of our community. Because we don't measure it—it's not in our national accounts.

Famously, I keep saying that if everybody stopped volunteering and started getting into prostitution and illegal drugs activity, GDP would rise. It's crazy! So I think that unmeasured part means we don't value it enough. It's a massively important part of our society, but because it's not measured or looked at, nobody's really thought about how we make it as efficient as possible.

How do we help unleash the potential that's there? Because when I look at charities and I talk to them, as we have for the Commission, we find that they are spending an awful lot of time and money on applying for grants. Couldn't we ask the grant providers to make it a bit easier and a bit more standardised? We find that there are a lot of government programmes to help small and medium-sized enterprises to be more productive and to think about how for example to use digital—to be web-based. And all those programmes aren't open to charities—and that's crazy.

And another part of it is why is it that philanthropy in this country seem to be rather different and in some cases much lower than places like, say, the United States. And we're looking at the incentives to philanthropy. There are some brilliant philanthropists in our society who are doing great things, but we need to think about why we aren't doing more, and we're looking at the whole tax position, things like Gift Aid and the like.

When I taught economics, we were taught there's a private sector and there are things that businesses don't do—the things that the state has to do, like defence, [...] the NHS and stuff like that, where you're not doing it for a profit. It was just that it was either public or private, but actually there's this massive part in between which is not done by the private sector or the public sector—which is done by communities, by voluntary groups, food banks. We saw it during COVID where you can see [...] the gaps—these things where the state or the private sector is just not filling really important needs that people have. That's where civil society comes in, that's where charities come in. And so we're trying in all of this work to work out how you value charities and how you make them fulfil their potential.

HH

For me as a charity trustee and as a social enterprise—I have both of those roles, and I've been a commissioner in the NHS in the past—I don't quite know, because it is civil society, the best way to go in terms of securing the future of our 40-year-old charity Being There (supporting people with life-limiting illness). Every year we have to wait with bated breath to find out whether our NHS contract is going to be renewed or not, which is a very unstable thing. What should the funding model be for the voluntary community and social enterprise sector?

GO'D

I would say the things that don't get funded are like the infrastructure; it's very hard when you're a charity to say, look, we're going to set up proper systems to manage our impact. People are saying, well, how much is going to the frontline? What people really should be asking is: What impact are you making or what difference? And quite often that requires you to set up systems to measure your impact.

HH

Yes, I came out of the NHS and the first thing I did was volunteer for Being There. I'd been trained by the New Economic Foundation on how to do a social return on investment (SROI). You shouldn't be doing a social return on investment on your own organisation, I realise that, but we were at that stage where I didn't know about our future. So we did a basic SROI based on the Cabinet Office guidance. Fortunately [our charity] measured a lot of really important things like how they avoided hospital admission for people with life-limiting conditions. And of course we could look up the proxy values easy enough for that, the social values; we presented that to the commissioners. And that was a game changer, I think, in terms of how that charity was viewed—that it was able to put a value on it. And since that time we've added it to our annual report. But these things are really difficult for small organisations and getting the support to do that because it costs money to have these evaluations done externally, doesn't it?

GO'D

Absolutely. I'm the chair of trustees at Pro Bono Economics, and we started off by just helping charities to measure their impact—exactly the things you talked about—for free. There's a limit to what we can do, and we're now trying not just to do that but to actually influence policy change, to try to make these things better. You're right, it's tough for a charity where quite often when you apply for grants it's difficult to get money in there for evaluation, for the infrastructure that you need to do these things. It's not as glamorous as some of the other things that you could spend money on. But it's really important. Social infrastructure and social capital are really undervalued. We are spending huge amounts on physical capital and we are very short on social capital.

HH

If you were the current cabinet secretary, what would be your advice on the future of social prescribing?

GO'D

It's a massive opportunity. You think of what's going to happen over the next few years. It's going to be really tough on public spending because there are commitments to spend a lot more on defence, and the world has become a more dangerous place, so that's really expensive.

We know on COVID that we've got a big backlog, so there's a lot more that we need to spend—and there's an ageing society, so we'll have to spend a lot more on health. All of these things start to mount up. So what you're looking for is opportunities to say, how can we do this more effectively? Social prescribing is a brilliant way of using […] that money more efficiently and using it in a way that prevents future failure. So it makes the problem less intense as you go further on.

[…] We are now borrowing a lot, and I understand why. But that comes from future taxpayers, it's just deferring tax, not anything else, so it's not going to get much easier for quite a long time. Long term we need to be working on how we solve these problems in a way that is much more about prevention than cure. Social prescribing, if it basically reduced our drugs bill […], getting people to exercise more—wouldn't that be brilliant? Or looking at the number of antidepressants prescribed … could we save a fair bit of money there?

HH

I haven't asked you about welfare reform. I'm a big fan of Darren McGarvey (2022), the author and rapper. […] Is there anything that can be done around welfare reform? Do you see any ideas that might support the idea that some people really aren't scrounges but their experience of claiming benefits quite often makes them very sick indeed?

GO'D

That's a longer-term issue, and the whole principle of job centres or the benefits system is to try to get people back into work, because we know that unemployment is a massive problem for wellbeing. People's sense of self-worth goes down. Obviously their income's down—it has all sorts of knock-on issues—so getting people into jobs is massively important—and to try to make sure that the system incentivises that.

Obviously they'll be an element in any welfare system when you're making sure that there isn't widespread fraud […] let's not back away from that, but yes we should be treating people with respect. I always say, how would you feel if you were the customer […], how do we encourage the individual that we're dealing with, that almost certainly is facing multiple problems and multiple difficulties—how do we help them make their lives better, improve their own wellbeing? And along the way that will hopefully mean that they reduced their cost to the state because we get them into good jobs and we stop them claiming benefits. This is not an easy one, I'll be honest with you.

HH

Is there anything else you'd like to say?

GO'D

There's interesting work coming out of the Bee Well study on gender identification issues which I think needs more exploring. There are curious things about age—we kind of go through this midlife crisis which people have documented. I think beginning to understand, analyse and research […] where people are beginning to feel that their lives are losing meaning. And I suppose the other thing is this whole concept of good work and what constitutes a good job and not just a job, and how we give people who are in jobs a sense of it being worthwhile.

I think we should accept the fact that AI is going to mean that a lot more jobs that are repetitive will be done by machines, and these are not just repetitive physical jobs but repetitive mental jobs like basic stuff on accounting and auditing, which may well be done by AI systems. So we need to think about the future, how do we make sure that there are opportunities for people to make a real difference, and I think the biggest area will be one that is close to you, which is social care, because people want to be looked after by people. We haven't yet got the robot that really replaces the nurse and a loving carer. [...] These are massively important jobs and yet are paid incredibly badly. So I think there's real opportunities there.

REFERENCES

Asimov, I., Silverberg, R., 1992. The Positronic Man. Bantam/Spectra, New York.

Crisp, N., 2020. Health is made at home, hospitals are for repairs: Building a healthy and health-creating society. SALUS Global Knowledge Exchange. Billericay.

HM Government, 2022a. The Green Book. Available from: https://www.gov.uk/government/publications/the-green-book-appraisal-and-evaluation-in-central-governent/the-green-book-2020 (Accessed 3 March 2023).

HM Government, 2022b. Levelling Up the United Kingdom. Available from: https://www.gov.uk/government/publications/levelling-up-the-united-kingdom (Accessed 3 January 2023).

List, J. 2022. The Voltage Effect. Penguin Business. Dublin.

McGarvey, D., 2022. The Social Distance Between Us: How Remote Politics Wrecked Britain. Ebury Press, London.

Office for National Statistics, 2024. Personal Wellbeing User Guidance. Available from: https://www.ons.gov.uk/peoplepopulationandcommunity/wellbeing/methodologies/personalwellbeingsurveyuserguide (Accessed 3 January 2023).

Organisation for Economic Co-operation and Development. Better Life Initiative: Measuring Well-Being and Progress. Available from: https://www.oecd.org/wise/better-life-initiative.htm (Accessed 3 January 2023).

The Law Family Commission and Pro Bono Economics, 2023. The Law Family Commission on Civil Society. Available from: https://civilsocietycommission.org/ (Accessed 10 March 2023).

Chapter 11

Primary Care, Health Creation and the Role of Social Prescribing

Merron Simpson and Hazel Stuteley

Introduction

The Health Creation Alliance (THCA) and C2 Connecting Communities (C2), the two organisations we lead, have been pioneering the development and practical approaches to community-led 'health creation' for several decades. Put simply, local service providers—NHS, police, education, housing, employment agencies, fire service, voluntary and community sector and local councils—work together as equal partners with local people, communities of geography or identity. Collectively, they tackle and remove barriers to wellness. Where there is parity of agency between communities and services, this consistently leads to transformative and lasting quality-of-life, health and socioeconomic outcomes (Fujiwara et al., 2016).

What Makes People and Communities Well?

Research backed by experience tells us, time and again, that lacking a sense of control and influence over our lives and immediate environments is a major cause of health inequalities, damaging health and social behaviours and leading to costly management of chronic illness and community breakdown (Wilkinson and Pickett, 2009).

Our experience over many years of working with our members tells us that much of this *is reversible* through health creation; a more precise version of the question might therefore be: *What makes people and communities well—and what is keeping them well?* Working backwards from experience leads us to a paradigm that is entirely different from the usual 'service paradigm' on which most national programmes and policies are based.

Control Shift: A Tale of Two Paradigms

THE SERVICE PARADIGM

The service paradigm starts with services and with the individuals who use those services. So, co-production is about designing *services with* people and communities; funded social prescribing link workers connect individual *patients* to the right *services* or local agencies; even personal budgets start from the perspective of diversifying individuals' experiences beyond the existing *service* provision.

All three examples—co-production, social prescribing and personal budgets—have elements of health creation within them and *will* improve lives. However, their *service* starting point makes it difficult to unlock the power to transform places and people's lives because this requires a shift in the locus of control and resources to communities and leaders with lived experience. This enables greater community control and many more interventions that are community and lived experience led.

THE HEALTH CREATION PARADIGM

Health creation starts with *people,* not services, and with what makes communities well.

It is aligned with concepts of 'human flourishing', describing a process where people and communities 'move towards health' through the constructive relationships with family, friends, teachers and others. This is a key argument made by Lord Nigel Crisp in his book, *Health Is Made at Home* (2020).

For many people the journey is difficult because they don't have constructive relationships in place through which they can gain confidence, become resilient and access the things they need, whether physical, social or emotional. Poverty, trauma and discrimination are the common backdrop to this, and all are found in high concentration within our most disadvantaged, very low-income communities where health outcomes are poorest.

THE ROLE OF HEALTH, SYSTEMS LEADERS, PUBLIC AND THIRD SECTORS IN HEALTH CREATION

Adopting health creation demands a shift in mindset and action. Insights from complexity science offer a compelling argument for viewing a community as a *complex adaptive system* (Mitleton-Kelly, 2006) with ability to transform and create 'new order'. Complexity science has been built into our approaches since 2004. The quality and nature of creating new relationships between local people and agencies are the key to success. This means that service providers and systems leaders look through a different lens and shift from 'calling the shots' to 'creating the enabling conditions' for individuals and communities to take control and self-organise. Health Foundation (2010). This call to action prefaced THCA's Health Creation: Coming of Age event (The Health Creation Alliance, 2022 online). This same approach features in systems leadership (Sorkin, 2016).

Far from being an additional thing for services to do, the evidence shows that over time, working to create the conditions for communities to take control lessens the burden on services. An example here is the Wigan Deal where power and control is shifted from the council to people (Naylor and Wellings, 2019). Health creation is an opportunity to improve wellness and economic productivity potential and to spend increasingly limited money in the most efficient way.

A Framework to Support A Transformation to Health Creation

Seven years ago, THCA (formerly the New NHS Alliance), supported by its growing membership and C2, set out to bring clarity to the core question: What makes people and communities well? This question led THCA to develop a powerful framework for health creation that can aid translation into practice in many contexts and guide a whole-system approach to enhancing health and addressing health inequalities.

We started by drawing on a broad range of wisdom gained from clinical, academic, sociological, economic and community leaders who have a long track record working to address inequality and transform health outcomes for people and place. We also dug deep, through myriad interactions with our diverse membership, to understand more about the conditions that have made communities well. We distilled the essence of this into a pithy framework and have since gathered significant supporting evidence.

The framework consists of four elements, expanded below:

- A definition of health creation as a process
- The three Cs that describe how that process happens
- The six features of health-creating practices, the condition-creating elements
- The four types of relationships to address the wider determinants of health and drivers of system transformation.

A DEFINITION OF HEALTH CREATION

Health creation is the process through which individuals and communities gain a sense of purpose, hope, mastery and control over their own lives and immediate environment; when this happens their health and wellbeing are enhanced.

(Hazel Stuteley OBE, 2014)

THE PROCESS—CONNECTIONS, CONFIDENCE, CONTROL

Building meaningful and constructive **Connections** between people increases **Confidence**, leading over time to greater **Control** over our lives and the determinants of our health.

These are the three Cs (3Cs) of health creation—Connections, Confidence and Control—describing a new way of conceptualising and drawing together a range of theories from Antonovsky, Frankl, Burns, Sen, Marmot and the Young Foundation (THCA, online). These have long been expressed in the health world by different names and are based on *salutogenesis* (Antonovsky, 1987), the ancient study of wellness, as opposed to *pathogenesis*, the study of disease, the latter reflecting the NHS predominant biochemical model of health since inception.

THE SIX FEATURES OF HEALTH-CREATING PRACTICES

Communities consistently tell us that there are six features that make the biggest difference to their health outcomes. All six define a health-creating dynamic in relationships between communities, service providers and decision-makers. The importance of getting the relationships right is expertly outlined by Hilary Cottam (2018, see Chapter 12).

Diligently embedding these six features into all our practices and relationships will drive change across systems. They are:

- listening and responding
- truth-telling
- strengths-focus
- self-organising
- reciprocity
- power-shifting

(Source: The Health Creation Alliance, https://the-healthcreationalliance.org/health-creation/)

THE FOUR TYPES OF RELATIONSHIPS

The challenge for Integrated Care Systems (ICSs) is to get all four relationship dynamics right:

- Between community members
- Between NHS and communities
- Between other local partners[1] and communities
- Between NHS and other local partners

Getting all these right enables emergence of new 'pathways' within a more diverse ecosystem of informal support and activity and formal services so that people and communities are much better able to access the things they need when they need them.

This framework of three Cs, six features and four relationships is a 'plumbline' against which any activity, innovation, service or approach can be measured. As one of THCA member recently said, *'If things are going right, the 6 features of health creating practices will be manifest'.*

Social Prescribing Can Be Health Creating

Social prescribing has seen a rapid rise and is a very welcome shift from the predominant NHS medical to a social model of health. However, it remains inherently within the service paradigm, starting with services and with patients using those services.

MANY ROLES BADGED AS 'SOCIAL PRESCRIBING'

Social prescribing has its roots outside the NHS in a range of advocacy, 'early help', 'navigator' and 'tenancy support' roles where people are supported to find their way around complex systems to find and get access to the things they need.

The Primary Care Network (PCN) contract of 2019 unleashed a new army of NHS-funded 'link workers' based in GP practices, whose role is principally to connect patients to community groups and statutory services that provide practical and emotional support. This provided both disruption and challenge to these pre-existing arrangements as clinicians set about developing a new social prescribing workforce and existing voluntary sector organisations already doing this work sought contracts with them to deliver. Initially, there were very different views on the best way to use this new resource to address patient needs, but over time the roles and relationships have evolved and settled down with increasing numbers of contracts managed through the voluntary sector.

In many places, an array of roles, purposes and employment arrangements now co-exist. There has also been a shift in the language used; many community groups have re-badged what they were historically doing as 'social prescribing' to access funding and to gain greater recognition by the NHS. The Bristol Somali Resource Centre (https://www.somalicentre.org.uk/) is an example of the latter; centre leaders describe what they offer to their community as 'social prescribing', even though they are not supported through NHS resources and the formal paid social prescribers refer people to them for assistance.

Social prescribing is varied, ranging from highly transactional referral mechanisms to highly relational community-building models. It is difficult to justify ascribing a single title to all the roles, models and approaches. This multiplicity could also be part of the reason the evidence that social prescribing improves health and reduces demand for health care remains comparatively weak.

---

[1]Other local partners include, for example, police, education, housing, employment agencies, fire service, voluntary and community sector and local councils.

SOME SOCIAL PRESCRIBING IS HEALTH CREATING

There are many examples of health-creating social prescribing enabling people to employ and enjoy their skills and passions through meaningful connection with others.

Our hypothesis is that where social prescribing works, a key reason is that *relationships are valued and the six features of health-creating practices are manifest within them,* the relationships the patient holds with their link worker, other agencies and, crucially, other community members. The six features are the 'active ingredients'; where they are not manifest, the outcomes will be poor.

FORMALISING HEALTH CREATION; A WORK IN PROGRESS

The Thriving Communities Programme, launched in November 2020 and led by the National Academy for Social prescribing (NASP), is a nod to the power of health creation.

Recognising the critical roles that voluntary, community, faith and social enterprise groups made to the COVID-19 response, it supports new partnerships, sharing of learning and innovation to improve and increase community activities working alongside social prescribing link workers. It was supported by a £1.8m fund; however, this is a drop in the ocean compared to the massive reductions in local government funding over the last decade that has reduced community capacity and hit low-income communities with the poorest health outcomes very hard. The evaluation is ongoing at the time of writing.

The Health Creation Framework provides a good investment and commissioning guide for Integrated Care Systems (ICSs) to create the enabling conditions and activities that support the development of solutions that are in line with community needs and ambitions. Running alongside this, population health data and the Core20PLUS5 approach (NHS England, 2021) help with prioritisation of communities for investment up to 2024. However, investment in relationship building and community-led activity will need to be long term to sustain health creation going forward.

A Big Problem Needs a Wholesale Solution

A WHOLESALE SOLUTION STARTS WITH A NEW SOCIAL CONTRACT

The chasm of health inequalities is ever widening, with real progress to address it evading us for many decades.

A 'wicked' problem of this size cannot be solved by social prescribing or the Thriving Communities programme alone. It requires a much more fundamental shift in how we *all* work, supported by a new social contract that redraws the power dynamic and creates equal partnerships of the people and communities experiencing health inequalities and those who make the decisions on how to address them. Enabling community and lived experience leaders to emerge and to inform and share in decision-making is the basis for fresh solutions to emerge and create a new ecosystem of possibility for individuals and communities to meet their needs, achieve their ambitions and thrive. A large part of the solution to health inequalities lies with the often-amazing people and communities experiencing them, enabled through the practice of health creation.

A new social contract must:

- Position communities that have the poorest health outcomes as equal partners, listened to as the experts, valued as proactive agents of their own destinies and invested in as health creators.
- Deliver a different dynamic between health and public services, voluntary and community sectors and local communities, with services and voluntary sector being equipped with skills in creating the enabling conditions for communities to self-organise and take action that creates health.
- Fundamentally redraw the dynamic between the public and politicians so that decision-making is genuinely shared with communities.

This cultural change has the power to transform health status, local environments and economic prospects (Fujiwara et al., 2016).

ICSs that adopt and embed health creation will actively forge new relationships with communities, inviting, nurturing and making space for their participation. They will develop a health-creating workforce, equipping them with the skills required to create the conditions for communities to self-organise and take action to address barriers to their collective health. They will play enabling roles guided by ongoing conversations so that solutions are jointly made in the spirit of equal partnership.

A health-creating ICS provides a new space for these conversations to take place given their new mandate to 'work with people and communities' (NHS England, 2022). It offers some autonomy over how money is spent and gives explicit permission for workforce and communities to innovate.

Our vision is based on long experience that this is how people and communities truly create their own health.

Health Creation Offers a Route to Whole-System Change

GREEN SHOOTS OF CHANGE

Health creation is happening everywhere in pockets. In some systems, elements are being consciously adopted and embedded into a range of practices, programmes, strategies and policies. In others, there are neighbourhoods and places that have been working to increase the collective voice and agency of communities for some time, although this has not yet been adopted system-wide.

Where health creation is starting to drive whole-system change:

- System leaders are actively identifying members of their workforce who are leading health creation at the frontline—including social prescribers—and are getting behind and supporting them to shift power and enable emergence of community and lived experience leaders.
- ICSs are investing a growing proportion of the overall budget to support relationship building, for example, through protected clinical time, and health-creating activity led by communities and lived experience leaders; formulae are being reworked to invest more in low-income communities.
- Health creation is understood as core to the success of population health management (Holmes, 2022), and the two are addressed as a package.

- Community-led neighbourhood partnerships are emerging, where communities are leading and local health and public services are responding.
- Community development that leads quickly to community-led development is leading to increased social capital, community confidence and community self-advocacy.

TOWARDS BUSINESS AS USUAL?

THCA's ambition and call to action for Integrated Care Systems is to recognise health creation as equally important as the treatment of illness and prevention of ill health and to adopt and embed it as a way of working to help address health inequalities, making it 'business as usual' across the whole system.

There is a long way to go before health creation becomes business as usual. National agencies and government need to play their part in creating the conditions for a wholesale systems shift. Hard-pressed communities often view the Department of Work and Pensions and the Home Office as creating a hostile environment, having no place in a health-creating society. Instead, government departments should consider:

- Adopting a 'health creation in all policies' approach—requiring an assessment of the impact of every new government policy on community health outcomes before adoption—would help to establish a health-creating ecosystem.
- Making health creation an explicit expectation in all relevant programmes and maturity matrices—such as population health management, Core20PLUS5 (priority populations and health conditions requiring accelerated improvement), Community Mental Health Transformation, primary care development—and providing an explicit narrative within programme descriptions on websites would help to make it a universal expectation.
- Adopting a national measure of social capital and requiring all areas to report against a simple social capital index such as the Collective Efficiency Scale (Stamford University, online) or Office for National Statistics indicators (2021).
- Passing a Community Power Act creating a statutory basis for the new social contract.

This call to action prefaced THCA's *Health Creation: Coming of Age* event (The Health Creation Alliance (2022, online)) series which showcased and explored how ICSs and their constituent parts should adopt and embed health creation as a way of working to reduce health inequalities. At the final London event of the series, attention turned to the role of social prescribing as a stepping stone to health creation. Dr Michael Dixon, GP, National Clinical Lead for Social Prescription, NHS England and Chair of the College of Medicine, said:

Social prescribing is the 'John the Baptist'. The real course is health creation. Social prescribing is a Trojan Horse to create health creation. Because social prescribing is about individuals and inequalities, as it builds up social capital, as it expands the volunteer sector, you begin to get all the virtuous circle that you require. I'm not saying social prescribing is the end, what you are doing here is actually the end game.

Conclusion

A pathogenic paradigm needs balancing with a health-creating or salutogenic paradigm. This is becoming recognised in UK health policy. Whilst some parts, particularly the 'curing' parts of the NHS, may still require more of a service-driven model, health creation enables 'flourishing' in individuals, communities and society that can be measured via indicators of social capital. THCA and C2 offer an underpinning framework, comprising three Cs, six features and four relationships that can fundamentally help to address health inequalities. We call for a new social contract between national, system and citizen leaders, based on this framework, that increases the power and agency of communities leading to new ecosystems of provision within which people can find the right solutions and pathways that lead to better health and wellbeing. Health creation is the next step for the social prescribing revolution.

REFERENCES

Antonovsky, A., 1987. Unravelling the Mystery of Health: How People Manage Stress and Stay Well. Jossey-Bass Publishers, San Francisco CA.

Cottam, H., 2018. Radical Help: How We Can Remake the Relationships Between Us and Revolutionise the Welfare State. Hachette UK, London.

Crisp, N., 2020. Health Is Made at Home, Hospitals Are for Repairs; Building a Health and Health Creating Society. Salus Global Knowledge Exchange, Billericay.

Fujiwara, D., Hotopp, U., Lawton, R., 2016. Lighting the way for C2 Connecting Communities. Social impact valuation of the Beacon Project 1995–2001. C2 Connecting Communities. Available from: https://c2connectingcommunities.co.uk/c2content/uploads/2020/12/C2_LightingTheWay_FINAL.pdf (Accessed 24 March 2023).

Health Foundation, 2010. Evidence scan: complex adaptive systems. Available from: https://www.health.org.uk/sites/default/files/ComplexAdaptiveSystems.pdf (Accessed 24 March 2023).

Holmes, J., 2022. What is a population health approach? King's Fund. Available from: https://www.kingsfund.org.uk/publications/population-health-approach (Accessed 17 July 2023).

Mitleton-Kelly, E., 2006. A complexity approach to co-creating an innovative environment. World Futures 62 (3), 223–239.

Naylor, C., Wellings, D., 2019. Lessons from the Wigan Deal. King's Fund, London. Available from:. https://www.kingsfund.org.uk/projects/lessons-wigan-deal (Accessed 23 March 2023).

New NHS Alliance, 2017. A Manifesto for Health Creation. Available from: https://thehealthcreationalliance.org/wp-content/uploads/2018/11/A-Manifesto-For-Health-Creation.pdf. Page 4.

NHS England, 2021. Core20PLUS5 (adults)—an approach to reducing healthcare inequalities. Available from: https://www.england.nhs.uk/about/equality/equality-hub/national-healthcare-inequalities-improvement-programme/core20plus5/ (Accessed 24 March 2021).

NHS England, 2022. Working in partnership with people and communities: statutory guidance. Available from: https://www.england.nhs.uk/publication/working-in-partnership-with-people-and-communities-statutory-guidance/ (Accessed 4 April 2023).

Office for National Statistics Indicators, 2021. Social capital in the UK 2020. Available from: https://www.ons.gov.uk/peoplepopulationandcommunity/wellbeing/bulletins/socialcapitalintheuk/2020 (Accessed 13 April 2023).

Sorkin, D., 2016. Systems leadership for beginners: what it is, how it works, and why it helps. Available from: https://www.national-voices.org.uk/blogs/systems-leadership-beginners-what-it-how-it-works-and-why-it-helps (Accessed 24 March 2023).

Stamford University. Collective efficiency scale. Available from: http://sparqtools.org/mobility-measure/collective-efficacy-scale/ (Accessed 13 April 2023).

The Health Creation Alliance. The roots of health creation. Available from: https://thehealthcreationalliance.org/the-roots-of-health-creation/ (Accessed 24 March 2023).

The Health Creation Alliance, 2022. Health creation: coming of age. Available from: https://thehealthcreationalliance.org/health-creation-coming-of-age/ (Accessed 24 March 2023).

Wilkinson, R., Pickett, K., 2009. The Spirit Level: Why More Equal Societies Almost Always Do Better. Allen Lane, London.

Chapter 12

Relational Welfare

Heather Henry

Introduction

Various authors and organisations have questioned whether a post-war welfare state is able to meet the challenges of 21st-century problems. Prominent amongst these is Hilary Cottam, a globally renowned designer, thinker and social activist who published a paper on relational welfare (2011) as a precursor to her book, *Radical Help* (2018a).

The relational welfare paradigm is about whether the welfare state is fit for purpose. It questions whether systems need to be fundamentally rethought to be more relational, focusing on building capabilities and recognising the pervasive influence of power and class as barriers for change. It is through this lens that we can examine how far social prescribing, linked to two foundational elements of the welfare state—health and social care—would fare if we revisited government's relationship with communities.

Cottam's paradigm is built on a series of her social experiments covering the whole life course from good early years and family life to ageing well. It starts with inviting people to describe what makes a good life and then using classic design principles of idea generation, prototyping, making changes and replication to build people's capabilities to enable them to flourish. Her conclusions are that the NHS needs to 'pivot', or to change course entirely, rather than to focus on fixing the current system.

What Is Relational Welfare?

'The welfare state is based on an outdated, transactional model, and needs to be replaced with something that is shared, collective and relational'.

(Cottam, 2011)

Cottam takes us through the history of the development of the post-war welfare state. Revolutionary in its time, it provided decent homes, social security and good education. The birth of the NHS followed, offering free access to health care for all for the first time. But the problems and needs that existed when the welfare state was born have changed, referred to in the Beveridge Report (1942) as the '5 giants' of want, idleness, ignorance, disease and squalor. Cottam gives us three reasons why the current welfare state is no longer appropriate:

1. Social challenges, such as obesity, an ageing society and globalisation, are entirely different in nature to the challenges of the 1940s and 1950s and need a different sort of response.
2. A crisis of care—we are unable to find or pay for kind and human care.
3. Increasing poverty and inequality, with inequalities greater than they have been since the 19th century.

The 'Factory' Model

Cottam argues that the welfare state, built in an era of command and control, mass production and hierarchies, represents an industrial system. The NHS, she says, functions like a factory where people move through the system from referral to assessment to treatment to discharge. This worked well in a post-war era dominated by short-term illnesses that could be fixed, like infections and broken bones, and when people often did not live long enough to develop problems of old age and conditions like diabetes were rare. The level of complexity of chronic illness is bound up with the social circumstances of people's lives—something that we recognise in social prescribing. Today, these complex issues cannot be cured or fixed, and they require a completely different skill set.

This factory model, says Cottam, reduces people to units who should behave in a certain way—the only trouble is, they don't.

'Factory' Updates

In their quest to make changes to the welfare system, successive governments have introduced reforms including the introduction of markets, the introduction of the private sector as a more efficient alternative and efforts to streamline services using 'lean' manufacturing models developed originally by the car manufacturer Toyota. A typical example of this would be in primary care. The coronavirus pandemic and the subsequent backlog of demand has forced general practice down a triage and remote consultation model. Whilst this may be more efficient, many, especially older adults with complex needs, feel that care is fractured and impersonal and a far cry from the more relational family doctor/pastoral care model of the past.

Over-Medicalisation

Cottam argues against over-medicalisation as described by Ivan Illich in his seminal work *Limits to Modern Medicine* (1976). Here, problems in our lives need medical 'repair', and little care is taken to support people to help themselves. This is described further by Cormac Russell in Chapter 16.

The 'Pivot'

Modern medicine, Cottam says, must pivot from trying to fix people with chronic conditions to supporting people to help themselves, a journey from medicalisation to socialisation and from 'patient' to person or community with their own agency to help themselves. She points to the mismatch between the help that is needed for complex care and what is on offer. One example that she gives is of an integrated diabetes service in Bolton, where the health behaviours of the patients were at odds with the services that had been designed to offer optimum care. In particular, she points to the health promotion messages that people with diabetes tried hard to circumvent so that they could move more quickly to the 'fixing', represented by insulin prescribing.

The admission of the need to pivot, however, is hard to swallow. It implies that the current NHS and social care models are not working, and that current leadership is failing. The question is then whether leaders have the emotional intelligence to both recognise that pivoting is needed and be willing to redesign how care is delivered.

The Proximity Gap

Both Cottam and the social commentator Darren McGarvey explain that some of the difficulties in designing the welfare state come from a lack of proximity and understanding between decision-makers and the people they serve. In his book *The Social Distance Between Us* (2021), McGarvey says:

Classes exist in parallel to one another with little meaningful interaction between them save for the power one class has over the other […]. Sadly, and in a society so divided by inequality, many are largely insulated from other social realities. In the absence of any lived experience, they rely on media, word of mouth and assumption in reaching conclusions about issues which fall outside their experiential wheelhouse and in the process grant politicians unfettered control over pressing social problems of which they too have a tenuous grasp.

Listening directly to those with lived experience and enabling them to help us redesign ways to create a good life is therefore critical.

Inequality

A misunderstanding by leaders of the inequality experienced by the hardest-pressed communities clearly compounds issues of poor health. But close on the heels of this lack of social proximity for many like McGarvey, outright class war is the corrosive impact of how the 'have nots' behave when they see this inequality. Cottam references the work of Wilkinson and Pickett, whose epidemiological studies, published in a book called *The Spirit Level* (2009), rocked public health opinion.

Using worldwide epidemiological data, Wilkinson and Pickett assert a causal link between those countries that have the biggest income gaps between the rich and the poor and an increase in a myriad of problems such as violence, mental illness and teenage pregnancies. They point to the 'pernicious effects that inequality has on societies: eroding trust, increasing anxiety and illness, (and) encouraging excessive consumption'.

The Spirit Level talks about the negative effect of social comparisons and how people naturally benchmark against others, find themselves wanting and make up for it by purchasing things they cannot afford to hide their perceived deficiencies. We can see this in young people who are image conscious and recognise how this may lead to things like excessive use of Botox and/or bulimia and anorexia. In one unequal rural community that I worked in, the town councillor said to me, 'If these people are so poor, then why do they always have the biggest tellys?' At the time I had no answer, but looking back I think that they were trying to keep up with others or even overcompensate for what they lack.

Cottam takes this theme of 'following the crowd' further, quoting work from Christakis and Fowler (2009) who found that illnesses such as obesity and back pain seemed to replicate through social networks. She takes this idea and thinks of whether it might work in reverse—could good health be spread similarly through social networks? Perhaps expectations of yourself change when you see others in similar or worse positions making positive changes.

My interpretation of this is a project that I supported called Salford Dadz (Robertson et al., 2015), part of a wider programme called Dadly Does It (Unlimited Potential, online), where fathers in Salford experiencing deep disadvantage were supported to find ways to improve their own wellbeing and consequently that of their children. Their solution was to create opportunities, though various 'dadly' activities like a dads' and children's Saturday club, to speak openly to each other about what troubled them. Healing started as soon as 3 weeks after initial involvement. Men saw these marvellous changes in their peers and began to get involved. Over a 2-year period, mental health issues reduced, dads slowly began to get meaningful employment or volunteering opportunities, and some child protection orders were no longer needed. But perhaps more importantly, the dads' public displays of fatherliness, such as the Father's Day fetes that they organised, changed the women's perspective of men in this town.

They were no longer useless; they made a positive contribution. And that changed the relationships between other fathers and mothers.

A Consumerist Model

Today's health care is perceived by the public as 'free, perfect and now', says Cottam. For every problem there will be a service, and that drives up demand. People are even encouraged to rate their doctor or NHS service online and seemingly forget that health and care is a shared endeavour.

Cottam says that in redesigning the system we are asking ourselves the wrong question. Rather than considering how this consumerist health and care system should change, we should ask how we can enable people to flourish, designing around the person, family or community rather than fitting their needs into the system.

A major barrier to doing this successfully is that the timescales involved before change can be measured are 10 years or more, whereas political timescales and the churn of leadership lead to inconsistency of purpose.

Framing the Wellbeing Conversation

Another barrier to the public's understanding of the development of social prescribing is the public's perception. The Health Foundation commissioned a review to firstly understand that people think that their health and wellbeing are a personal responsibility (Health Foundation, 2019). In the second stage of this work, the Health Foundation published a toolkit (Frameworks Institute, 2022) on how we might reframe the conversation about the social determinants of health. This consists of five recommendations on how to frame the wellbeing conversation:

- Show why the change matters, emphasising that lives will be cut short.
- Harness the power of explanation about how the world around us shapes our health.
- Show that change is possible, addressing fatalistic health beliefs.
- Use certain arguments, like the impact of the pandemic, with caution, as they can decrease support for policy changes.
- Use data in context – metaphor is useful.

These reports will support leaders wanting to communicate about why social prescribing will support wellbeing.

The Central Role of Relationships

What we really need, says Cottam, is a relational model of welfare. By this she means:

- Collaboration—to create new ideas
- Participation—become active agents of change
- Getting to know one another and forming trusted longer-term relationships
- Professionals in chronic and complex care shifting from solving problems to 'listening, challenging and supporting a process of discovery and transformation'.

Some parts of the health and care system have recognised this and are beginning to understand that integrated care, person and community-centred care, and public health need systems leadership. This is more about taking a 'balcony view' of what is happening and spending time fostering relationships across the system. The skills required relate to an understanding of complexity theory, whereby setting the right conditions for change is fundamental to enabling complex adaptive systems (families and communities) to self-organise, rather than practising traditional command-and-control leadership. There needs to be new alliances built between state and society, Cottam argues. Her calls echo those of Nigel Crisp (2020), former chief executive of the NHS, that health should be made at home and that 'hospitals are for repairs'.

Lessons in Life Satisfaction

Moving on from the relationships between system leaders, Cottam looks at how relationships also enable people to flourish. She points to a famous longitudinal study that is still tracking the lives of male sophomore students at Harvard university (and later with the addition of inner-city men in Boston) more than 80 years later (Vaillant, 2012). The main conclusion is that it is the warmth and quality of the men's long-term relationships that lead to better life satisfaction and longer lives. In her various experiments, Cottam finds that when developing and sustaining relationships are built into the design of her social experiments, people fare

better over time than if they are, for example, given talking therapy or drugs.

Resources

Health and care have become predicated on a scarcity of resources, says Cottam. She argues that, with 80% of resources and staff time consumed in non-client-facing work, it is massively bureaucratic. The first of a series of five social 'experiments' that are described in Radical Help start with a 'troubled' family from Swindon, whose lives are in chaos. Such families, says Cottam, cost the state an average of £250,000 a year. This is spent on 'control and restraint' rather than to offer positive opportunities for the family.

Cottam and her team conduct a social work experiment, named 'Life', reversing this 80:20 ratio. Here, the family choose the staff with whom they would like to work. These staff are chosen because they are intuitive, won't talk down to families and won't go soft on them either. The staff are allocated a sliver of this £250,000 and support the family to decide how the money should be spent. The families are given the power to 'build their own way out' (Cottam, 2018a).

Steps to 'Life'

The 'Life' experiment included the following steps:

- Families accept the invitation to participate.
- They build relationships with team members so that they open up.
- Together, they develop a plan that gives the family members purpose and reason.
- Work starts to build the families' capabilities.
- The team then supports opportunities identified by the family members themselves to change their lives.
- A planned exit occurs once broader relationships have been built with work, schools and the wider community.

Cottam reports that it took an average of 18 months for the participants of 'Life' to work through these steps. Crucially, it was the families themselves who were given the power and control over the process, with the staff offering support so that family members became more and more capable of managing their own lives. Developing a plan gives purpose and reason, and it has practical steps for families to try out. A precursor to this was the building of trusting relationships between the staff and the families and between the families themselves. This was developed by, for example, going for a meal at McDonald's followed by paintballing together—a basically human, rather than transactional, process.

Capabilities

So, in this relational welfare model, the focus moves from cure or care to building people's capabilities so that they can live the life they desire. Cottam relates this to the Aristotelian ides of human flourishing, or eudaimonia. Working with families, Cottam's team identified four types of capabilities:

- Work and learning
- Health and vitality
- Community
- Relationships

In addition, family members also talked about the importance of how they felt about themselves and the importance of love.

The families interrogated this framework of four capabilities to help them build their visions and steps towards a better future.

Interpretation for Social Prescribing

Cottam's paradigm overlaps with the broad principles and of language of social prescribing, particularly around 'what matters to me'.

In England, there is a workforce development framework (NHS England, 2023) that also contains a competency framework for social prescribing link workers (SPLWs). This framework has four competency areas:

- Competencies to engage and connect with people
- Competencies to enable and support people
- Competencies to enable community development
- Competencies for safe and effective practice

This enables comparison between the relational welfare paradigm and the predominant personalised care paradigm outlined in Chapter 8.

FLOURISHING

Health and care systems are concerned with physical and mental health and wellbeing, whereas the language of Cottam is about flourishing or eudaimonia, meaning living

well and being happy. We can argue whether they mean the same thing, but in health and care, people are defined by their needs and a desire to address them, whereas Cottam's paradigm is firmly rooted in the interconnectedness of four capabilities of work, health, community and relationships to enable people to live their best life.

RELATIONSHIPS

Central to Cottam's paradigm is the importance of building and sustaining relationships along the life course—both with the worker and with the wider community. One of the differences here is that the relationships in the personalised care paradigm focus mainly on the individual rather than the wider community.

The goal for Cottam is much broader in terms of helping people to develop wider positive relationships with family, friends and communities that are long term and supportive. Although you may expect that the SPLW supports people to form relationships with these wider assets, it is not explicit, and timescales for doing so are often short due to the pressure of the number of referrals to their services.

CAPABILITIES

Capabilities matter in both a person- and community-centred paradigm and a relational welfare paradigm. They are defined by NHS England as 'patient activation', meaning 'the knowledge, skills and confidence a person has in managing their own health and care' (NHS England, 2023), rather than a wider sense of flourishing supported by the four capabilities of community, relationships, health and work.

There are also capabilities in relational welfare around strengthening the bonds between people and communities rather than between people and organisations. Cottam calls this 'collective capability' and describes it as 'our collective bonds that create the conditions for flourishing', saying that 'we can only sustain change in good company' (Cottam, 2018b). By contrast, in the person- and community-centred paradigm there is a wider role for the SPLW in 'patient and public involvement' and co-production to support service planning, design and delivery. Whilst both involve partnership between the people that live somewhere and the people that work somewhere, there is a clear difference in emphasis: one on self-sufficiency and the other on designing services to continue to meet need.

PLANS

Plans are central to Cottam, to galvanise action. Plans offer that vision for a better life—and indeed, the SPLW competency framework includes the development of a 'personalised care and support plan'. However, the language is personal and individual whereas much of Cottam's work focuses on planning with, or in the context of, communities: for example, of young people, of older people, of families and of neighbourhoods. Understanding the history and culture and communal needs of those communities is undoubtably important. Emotionally intelligent SPLWs will of course be aware of this, but it is not yet explicit within their competencies.

POWER AND CONTROL

Coaching and facilitation, that is, letting the person lead, are ways that Cottam enables people to have power and control. There is much in the NHS competency framework and indeed within personalised budgets about ways to coach and facilitate, including understanding of behavioural models and motivational interviewing. It is unlikely, however, that there is the same level of flexibility and freedom to act, within the budgets, risk assessments, rules and regulations of current systems.

Conclusion

Social prescribing offers a significant change to the health and care system, nested as it does in the front of the NHS—in primary care. It bears some comparison to Cottam's ideas of relational welfare and of human flourishing. There is hope here for building people's capabilities to live a good life rather than focusing on fixing individual health problems.

Relational welfare contains many of the components identified in Chapter 3 on the evidence for what contributes to wellbeing: people need to have personal resources (or capabilities) to be able to cope with problems. Relationships are central, and this in turn helps the self-determination—or power and control—needed to enable people to help themselves.

The question remains as to whether the wider system can 'pivot' further in the light of this knowledge of the importance of relationships, or whether the public and successive governments will stay wedded to a transactional, consumerist, care and cure model.

Such a pivot will require successive governments over a much longer term to accept design principles to guide it, so that hospitals focus on repairs—and health, or better still, flourishing, is truly made at home. Governments will then have to commit to that partnership with the people with lived experience of complex need and inequalities and overcome generations of a lack of proximity, so that policy is no longer determined by politics and class. And even more challenging might be how to explain the pivot to a consumerist public so that they understand how health and care is changing.

REFERENCES

Beveridge, W., 1942. Social Insurance and Allied Services (The Beveridge Report) HMSO. London.

Christakis, N., Fowler, J., 2009. Connected: The Surprising Power of Our Social Networks and How They Shape Our Lives. Little, Brown and Company, New York.

Cottam, H., 2011. Relational welfare. Soundings. 48, 134–144.

Cottam, H., 2018a. Radical Help: How We Can Remake the Relationships Between Us and Revolutionise the Welfare State. Virago Little Brown, London.

Cottam, H., 2018b. The pivot: changing our relationship with the health system. The King's Fund, London Available from: https://www.kingsfund.org.uk/insight-and-analysis/blogs/pivot-changing-our-relationship-health-system (Accessed 1 March 2024).

Crisp, N., 2020. Health Is Made at Home, Hospitals Are for Repairs: Building a Healthy and Health-Creating Society. Salus, Billaricay.

FrameWorks Institute, 2022. A Matter of Life and Death: Explaining the Wider Determinants of Health in the UK. FrameWorks Institute, Washington, DC. Available from:. https://www.health.org.uk/publications/how-to-talk-about-the-building-blocks-of-health (Accessed 10 July 2023).

Health Foundation, 2019. Reframing the conversation on the social determinants of health. Available from: https://www.health.org.uk/publications/reports/reframing-the-conversation-on-the-social-determinants-of-health (Accessed 1 September 2023).

Illich, I., 1976. Limits to Medicine: Medical Nemesis—The Expropriation of Health. Marion Boyars, London.

McGarvey, D., 2021. The Social Distance Between Us: How Remote Politics Has Wrecked Britain. Ebury Press, London.

NHS England, 2023. Workforce development framework: social prescribing link workers. Available from: https://www.england.nhs.uk/publication/workforce-development-framework-social-prescribing-link-workers/ (Accessed 10 July 2023).

Robertson, S., Woodall, J., Hanna, E., et al., 2015. Salford Dadz: year 2 external evaluation. Project Report. Unlimited Potential. Available from: https://eprints.leedsbeckett.ac.uk/id/eprint/1728/ (Accessed 10 July 2023).

Unlimited Potential. Dadly Does It. Available from: https://www.unlimitedpotential.org.uk/enterprise/innovation-projects/dadly-does-it (Accessed 10 July 2023).

Vaillant, G., 2012. Triumphs of Experience, the Men of the Harvard Grant Study. The Belknap Press of Harvard University, Cambridge, MA.

Wilkinson, R., Pickett, K., 2009. The Spirit Level - Why Equality is Better for Everyone. Allen Lane, London.

Chapter 13

Summary Section 2 Paradigms

Heather Henry

The first part of this book summarised the history of social prescribing and how far we have got in turning the health and care sector's 'super tanker' from a focus on health to one around wellbeing. The general view is that social prescribing represents an important and positive development. But the question now is what comes next.

The second section of this book therefore goes on to set the scene further: social prescribing has emerged from the comprehensive NHS model of personalised care paradigm or world view. Here, the focus of health and care broadens from a biomedical to a psychosocial view that stretches into community development, experienced-based design, workforce development and more.

But there are many competing world views and visions for where the welfare state is or should be heading and what this means for citizen wellbeing. It is important to consider a range of paradigms at this juncture to see what they may be able to contribute to the development of social prescribing going forward.

The contributors drawn together here do not offer an exhaustive collection of potential paradigms, but they are perhaps some of the most well known or vocal. An overview of these paradigms will also help you to interpret the contributions in the sections that follow on the perspectives and practice of social prescribing.

Commonalities

There are several commonalities between the paradigms presented. For example:
- A focus on what makes people well rather than what prevents them from being ill—a move from a pathogenic to a salutogenic or health-creating society, with some going further and talking about 'flourishing'
- Power and control shifting towards communities
- A trust and relationship-driven focus rather than remote industrialised care
- Participation and interdependence rather than a passive, individual approach
- A recognition and celebration of strengths and assets rather than just needs
- The development of confidence and capabilities to self-care

The Economic View

Social prescribing deals with the aftermath of structural inequalities, so perhaps we should start with a conversation about the way that governments operate. From here we can envisage how policies that may support wellbeing may develop.

Levelling up to address widening inequalities is very current in national policy, and within this is the priority to improve healthy life expectancy and wellbeing (HM Government, 2022). Lord O'Donnell, an economist and former cabinet secretary, offers his world view, which is that the ultimate goal of governments is not just about economic success but must include how to support citizens to have worthwhile, satisfied and high-quality lives. After all, healthier and happier people make for a more economically active society—a potentially virtuous circle. He makes the case for measuring 'growth' in national wellbeing, and not just economic output, as a measurable goal of a country's progress. He sets out the progress made in measuring subjective wellbeing and argues that it should be prioritised above hard data like exam results. These are important signs that thinking on the role of the welfare state and public policy is changing.

There are two movements supporting these ideas: the Wellbeing Economy Alliance and the Wellbeing Economy Governments, the latter garnering international support. According to Mason and Büchs, (2023), the barriers to the wider adoption of the paradigm of a wellbeing economy are:

- The dominance of neoclassical economics training within policymaking institutions
- Siloed short-termist approaches to policymaking
- The role of vested interests

Alongside this are related economic movements that seek to improve the financial wellbeing of communities. Such ideas help social prescribing leaders to connect the dots between social movements to enhance community wellbeing. The first is 'community wealth building', defined as 'an approach to economic development that changes the way that our economies function, retaining more wealth and opportunity for the benefit of local people' (Centre for Local Economic Strategies; https://cles.org.uk/the-community-wealt-communih-building-centre-of-excellence/).

The Centre for Local Economic Strategies (CLES, 2020) states that 'in the UK, the 5 richest families own more wealth that the poorest 13 million people'.

To build community wealth, we need to:

- Make labour markets just and fair
- Change how public institutions spend their money so it benefits communities and grows local social enterprises
- Enable local land and property to generate wealth for local people
- Develop a more inclusive economy with democratic and inclusive ownership
- Support financial institutions to work for local people, places and the planet

The NHS itself, reputed to be the fifth largest employer in the world (BBC, 2012), has a huge opportunity through its land, job opportunities and spending power to enable local people to improve their wellbeing. NHS and other non-profit public-sector organisations like universities are called 'anchor institutions' for this reason, because they can anchor and build on the wealth of the communities that they serve. So helping people back into employment, paying them a fair wage, using local contractors where possible and supporting the development of social enterprises who trade rather than accept aid all create sustainable money in local pockets.

The Public Services (Social Value) Act became law in 2013. It requires people who commission public services to think about how they can also secure wider social, economic and environmental benefits. It encourages commissioners to talk to their local provider market or community to design better services and find new and innovative solutions to difficult problems (HM Government, 2021). In social prescribing terms, the Social Value Act is a lever to build community power and start to address poverty.

There are also many barriers to VCSE organisations entering into public procurement, which has encouraged the Department for Digital, Culture Media and Sport (2022) to analyse progress and support procurement in this sector. It estimates a growth potential of around £5billion in contracts let in health and social care—one-quarter of the c. £20-billion market.

Laws have existed for many years to support 'asset transfer' of buildings and/or land from public authorities, usually the local authority, to community organisations. Local authorities can sell an asset at less than full market value where this would support a use that brings social, economic or environmental benefits to the community.

A movement has been emerging across the UK around lending to social entrepreneurs whose ideas have been rejected by traditional banks. This is based on the ideas of Muhammad Yunus, a Bangladeshi social entrepreneur and banker who developed the idea of 'microfinance': loaning very small amounts to local people trying to improve their lives and that of people around them. Alongside this is support for what are termed self-reliant groups (SRGs): where a group of friends come together for tea and a chat and each save £1 a week. As it builds, this money can then be loaned to members experiencing hard times. The SRG can be supported to share skills and learn together. Some are then given help to start a small business to bring in much-needed income. Examples of organisations supporting SRGs and microfinance in the UK include Purple Shoots, based in Wales (purpleshoots.org); WEvolution, based in Scotland (wevolution.org.uk); Church Action on Poverty, a national charity; and Trustleeds, based in Leeds (trustleeds.org.uk).

Community wealth building, asset transfer and anchor institutions are all part of a wider movement called welfare economics, which is the study of how the allocation of resources and goods affects social welfare.

Behavioural Science

Like several other contributors, O'Donnell refers to the importance of understanding how behavioural science and complex systems, like communities, work, rather than assuming that people are robots who will always behave in a certain way. To be successful, social prescribing requires a deep understanding of psychology. This is helping social prescribing to move away from just offering exercise on prescription, for example, and starting instead with an understanding of the barriers to improving someone's wellbeing.

Health professionals are taught about models that help them to understand how the health beliefs of their patients affect what they do. Hochbaum's (1958) model is perhaps one of the most well-known models (Box 13.1).

Time has helped us to enhance the understanding of beliefs and behaviour since Hochbaum in 1958. The Behavioural Insights Team (BIT) that O'Donnell mentions has developed some simple tools for leaders to use. One such tool is called the EAST framework (Service et al., 2014), which enables Easy, Attractive, Social and Timely access to support. If you look closely, you can spot how EAST plays out in Cottam's social experiments in her book *Radical Help* (see Chapter 12); for example, she invited workless people to step through a makeshift door in a South London Jobcentre emblazoned with 'Get yourself out of here!'—easy and attractive. Next came arranging for people who did step through the door to meet socially and start to develop the soft skills needed by employers, such as communication. Cottam did this by firstly arranging exercise sessions in the park and then, as participants bonded as a group, inviting them to do small voluntary projects. In terms of time, people were conditioned by the Jobcentre system to turn up because they thought that they had to. But in the EAST framework it is normally about arranging a suitable time and place that is convenient to people rather than the service. An example might be when the NHS brought COVID-19 vaccinations into community spaces.

A second tool from BIT is the barrier identification tool (BIT, online), which is based on the work of Mitchie et al. (2014), who developed the COM-B model. This proposes that for someone to engage in a particular behaviour (B) there may be barriers to overcome: they must be physically and psychologically able (Capable) and have the social and physical opportunity (O) to do the behaviour and, in addition, be motivated to take the desired action more than any other competing action (M—the want or need to do the behaviour).

The COM-B model has been developed as part of a larger system of behaviour called the behaviour change wheel (BCW) (Michie et al., 2014). This tool helps leaders to move from a behavioural analysis of the problem to the actual design of the intervention.

BOX 13.1 HOCHBAUM'S HEALTH BELIEF MODEL (1958)

People will take action to prevent, screen for, or control a condition of ill health if:
- They believe they are susceptible to the conditions.
- They believe the condition and the consequences are severe.
- They perceive that taking an action has some benefit in terms of reducing the threat, as well as other benefits.
- They perceive that the barriers to taking the action are low.
- There are cues to action or triggers.
- The person believes that he/she can do the behaviour that will produce the desired outcome, i.e. self-efficacy

An Enabling State

So exactly how is public policy and views on the role of the welfare state changing and how does this fit with the paradigms presented here?

The Wanless report (2004), an independent assessment of the health service's likely future needs and likely cost over the next 20 years, presented and analysed various scenarios for the future. Wanless recommended that high levels of public engagement are needed to keep people well and manage rising demand—the 'fully engaged scenario'—something that did not materialise.

In 2013 and again in 2018, the Carnegie Trust undertook a policy and evidence review of public services by examining publications spanning the UK and Ireland (Wallace, 2013, 2018). From this analysis, Carnegie identified a movement from the current welfare state to what they termed an 'enabling state'. They defined this as 'a challenging new relationship between citizens, communities, and the state. In the enabling state more is expected, and indeed demanded of citizens, families and communities to contribute to their own welfare and wellbeing' (Wallace, 2013).

Their 2013 analysis spoke of a 'piecemeal, sporadic and often a nonspecific approach' to an enabling state that lacked a public narrative or vision meaning that 'fat wallets and sharp elbows' might further increase inequality.

Communicating Paradigms

The Carnegie Trust also noted that the language used to explain the enabling state was not settled, meaning that it could be interpreted and adopted by public service professionals in different ways, or not at all. This is reflected in the paradigms presented here, where contributors' ideas link to an enabling state using differing language and frames. Some paradigms also refer to the importance of communicating changes in public policy both to workers and citizens. We shall look at how we communicate changes later in the book.

Emerging Themes

From their 2013 analysis, the Carnegie Trust (Wallace, 2013) identified six emerging themes:

1. Empowered citizens and communities: where an enabling state would help citizens to unlock their capacity and support, for example, the transfer of assets into community ownership and the delivery of services.
2. Co-production of public services using, for example, citizens' lived experience or local democratic processes.
3. Communities addressing difficult problems where the state has previously been least successful, like loneliness or mental health issues.

4. Creating a level playing field, where an enabling state recognises and responds to differences that exist in individual and community capacity to reduce inequalities.
5. A joined-up and holistic preventative approach to service delivery
6. Shared responsibilities for improving individual and collective wellbeing between all parts of society: individuals, civil society, business and the state

Progress

Five years later, Carnegie reviewed progress in England, Scotland, Wales and Northern Ireland, discovering much progress on policy developments such as the passing of the Community Empowerment (Scotland) Act 2015, which supports and promotes community asset ownership (Wallace, 2018).

In England, The NHS Five Year Forward View (NHS England, 2014) stated a commitment to 'engage with communities and citizens in new ways, involving them directly in decisions about the future of health and care services'. The NHS, it says, would encourage volunteering and create stronger partnerships with the voluntary and charitable sector, recognising their understanding of communities and their ability to reach them in ways that the NHS cannot.

A year later, Public Health England and NHS England started a project called 'Working with communities: empowerment evidence and learning'. The stage 1 report (South, 2015) recognised that 'community life, social connections and having a voice in local decisions are all factors that underpin good health.' The report (South, 2015) outlined a 'family of community-centred approaches':

- Strengthening communities—building community capacity to take action on health and the social determinants of health
- Volunteer/peer roles—enhancing individuals' capabilities to provide advice, information and support or organise activities around health and wellbeing in their or other communities
- Collaborations and partnerships—working in partnership with communities to design and/or deliver services and programmes

- Access to community resources—connecting people to community resources, information and social activities

Within this family, social prescribing might be best associated with accessing community resources, but as some contributors in this book identify, many go well beyond this and into community building. South (2015) outlines a plethora of interconnected roles within this family of approaches, such as health trainers and peer educators, making sense of the confusing array of roles and titles that can make navigating wellbeing services so complex.

Framing

The way societal shifts are framed, says Carnegie, can help us to interpret paradigm shifts. They describe frames as deep values that help us to make sense of the world (Wallace, 2013). Examples include:

- Self-interest versus common interest, with the former revolving around extrinsic reward and the latter with intrinsic reward
- 'Strict father' (authoritarian government) versus 'nurturing parent' (government supporting social justice)
- Elite governance in the hands of the few versus participatory democracy with citizen power

Tipping Point

Progress remains slow, and so to achieve the paradigm shift towards an enabling state, Carnegie suggests that we look to Malcolm Gladwell's (2002) ideas about when and how ideas reach tipping point: *'the moment of critical mass, the threshold, the boiling point'*. Gladwell identified some key people and concepts to help achieve this:

- The 'Law of the Few'—those with a rare set of gifts
- 'Connectors', who make links between different actors
- 'Mavens', who have detailed information on concepts
- 'Persuaders', who bring others on board.
- The 'Stickiness Factor'—The search for the right language to describe the paradigm shift and to make it stick in the mind

- The 'Power of Context'—the environment in which the message or idea is delivered can have a huge impact on whether enough people adopt and spread it to create an 'epidemic'

Perhaps we began to see the beginnings of an enabling state using the power of context during and immediately after the COVID-19 pandemic, when the power of community to help itself become more obvious and with it the role of the social prescribing link worker. Many acted as connectors, and some identified mavens and persuaders within individual communities (NHS England, 2020).

Carnegie points to a 'gathering storm of social, environmental and economic pressures' on public services that are driving thoughts towards a new way of working. This is matched with citizens' growing expectations of autonomy, influence and choice over services received and the evidence that having control over your life and agency to change it are important in making people well (Wallace, 2018).

Human Learning Systems

Perhaps it is a moot point to introduce another concept, that of 'human learning systems' (HLS, https://www.humanlearning.systems/), as a way for public services to think in order to create the conditions to enable new and better ways of working to flourish. Planning and organising public services is called 'public management'. It is generally characterised by a 'new public management' approach of '3 Ms'—markets, managers and metrics—characterised by a focus on customers, efficiency and the use of private sector management tools. New public management, say the proponents of HLS, is slow to learn and adapt because it is fundamentally about control (Brogan et al., 2021).

In contrast, HLS acknowledge that many of society's problems are messy and complex, echoed by the problems of people signposted to social prescribing. Here, there is no straight line between the causes and the effects, making problem solving complex. This may mean, for example, that there is no one best way to develop social prescribing systems—it depends on the people and the situation—and this may vary between communities and cultures (Box 13.2).

BOX 13.2 THREE KEY CHALLENGES OF COMPLEXITY

Variety—Everyone's lives are different. People's strengths and needs are different. As a result, what a 'good outcome' for people, and how it is achieved, looks different for each person.

Change—A complex world is an ever-changing world. What works in public service today will not necessarily work tomorrow. What works for one person or one place will not necessarily work for another.

Lack of control—Complex systems are beyond our control. The outcomes that we seek are influenced by a range of people, organisations and structures—public, private and civil society—which are beyond the direct control of Government, either central or local.

From https://www.humanlearning.systems/overview/.

Complexity science is used within HLS to help us understand what is happening, and it recognises that some problems may not be 'solved' but may instead be held in 'dynamic equilibrium', maintaining a balance in a natural system, despite it being in a constant state of change.

Health and care leaders are now recognising the difference between complicated and complex. In complex situations, leaders must feel their way, identifying 'unknown unknowns' and then probing, sensing and responding – building social prescribing from the ground up (Snowden and Boone, 2007). There may be no straightforward solutions, such as signposting someone to a community group, but instead there is an enabling state of human learning, kindness and compassion, backed by an understanding of design skills and built with an awareness of a community's history and culture.

Complexity science is visible within many of the preceding paradigms, such as health creation and relational welfare www.humanlearning.systems. HLS consists of three interconnected ideas:

- Human: relational working that understands and responds to human beings
- Learning: testing, failing and making changes— the primary task of leaders is about creating effective learning environments
- Systems: real outcomes are created by actors collaborating in healthy systems

Lenses to Analyse Perspectives

These themes, frames and progress towards tipping points will all help us as we move forward to Section 3, where we examine social prescribing from a range of perspectives. Again, these perspectives are not exhaustive. Some are critical, some supportive, some dispassionately analyse social prescribing at its face. But each will present another piece of information on which to help local and national leaders, practitioners, and citizens to put wellbeing at the heart of decision-making.

REFERENCES

BBC online, 2012. Which is the world's biggest employer? Available from: https://www.bbc.co.uk/news/magazine-17429786 (Accessed 23 August 2023).

Brogan, A., Hawkins, M., Eichstellar, G., Hesselgraves, H., Nurre Jennions, B., Lowe, T., Plimmer, D., Terry, V., Williams, G., 2021. Human Learning Systems: Public Service for the Real World. Available from: https://realworld.report/ (Accessed 3 January 2024).

Centre for Local Economic Strategies, 2020. Community Wealth Building. YouTube. Available from: https://youtu.be/LNVfKpV-lyvY (Accessed 23 August 2023).

Department for Digital, Culture Media and Sport, 2022. The role of Voluntary, Community, and Social Enterprise (VCSE) organisations in public procurement. Available from: https://www.gov.uk/government/publications/the-role-of-voluntary-community-and-social-enterprise-vcse-organisations-in-public-procurement/the-role-of-voluntary-community-and-social-enterprise-vcse-organisations-in-public-procurement#section-4-current-participation-in-public-procurement (Accessed 1 September 2023).

Gladwell, M., 2002. The Tipping Point: How Little Things Can Make a Big Difference. Back Bay Books, New York.

HM Government, 2021. Social Value Act: information and resources. Available from: https://www.gov.uk/government/publications/social-value-act-information-and-resources/social-value-act-information-and-resources (Accessed 23 September 2023).

HM Government, 2022. Levelling up the United Kingdom. Available from: https://www.gov.uk/government/publications/levelling-up-the-united-kingdom (Accessed 4 September 2023).

Hochbaum, G.M., 1958. Public Participation in Medical Screening Programs: A SocioPsychological Study. U.S. Dept. of Health, Education, and Welfare, Washington, DC.

Mason, M., Büchs, M., 2023. Barriers to adopting wellbeing economy narratives: Comparing the Wellbeing Economy Alliance and Wellbeing Economy Governments. Sustain. Sci. Pract. Policy. 19 (1), 2222624. https://doi.org/10.1080/15487733.2023.2222624.

Michie, S., Atkins, L., West, R., 2014. The Behaviour Change Wheel: A Guide to Designing Interventions, 1st ed. Silverback, London.

NHS England, 2014. Five year forward view. Available from: https://www.england.nhs.uk/wp-content/uploads/2014/10/5yfv-web.pdf (Accessed 21 July 2023).

NHS England, 2020. Social prescribers' key role in coronavirus support. Available from: https://www.england.nhs.uk/northwest/2020/06/05/social-prescribers-key-role-in-coronavirus-support/ (Accessed 30 August 2023).

Service, O., Hallsworth, M., Halpern, D., 2014. EAST: Four Simple Ways to Apply Behavioural Insights. The Behavioural Insights Team, London.

Snowden, D.J., Boone, M.E., 2007. A leader's framework for decision making. Harvard Business Rev 85 (11), 68–76. https://hbr.org/2007/11/a-leaders-framework-for-decision-making.

South, J., 2015. Health and wellbeing: A guide to community-centred approaches. Public Health England. Available from: https://www.gov.uk/government/publications/health-and-wellbeing-a-guide-to-community-centred-approaches (Accessed 13 February 2023).

Wallace, J., 2013. The Rise of the Enabling State: A Review of Policy and Evidence Across the UK and Ireland. Carnegie Trust.

Wallace, J. (Ed.), 2018. The Enabling State: Where Are We Now? Review of Policy Developments 2013–2018. Carnegie Trust.

Wanless, D., 2004, Securing good health for the whole population. Final report. HM Treasury, London.

Perspectives

Chapter 14

Social Prescribing With Children & Young People

Dawn Mitchell and Paul Jarvis-Beesley

Introduction

Readers are likely aware of the growth in popularity and availability of social prescribing in the last 5 years or so. It is reasonable to presume that this growth has been evenly spread, with all sections of our population having equal access to a link worker. One might even expect that extra effort has been put into reaching those who have the poorest mental health and the least access to support in the first place (*The Lancet*, 2020). It may come as a surprise, therefore, to learn that social prescribing for children and young people has lagged far behind the provision for adults. Services for children and young people are still few and far between. But commissioners, practitioners and researchers alike are now alert. Social prescribing for children and young people is happening—more than you think but not as much as we'd like.

Case Study

When Jared was 13, his parents separated. Both his parents had two part-time jobs each, earning very low incomes. A highlight of his week was a trip to the local climbing wall with his Dad every weekend. After the separation, Jared stayed with his Dad but his brother moved in with their Mum. When his Dad's new partner moved in, things changed. The climbing stopped, he spent more time on the street, started using cannabis and alcohol, gained weight and lost confidence. By 15, he'd had a number of reprimands and was in line for an antisocial behaviour order (ASBO) when a police community support worker (PCSO) who recognised him from the climbing wall referred Jared to the local youth link worker instead. The worker came to see Jared at home three times. She helped Jared to discover that he really missed his brother, as well as

the climbing. Together, they arranged with the family for the two boys to spend regular time together. And while Jared's dad no longer wanted to go climbing, the link worker paid for Jared to join the local club. Jared lives in Sheffield where a Youth Social Prescribing programme has been running since October 2018.

Complex Challenges

Children and young people live complex lives, facing multiple psychosocial, physical, economic and cultural challenges on a daily basis. This is especially true of young people living with vulnerabilities due to disability, discrimination and socio-economic circumstances. The COVID pandemic exacerbated already high levels of stress, anxiety and mental ill-health amongst 8- to 25-year-olds (The Health Foundation, 2022). It is accepted that 'starting young' is the best way to transform life chances and build brighter futures (Early Intervention Foundation [EIF], 2022; Public Health England [PHE], 2021).

The drivers for children and young people's mental health and wellbeing are complex. They include a range of home-, school- and work-based risk factors, as well as lifestyle factors, social networks, cultural challenges and personal circumstances (Mental Health Foundation, 2022). What affects a young person at a given point in time regularly changes. In a system designed predominantly for adults, it can be hard for a young person to recognise they need help, let alone know to whom they might turn (Bush, 2016).

'No Wrong Door'

Pioneering youth agencies and children and young people's services in some parts of the UK have adopted a 'no wrong door' approach. The idea is to provide a team of multi-skilled workers able to support struggling young people through adolescence and into adulthood. The charity StreetGames founded the Social Prescribing Youth Network (SPYN) about which we will talk more below. It advocates the '5 Rights' when it comes to delivering safe and developmental social activities: Right Place, Right Time, Right Price, Right Style and, perhaps most importantly of all, Right People (StreetGames, 2017). Most adverse childhood experiences are social, rather than medical, determinants of future health. So it makes sense that a response that is social in nature, such as social prescribing, is likely to help.

Integration and Collaboration

What are the options when looking for the best way to support children and young people with their mental health and wellbeing, and how does social prescribing fit in? At one end of the spectrum, there is a 'minimum standards' approach, also referred to by some as 'ticking boxes'. While there is a clear merit in universality, the restraint on local creativity and ambition can result in disconnected services at system level and a proliferation of pilot schemes. Such pilots, predominantly in the public and voluntary sectors, give the illusion of providing inclusive and universal support but, in reality, may represent a race to the bottom. At the other end of the spectrum, properly integrated services with multi-disciplinary teams collaborating to deliver the best possible outcomes for children and young people are transforming lives. We have seen examples of this in action in Sheffield, Luton, Brighton & Hove, London, Manchester and Cumbria (Bertotti et al., 2020).

Social Prescribing Youth Network

Just as the schemes mentioned above have provided life-enhancing connections for young people who were feeling disconnected from their communities, so we, in turn, as professionals, need to connect these local schemes to create a national movement. That is where the Social Prescribing Youth Network comes in.

We, the authors of this chapter, are community-based researchers, frontline practitioners and collaborators with academia. Our interest is in providing the best possible support for children and young people and, at the same time, building the evidence base. That means finding what it is about social prescribing that works, where it is being offered and by whom (the 5 Rights mentioned above) so that we can share it with others. As founders of the Social Prescribing Youth Network, we declare our bias! We naturally want to present the work in a positive light but we also have good, objective reasons to be optimistic.

We have seen firsthand how making a dedicated youth link worker available in the right place can have a transformational effect. Having set up social prescribing schemes in four English cities in September 2018, we asked the health and social care researchers at the University of East London to evaluate it over 30 months. In all, 520 young people aged 14 to 25 received help (42.6% male, 52.7% female, 1.8% preferred not to say, 3% self-described). Three hundred and ten health care and other professionals were involved in making and receiving referrals; 340 referrals were made into 48 different services and activities (StreetGames, 2020).

Using 'before and after' validated questions, researchers found statistically significant increases in personal and mental wellbeing, a decline in loneliness and increases in physical activity. The economic evaluation showed a social return on investment (SROI) of £5.04 for every £1 spent—as it happens, nearly double the average SROI for adult social prescribing (Bertotti et al., 2020).

The Critical Role of the Youth Link Worker

The youth link workers are the right people. The right style is also critical. Young people told us that as well as visiting their GP, they are equally if not more likely to seek help from peers, teachers, youth workers, school nurses and even community safety officers. All of these frontline professionals are able to refer a young person to a link worker, where youth social prescribing is available.

Thinking of the right price and recognising that VCSE services and activities are not without cost, each link worker has a budget to spend on their prescriptions. On average, this was no more than £120 per young person—a little goes a long way.

On the qualitative side, young people, interviewed by trained peer researchers, talk about the informality and 'no pressure, no agenda' nature of the link worker support giving them confidence and autonomy they previously lacked. One young person summed it up like this: 'If someone had bought me a pair of football boots two years ago, I would never have needed therapy'.

The 'right time' is that moment when a young person themself makes a help-seeking move. At that point, through youth social prescribing, the asset-based and person-centred approach kicks in. From the moment the referral is made, the child and family, or independent young person, who is making an appointment to see their link worker is reassured that their choices and shared decision-making are paramount. One young person said: *'I feel like, if you've come to this place you've probably got something you want to talk through that might take time to resolve so it's not just fix it, it's a good kind of place where you can keep coming back'*.

Inequalities in Provision

Social prescribing is having a heyday, and for good reasons. But children and young people are missing out—again. NHS England describes Social Prescribing as an 'all-age' service (NHS England, 2020), but its availability is far from evenly distributed across our age groups. This is partly down to local decision-making and partly down to national priorities and guidelines. Pioneers in children and young people's social prescribing have paved the way, and new services are appearing monthly.

It is our poorest and most underserved young people who have come out worst, not just from the COVID pandemic but from the decade of austerity that preceded it. Professor Sir Michael Marmot and the Health Foundation lay out the stark facts for our underserved communities: infant mortality is back on the rise, having previously levelled out; the difference in the number of children receiving free school meals who are permanently excluded from school compared with those who aren't receiving free school meals is growing again, having previously shrunk; and violent youth crime is on the increase (Institute of Health Equity, 2020).

So why do we remain optimistic? Partly due to the countless examples of transformational change we have witnessed delivered by the undersung heroes in our local communities—heroes such as coaches, artists, volunteers and youth leaders who have turned around young lives against the odds. And partly due to the increasing inclusion of the Voluntary & Community Sector in strategic planning for youth health and wellbeing, signalling, as it does, a swing towards more asset-based thinking, which is a good thing (National Council for Voluntary Organisations [NCVO], 2020; NHS England, 2021).

To aid that strategic planning, SPYN provides a 'free to join' network that brings together practitioners, commissioners and researchers. It produces a range of freely available resources, including guidelines for setting up new schemes, case studies, evaluations and even a template job description and person specification for recruiting a youth link worker. All are produced with the aim of increasing the availability of social prescribing for children and young people to the point of universality (StreetGames, 2021).

For those wishing to see youth social prescribing introduced or developed in their area, here is a starting checklist of what you could look for.

Locally Trusted Organisations (LTOs)

LTOs are youth clubs, community organisations, housing associations, charities and others that have multiple primary purposes (sport, art, training, debt relief, food bank etc) and enjoy an enviable reach into their neighbourhood, with many acting as the 'lifeblood' of their community. They have 'earned their spurs' and are trusted by those whom other agencies find hard to reach. LTOs deliver 'prescribed' activities but may also host the youth link worker and/or coordinate the whole scheme. LTOs are critical to the provision of youth social prescribing. Most areas have a directory or a forum for finding and communicating with LTOs. The local authority or local Council for Voluntary Services, or equivalent, are good places to start.

Youth Link Worker (YLW)

YLWs combine an aptitude and passion for working developmentally with young people, with a knowledge of local assets and activities and an ability to network and collaborate with other agencies. As the first point of contact after a referral has been made, the YLW builds trust with the young person, or child and family, works with them to structure the support sessions and, without any agenda, begins the process of helping their client to make the connections in their community that they need for their immediate and longer-term wellbeing. The YLW may be based in primary care, education or a youth and community setting. Wherever they are based, or hosted, they are usually mobile, able to meet with young people at home, in a café or other local venue. As word spreads, the presence of a YLW in a particular locality can trigger a young person to seek help early rather than wait and allow a problem to get worse.

Referral Pathway

Unlike adults, young people do not usually frequent their GP surgery when seeking help. Some do, of course, but the majority seek help from peers, family members, teachers, youth workers and other support workers. For this reason, a referral pathway for children and young people's social prescribing usually enables a wide range of frontline professionals, including community safety officers, to make referrals to the YLW. Following a period of direct support from the YLW, the young person or family may then be referred on to a provider of services or activities, usually in the voluntary or community sector, that they have chosen as matching their needs at that time. This could be sports, arts, volunteering, lifestyle coaching, debt relief, housing, employment training or pretty much anything else. It must also be remembered that social prescribing is not always the answer. Sometimes, young people seeking social support do in fact have medical needs. In these cases, the YLW can support a reluctant or under-confident young person to access their GP. Many GPs are doing fantastic work to make themselves more accessible to young people and overcome traditional barriers.

Conclusion

YLWs describe deep satisfaction in being able to help young people discover new opportunities and experiences that build their social capital and affect their future prospects. It is also a highly demanding and, at times, stressful role. A commitment to supporting the YLW with managerial and perhaps even clinical supervision, within a strong and connected system of commissioners, referrers and providers, is critical. Getting the '5 Rights' right takes time. It does not happen overnight, and mistakes are made. Being able to talk about mistakes, as well as successes, at whatever level is a sure sign of a working and learning collaboration. At a functional level, how social prescribing for young people is described, promoted and organised locally will have a huge impact on its effectiveness. Who are the best people to help with this? Young people themselves, naturally.

REFERENCES

Bertotti, M., Frostick, C., Sharpe, D., Temirov O., 2020. A two-year evaluation of the young people social prescribing (YPSP) pilot. Available from: https://repository.uel.ac.uk/item/88x15 (Accessed 5 August 2022).

Bush, M., 2016. Beyond Adversity: Addressing the Mental Health Needs of Young People Who Face Complexity and Adversity In Their Lives. Young Minds, London.

EIF (Early Intervention Foundation), 2022. What is early intervention. Available from: https://www.eif.org.uk/why-it-matters/what-is-early-intervention (Accessed 6 October 2022).

The Health Foundation, 2022. Children and young people's mental health: COVID 19 and the road ahead. Available from: https://www.health.org.uk/news-and-comment/charts-and-infographics/children-and-young-people-s-mental-health (Accessed 6 October 2022).

Institute of Health Equity, 2020. Build Back Fairer: The COVID 19 Marmot Review. Available from: https://www.instituteofhealthequity.org/resources-reports/build-back-fairer-the-covid-19-marmot-review (Accessed 6 October 2022).

The Lancet, 2020. Child Mental Health Services in England: a continuing crisis. Available from: https://www.thelancet.com/journals/lancet/article/PIIS0140-6736(20)30289-0/fulltext (Accessed 6 October 2022).

Mental Health Foundation, 2022. Children and Young People. Available from: https://www.mentalhealth.org.uk/explore-mental-health/a-z-topics/children-and-young-people (Accessed 6 October 2022).

NCVO, 2020. Creating Partnerships for Success. Available from: https://www.ncvo.org.uk/news-and-insights/news-index/creating-partnerships-success/#/ (Accessed 6 October 2022).

NHS England, 2020. Social Prescribing and Community-based Support: Summary Guide. Available from: https://www.england.nhs.uk/wp-content/uploads/2020/06/social-prescribing-summary-guide-updated-june-20.pdf (Accessed 6 October 2022).

NHS England, 2021. Building strong integrated care systems everywhere. Available from: https://www.england.nhs.uk/wp-content/uploads/2021/06/B0905-vcse-and-ics-partnerships.pdf (Accesssed 6 October 2022).

PHE (Public Health England), 2021. Best Start in Life and Beyond. Department of Health, London.

StreetGames, 2017. Insight into Action: Lessons from the Doorstep Sport Club Programme. StreetGames, Manchester.

StreetGames, 2020. Social prescribing in practice. Available from: https://network.streetgames.org/sites/default/files/Youth%20 Social%20Prescribing%20in%20Practice%20Report%20 2021%20Updated.pdf (Accessed 6 October 2022) England.

StreetGames, 2021. Resources for children and young people's social prescribing. Available from: https://network.streetgames.org/ resources/young-peoples-social-prescribing-resources (Accessed 6 October 2022).

Chapter 15

An Ethnographic View of General Practice

Bethan Griffith

Introduction

This chapter is based on in-depth ethnographic field-work undertaken at two primary care sites in North East England between October 2018 and June 2019. Both sites had been able to access a local social prescribing intervention since 2015. I observed routine consultations between practice staff and patients, paying particular attention to how patients eligible for social prescribing were identified, how the intervention was talked about and how patients responded to the offer of referral. Observations were recorded in detailed ethnographic field notes. I also conducted 13 semi-structured, audio-recorded interviews with GP practice staff, link workers, patients and local stakeholders. Here, I reflect on my findings based on analysis of the field notes and interview transcripts.

The relationship between UK primary care and social prescribing goes back many years. A spectrum of social prescribing models has emerged, from those that are lighter touch and more transactional to those that are more holistic and relational (Calderón-Larrañaga et al., 2021; Kimberlee, 2015). Likewise, the relationships between primary care staff and social prescribing at a local level has been quite differentiated, with concerns about a lack of engagement by GPs resulting in lower-than-expected referral rates to social prescribing link workers (Moore et al., 2022). Difficulty embedding link workers within primary care has been linked to the challenges of working across professional boundaries (Bertotti el al., 2018; Aughterson et al., 2020; Fixsen et al., 2020; Tierney et al., 2020). Nevertheless, social prescribing link workers are integral to recently introduced primary care networks, with plans to significantly increase the number of link workers operating in the NHS (NHS England, 2019). It is therefore important to understand how primary care staff attach meaning to social prescribing.

The Primary Care Context

Former president of the Royal College of General Practitioners Iona Heath has spoken of the messy reality of the 'multiple, interacting and compounding problems' for which individuals attend their GP surgeries (Heath, 2015), which might make the term *routine* care sound somewhat reductive. Yet, for want of a better word, I observed staff delivering *routine* care in areas of significant socio-economic deprivation. The multiple challenges facing primary care are well documented elsewhere and include workforce pressures, increasing demand, increasing complexity and higher expectations, all of which contribute to unsustainable workloads (Baird et al., 2016). These challenges were evident during the fieldwork and are only likely to have worsened since fieldwork ended and the COVID-19 pandemic struck (Kings Fund, 2022). Clinical and social complexity were commonplace, and patients were often seeking care from disadvantaged positions, revealing tensions in how care unfolded. Anthropologist Annemarie Mol has described two competing logics of choice and care (Mol, 2008). A logic of choice promotes the idea that patients have options from which they can choose, promoting personal responsibility and self-management. Whilst this logic of choice is common in health policy, it often fails to recognise the complex, uncertain and ongoing nature of chronic disease, favouring a series of bounded transactions. A logic of care, on the other hand, is necessarily open ended as it attends to complexity and the unpredictable nature of disease whilst privileging the practicalities of daily life. Staff drew differentially on these competing logics as they attempted to balance the often fragile reality of patients' lives with the technical and bureaucratic requirements of treating disease and satisfying contractual targets (Mol, 2008; Kleinman, 1988, 2019). Dan, for example, was a patient with complex mental health issues who *'never attended'*. His doctor had tried to visit him at home, but he was always out. His family were refusing to care for him, as he would not look after himself or his flat.

When Dan came in, he smelt strongly of tobacco and urine. He had a long yellowing beard and heavily nicotine-stained fingers with blackened fingernails. 'We haven't seen you for a while', said Dr Michael. 'Aye, I don't like doctors, doctor', Dan replied. He said he had come with his chest and had some urine symptoms. A friend had had prostate cancer, he added.

After Dan left the room to go and provide a urine sample, Dr Michael commented:

'If I had 45 minutes I could do everything he needs. I want people to know, people say they work in inner city medicine but it's not like this'. Dan returned having been unable to manage a urine sample. Dr Michael talked him through what was needed. He would need blood tests [the doctor said], before Dan added he had lost weight. Dr Michael picked up the phone to ring the nurse who agreed she would squeeze the patient in straight away for bloods. 'I can't stay now', said the patient. 'I have an appointment'. 'OK, but you will come back?' asked the doctor. The patient left with a script for antibiotics, assuring Dr Michael he could return for all the other necessary tests.

Field Notes_Dr Michael_20.11.18

Whilst Dan might appear not to engage, despite his apparent fear of having prostate cancer, there is also evidence of organisational constraints to care. The attempted home visit and the *squeezing* him in for a blood test demonstrate flexibility and adaptability that are inherent in a logic of care (Mol, 2008). However, Dr Michael's routines were also shaped by the bureaucratic and contractual requirements within which he was operating. *'Everything he needs'* likely included

further investigation of Dan's urinary symptoms but could also allude to the routine information and measurements needed to secure contractual payments by attending to all the *'alerts and reviews'* Dr Michael told me were on the computer system. The interaction of such different priorities has long shaped the clinical reality in health care encounters (Kleinman, 1988), but in this example, Dan's complex social circumstances make their reconciliation particularly challenging. The lived reality made it difficult to pay attention to context and the 'fleshiness and fragility of life' (Mol, 2008, p. 13).

It was amongst these care practices, with their tensions and contradictions, that social prescribing was becoming embedded. Staff drew on these experiences when talking about the intervention, with Dr Michael commenting, 'Where social determinants of health are every day and very obvious, a more comprehensive kind of response has always been an attractive idea for general practitioners' (Interview_Dr Michael).

Dr Michael went on to talk about a *'person next door'* approach in a way that constructed social prescribing as an undifferentiated response to the lived reality of patients with complex clinical needs and increasingly challenging social circumstances.

However, a logic of choice was not absent from practice or in understanding social prescribing. Staff drew on both logics of care and choice, which could generate tensions and contradictions, simultaneously constructing social prescribing as a behaviour change intervention with potential financial savings:

I think the logic model was, essentially we need to do something to change the behaviour of people with long-term conditions so they're better able to take control of their lives. If they're better able to take control of their lives, do they then have less impact on secondary care and less need for secondary care services?

(Interview_Dr Andrew)

These different ways of talking about social prescribing resonate with existing research, highlighting the varied experiences of social prescribing and the potential for unintended consequences and lifestyle drift that deviate from policy aims (Chng et al., 2021; Gibson et al., 2021; Griffith et al., 2022). Calls for a care-based framing of social prescribing, that promotes a relational model of link working, caution against a focus on personal responsibility and choice when complex social circumstances and structural constraints mean that choice becomes little more than an illusion (Calderón-Larrañaga et al., 2022; Griffith et al., 2022; Henwood et al., 2011). What did become clear was that these varied understandings, or framings, of social prescribing were not static. Through observing staff interacting with the local practicalities and materialities of the intervention, we saw how the meanings attached to social prescribing were being constantly re-negotiated within these competing logics of choice and care (Latour, 2000; Mol, 2002).

Social Prescribing in Practice: Referral and Engagement

Dr Anne was well informed about social prescribing and clearly in favour of 'it'. She drew differentially on her experiences of working with the local community and her personal political beliefs to understand it as an alternative to *'medicalising everything'*. One morning she saw James, a young man in his 20s whose mother had died some years ago. He described how he spent all day playing computer games and that his only friends were online. James was diabetic and clinically obese. He was also anxious and worried about his heart. He had recently changed his diet but did not exercise:

Dr Anne told him she had 'a conundrum'—he was worried about his heart, but the things he could do for his health, like exercise and manage his diabetes, he didn't want to do…. 'Are we helping by giving a sick note?' she asked [after James had left the room], then added that all it did was let them know if they had to reschedule appointments with a work coach they wouldn't get sanctioned. 'I know he'll be playing [computer games] all day' [she said], adding that he had not made the connection between his actual health and his health anxiety. He was probably someone who would benefit from the social prescribing model [she said], adding, 'He needs someone to go with him'.

(Field Notes_Dr Anne_17.01.19)

I could see that Dr Anne was frustrated and saw potential in a model of social prescribing that could offer undifferentiated support rather than simply *signposting* James to a service he might not attend (White et al., 2022). He would also have to be eligible. In this instance, James was too young, as only those aged 40 to 74 with certain long-term conditions could be referred to this particular intervention. In this way, the practicalities of the intervention did not address the sense of futility that Anne linked to wider political and structural changes in the locality:

After [the last] patient had left … We discussed local health inequalities. The North, she said, always did badly when the Tories were in. The loss of industry meant there was no structure, no career path. You could spot deprivation, she added, wherever there was a [bakery] 'outlet' store, it's cheap, she added, all people can eat is rubbish food.

(Field Notes_Dr Anne_17.01.19)

When staff identified patients like James, who needed relational, undifferentiated support, they were not always eligible. In contrast, patients who *were* eligible frequently had reminders in their digital notes encouraging staff to offer referral, even if the patients did not obviously need it. This could result in the intervention being 'sold' in a transaction. One of the highest referrers was Ivy, a Health Care Assistant. She performed many of the routine chronic disease reviews and frequently came across reminders in the patient notes to offer social prescribing. On one occasion, she jokingly regretted that she did not work on commission, comparing her experience to that of working in sales. Her approach to referral drew on different aspects of social prescribing from help with gym membership to the prospect of securing more income, depending on her knowledge of the patient. One morning, as I sat in with Ivy, a female patient was due for a blood pressure review. Her hypertension qualified her for referral, Ivy noted, before calling her in:

The patient had come from work and was in a uniform; Ivy acknowledged that she worked hard. She then went on to tell her about [the social prescribing intervention]. 'Because of your long-term conditions,' she said, 'you're entitled to referral'. The patient said she would have to leave it. Ivy said how they would help her to understand her condition 'just affects mind set and gets the [patients] to change that'. She then said they could help with benefits. 'I know what you're saying', the patient replied, before telling Ivy that she and her husband were working. 'You're entitled to nothing if you work', Ivy replied. The patient then told us she was joining a gym in the New Year with her daughter. Ivy then said that the [intervention] might help with this, as gyms could be expensive and they might help get her membership. 'Why don't you let them ring you?' she finished. 'There's no harm in a phone call'.

Fieldnotes_Ivy_HCA_12.12.18

Such reminders were not always successful. Staff acknowledged that if there were multiple reminders in a patient's notes, then clinical conditions, such as asthma, would be prioritised for discussion.

Such contradictions and tensions could limit the scope for engagement despite a clear enthusiasm for the concept of social prescribing and shaped how referral might be offered:

The discussion then moved to different referral techniques after [the nurse] said that often, when she mentioned [the intervention], patients 'didn't want to know'. A GP asked how people raised it in consultations. The nurse said she asked if people needed help, if they were socially isolated or needed help with forms. The same GP joked that if you say 'do you want to exercise or lose weight', the answer will always be no, but you can say instead 'we have this fantastic service—we can change your blood pressure tablets but these people can talk to you about all the other things that are important to you'. A different GP agreed enthusiasm was important, but for that you need a feedback loop to know it was working.

(Field Notes_Practice Meeting_07.11.2018)

It was not, however, a simple case of remembering to refer. There were examples where staff took an active decision *not* to refer, or patients declined. For some patients with long-term conditions the complexity of their social circumstance made referral difficult for both the member of staff and the patient. There might be clinical barriers, with the need to 'sort out' complex medical problems first, or social barriers that positioned patients in a web of challenging circumstances that made staff reluctant to disrupt continuity. Hannah, for example, had recently been seen

in A&E with a drug overdose. She had a history of domestic violence and had moved frequently. She had back problems as well as hepatitis C and liver cirrhosis. More recently, she had developed gynaecological symptoms that needed investigation. Her doctor explained she had '*too much going on*' to be referred, despite recognising the potential benefits of having a link worker. Patients who declined the offer of referral often cited a lack of time or a reluctance to meet with someone they did not know.

Understanding Social Prescribing Over Time: Feedback and Collaborative Working

Overall referral practices were varied, and more nuanced than previously described, drawing on both the logics of choice and care, that were shaped over time. They illustrate how staff were presented with a range of 'practicalities, materialities and events' (Mol, 2002, pp. 8–12) that shaped how they made sense of social prescribing, including their existing work routines and the local model of delivery.

For primary care, social prescribing was at once a way to free up staff time and to give patients time with a link worker to address what mattered to them. We have seen how staff deliberated over whether it was the right *time* to refer, with clinical, and sometimes social, problems needing attention *before* referral. The imagined future gains of social prescribing could be overshadowed by the immediacy of patients' complex lives. Furthermore, institutional and contractual timescales, such as clinical target cycles, could be prioritised over referral to social prescribing.

Over time, it appeared that this particular intervention had drifted increasingly towards a more transactional, behaviour-change model (Gibson et al., 2021, 2022; Griffith et al., 2022). This could put it out of sync with the *unfinished nature of care* (Kleinman, 2019) delivered by primary care staff, who would continue to see patients long after they had been discharged from the intervention.

Dr Ryan, for example, had established relationships with patients over many years. Sue was one such patient. She came one day to discuss her worsening diabetic control. She attributed it to '*stress, money, letters about debt*'. She had three grandchildren that she cared for whilst her daughter worked. She was also concerned about stomach symptoms that might be cancer and about her boiler, which might be faulty:

When he'd finished typing, Dr Ryan turned and asked about [social prescribing]. Sue said she'd seen them but they'd told her she was getting too much money. 'Really', Dr Ryan offered sceptically. 'Now things have changed', he offered, 'why don't we try again?'

(Field Notes_Dr Ryan_12.02.2019)

After the patient left, Dr Ryan completed a suspected cancer referral, pausing to reflect:

'Yeah, she was half an hour', before adding, 'she really had no money though, she really, really struggles'.

(Field Notes_Dr Ryan_12.02.2019)

This encounter is likely to have shaped how Dr Ryan understood the intervention, with it not appearing to have met the patient's needs on this occasion. It resonates with the earlier excerpt where one GP told colleagues, '*You need a feedback loop to know it was working*'. Yet, increasingly primary care staff did not get official feedback. Janet, a link worker, described during interview how providing feedback had become harder as their caseloads grew, adding that now they '*don't tell the doctors anything unless there's an issue*'. This meant staff relied on patients recounting their experiences of the intervention when making sense of what it offered. This could overlook some of the benefits that link workers attributed to the intervention and could shape meaning in unanticipated ways.

Attributing Value to Social Prescribing Over Time

Much of Janet's wider reflections drew on time; as she took a long-term view of social prescribing, she continued:

I think social prescribing works to make people happier and healthier in the long run. It's not overnight, you know, it's hard work getting people to trust you and then to listen to what you say.

(Interview_Janet_Link worker)

Indeed, its relationship with time was an important part of the imagined value of social prescribing, with improved health outcomes and easing of system-level pressures all being suggested as future gains. For patients, it might be simply that '*before*' they did not do something and '*after*' they did, like going out for a coffee once a week.

Yet, value was also tied up in the history of social prescribing and could vary between different actors and institutions (Graeber, 2001). From a primary care perspective, one local GP stakeholder recalled the early days of the intervention, commenting:

I suppose it was partly from the perspective of a GP, having been a GP [for years], in terms of what you see turning up in the GP surgery you think is significantly socially determined. What happens to people outside of their strictly biomedical parameters has more impact on their lives, their health and their wellbeing than anything you do at the doctors.

(Interview_Dr Andrew)

This account placed value on addressing the social determinants of health and resonated with both early accounts of social prescribing and subsequent social prescribing policy (Brandling and House, 2009; NHS England, 2019). However, it overlooked some of the tensions that have since emerged in the literature, including concerns about the extent to which social prescribing can address inequalities in health without considerable wider investment (Chng et al., 2021; Gibson et al., 2021; Griffith et al., 2022). It was also not the only way that social prescribing was understood locally. At the time of the fieldwork, social prescribing was becoming a significant part of NHS policy (NHS England, 2019). Rachel, a local community-sector stakeholder, understood social prescribing through a community development lens. She reflected on recent changes as she recalled how the local landscape had evolved:

I think that social prescribing was embedded in the voluntary sector … it was very driven by the voluntary sector and … my perception of what happened two years ago was that they were trying to reach out to the statutory providers to say, 'This is what we can offer you'. Over the past two years the tables have totally turned and now what we have is, we have … an emerging NHS-driven agenda, very much linked to health and non-clinical interventions, and what I see emerging is a disparity in a sense between the voluntary sector and the NHS driven agenda.

She later continued:

I refer to NHS England as the big boys, and the big boys have realised, 'Oh, I think this is a good thing that we need to start pushing', and once they start pushing and they formalise it, it's become that non-clinical rather than that community asset, community development and grass roots. I think that's when you start seeing the shifting sands, and I think the voluntary sector becomes that little bit precious about wanting to hold on and not wanting to change.

(Interview_Rachel_Social Prescribing Stakeholder)

Rachel went on to describe how local community groups were under increasing pressure to satisfy the choice-driven metrics of the NHS, which did not always align with their own ways of capturing impact and value. The NHS emerged more '*robust*', as Rachel put it, than the voluntary sector, which could undermine collaboration. This drew attention to the incommensurable value constructs of different actors and institutions prompting questions about which ones are becoming privileged.

Conclusion and Reflections

Through 8 months of in-depth ethnographic fieldwork with primary care teams and social prescribing stakeholders, I was able to trace how meaning was becoming attached to social prescribing locally. Meanings were not static and were continually reshaped by local materialities and practicalities, which could limit opportunities for engagement, despite enthusiasm for social prescribing in general.

Much of the value of the intervention was understood through time, both the imagined future gains and the historical drivers. Incommensurable constructs of value could lead to tensions between different actors and institutions and could undermine collaboration if some value constructs were perceived to dominate.

Since the fieldwork was completed, there has been significant changes to the context in which social prescribing is delivered. During the COVID-19 pandemic, link workers took on a range of activities in response to emerging challenges. Their varied experiences during this time have prompted questions about the scope of link working, the nature of '*good*' social prescribing and its relationship with primary care (Fixsen et al., 2022; Morris et al., 2022; Westlake et al., 2022). Link workers are now integral to new Primary Care Networks (NHS England, 2019), but, alongside the pandemic, a '*toxic cocktail*' of austerity, Brexit and the social care crisis has placed unsustainable pressures on the NHS (Patton, 2022, p. 175). This could compound the challenges of integrating link workers into frontline teams (Baird et al., 2022). The pandemic and '*diminished resources*' have also affected third-sector organisations, limiting some community services and further increasing the patchy diversity of social prescribing landscapes (Fixsen et al., 2022).

It will be important to recognise how collective understandings of social prescribing continue to evolve through the emerging materialities and practicalities of these post-pandemic landscapes, paying close attention to the competing priorities of different actors and institutions.

REFERENCES

Aughterson, H., Baxter, L., Fancourt, D., 2020. Social prescribing for individuals with mental health problems: A qualitative study of barriers and enablers experienced by general practitioners. BMC Fam. Pract. 21, 194.

Baird, B., Charles, A., Honeyman, M., Maguire, D., Das, P., 2016. Understanding Pressures in General Practice. King's Fund, London.

Baird, B., Lamming, L., Bhatt, R., 2022. Integrating Additional Roles into Primary Care Networks. King's Fund, London.

Bertotti, M., Frostick, C., Hutt, P., Sohanpal, R., Carnes, D., 2018. A realist evaluation of social prescribing: An exploration into the context and mechanisms underpinning a pathway linking primary care with the voluntary sector. Prim. Health Care Res. Dev. 19, 232–245.

Brandling, J., House, W. 2009. Social prescribing in general practice: Adding meaning to medicine. Br. J. Gen. Pract. 59(563), 454–456. doi:10.3399/bjgp09X421085 (Accessed 3 January 2024).

Calderón-Larrañaga, S., Milner, Y., Clinch, M., Greenhalgh, T., Finer, S., 2021. Tensions and opportunities in social prescribing: Developing a framework to facilitate its implementation and evaluation in primary care: A realist review. BJGP Open 5 (3).

Calderón-Larrañaga, S., Greenhalgh, T., Finer, S., Clinch, M., 2022. What does the literature mean by social prescribing? A critical review using discourse analysis. Sociol. Health Illn. 44(4–5), 848–868. doi:10.1111/1467-9566.13468.

Chng, N.R., Hawkins, K., Fitzpatrick, B., O'Donnell, C.A., Mackenzie, M., Wyke, S., Mercer, S.W., 2021. Implementing social prescribing in primary care in areas of high socioeconomic deprivation: Process evaluation of the 'Deep End' community links worker programme. Br. J. Gen. Pract. 71 (713), e912–e920.

Fixsen, A., Seers, H., Polley, M., Robins, J., 2020. Applying critical systems thinking to social prescribing: A relational model of stakeholder 'buy-in'. BMC Health Serv. Res. 20 (1), 1–13.

Fixsen, D.A., Barrett, D.S., Shimonovich, M., 2022. Supporting vulnerable populations during the pandemic: Stakeholders' experiences and perceptions of social prescribing in Scotland during Covid-19. Qual. Health Res. 32 (4), 670–682.

Gibson, K., Pollard, T.M., Moffatt, S., 2021. Social prescribing and classed inequality: A journey of upward health mobility? Soc. Sci. Med. 280, 114037.

Gibson, K., Moffatt, S., Pollard, T.M., 2022. 'He called me out of the blue': An ethnographic exploration of contrasting temporalities in a social prescribing intervention. Sociol. Health Illn. 44 (7), 1149–1166. doi:10.1111/1467-9566.

Graeber, D., 2001. Toward an Anthropological Theory of Value: The False Coin of Our Own Dreams. Springer.

Griffith, B., Pollard, T., Gibson, K., Jeffries, J., Moffatt, S., 2022. Constituting link working through choice and care: An ethnographic account of front-line social prescribing. Sociol. Health Illn. 45 (2), 279–297. doi:10.1111/1467-9566.13569.

Heath, I., 2015. Arm in arm with righteousness. Philos. Ethics Humanit. Med. 10 (1), 1–4.

Henwood, F., Harris, R., Spoel, P., 2011. Informing health? Negotiating the logics of choice and care in everyday practices of 'healthy living'. Soc. Sci. Med. 72 (12), 2026–2032.

Kimberlee, R., 2015. What is social prescribing? Adv. Soc. Sci. Res. J. 2 (1).

Kings Fund, 2022. Submission to the health and care select committee inquiry into the future of general practice. Available from: kingsfund.org.uk (Accessed November 2022).

Kleinman, A., 1988. The Illness Narratives: Suffering, Healing, and the Human Condition. Basic Books.

Kleinman, A., 2019. The Soul of Care: The Moral Education of a Husband and a Doctor. Penguin.

Latour, B., Daston, L. (Eds.), 2000. Biographies of Scientific Objects. University of Chicago Press.

Mol, A., 2008. The Logic of Care: Health and the Problem of Patient Choice. Routledge.

Mol, A., 2002. The Body Multiple: Ontology in Medical Practice. Duke University Press.

Moore, C., Unwin, P., Evans, N., Howie, F., 2022. Social prescribing: Exploring general practitioners' and healthcare professionals' perceptions of, and engagement with, the NHS model. Health Soc. Care Community. 30 (6), e5176–e5185. doi:10.1111/hsc.13935.

Morris, S.L., Gibson, K., Wildman, J.M., Griffith, B., Moffatt, S., Pollard, T.M., 2022. Social prescribing during the COVID-19 pandemic: A qualitative study of service providers' and clients' experiences. BMC Health Serv. Res. 22 (1), 258.

NHS England, 2019. NHS Long Term Plan. Available from: www.longtermplan.nhs.uk (Accessed 16 October 2023).

NHS England, 2019. Universal Personalised Care: Implementing the Comprehensive Model. NHS England, London.

Paton, C., 2022. NHS Reform and Health Politics in the UK Revolution, Counter-Revolution and Covid Crisis. Springer Nature, p. 175.

Tierney, S., Wong, G., Roberts, N., Boylan, AM., Park, S., Abrams, R., et al., 2020. Supporting social prescribing in primary care by linking people to local assets: A realist review. BMC Med. 18, 49. https://doi.org/10.1186/s12916-020-1510-7.

Westlake, D., Elston, J., Gude, A., Gradinger, F., Husk, K., Asthana, S., 2022. Impact of COVID-19 on social prescribing across an integrated care system: A researcher in residence study. Health Soc. Care Community. 30, e4086–e4094. https://doi.org/10.1111/hsc.13802.

White, C., Bell, J., Reid, M., Dyson, J., 2022. More than signposting: Findings from an evaluation of a social prescribing service. Health Soc. Care Community. 30 (6), e5105–e5114. doi:10.1111/hsc.13925.

Chapter 16

Social Prescribing: A Panacea or Another Top-Down Programme?

Cormac Russell

Introduction

Social prescribing is at best a misnomer and at worst a counterproductive and disabling term. We ought instead to speak of doctors as potential 'participation advocates' who can work in partnership with key allies. Doctors also engage in medical proscription: that is, they prevent inappropriate medicalisation of social and physical issues.

Nevertheless, as broadly practiced in the UK, social prescribing is too focused on referrals to the voluntary, community and social enterprise (VCSE) sector and thereby falls short of supporting socially isolated individuals to become participating, interdependent members of their communities.

Consensual Human Exchange

Far too many referrals are to programmes or structured services run by salaried strangers rather than to nearby neighbours interested in fostering reciprocal relationships in which people are received and celebrated for their 'gifts'. McKnight (2012) explains that care is the freely given gift of the heart. It is not an institutional intervention or a service (though both are important); it is a consensual human exchange that cannot be prescribed. Those who linger in waiting rooms need a life, not just a service. They yearn for belonging: the experience of unforced and unpaid-for acceptance, what most call *care*. That gift—the gift of care—which cannot be bought, managed, scaled up or otherwise commissioned, is the antidote to loneliness and the elixir of life.

The current shortcomings in social prescribing are therefore inevitable because too much emphasis and expectation are placed on the doctor and VCSE organisations and not enough support and animation are offered to the associational or civic life of communities themselves. Even with the support of community organisations, unless they move beyond referrals to VCSEs and instead encourage resident relationships and local associational life, they will fail in their duty of care to those who have been pushed to the margins.

I acknowledge the positive intentions underpinning social prescribing, and early research is finding that it enhances people's lives in relative terms. But these results must be considered for what they are: relative to the alternatives. On the one hand, what would have happened if beneficiaries had been medicalised instead of referred to social activities? On the other hand, what would have happened if they had experienced enhanced community practices and a more progressive social perspective in line with the Peckham experiment (see Chapter 2)—albeit with a more modern twist?

The Ethical Role of the Doctor

The role of the doctor can be fulfilled not solely through prescription or referral but through relationship building, advocating for pathways to citizenship and ending the medicalisation of socioeconomic and political issues.

Because I will be comparing terms such as *prescription* and *proscription* and *genuine participation* and *liberation*, I start here with a few working definitions:

PRESCRIPTION

1. an instruction written by a medical practitioner that authorises a patient to be issued a medicine or treatment
2. a recommendation that is authoritatively put forward

PROSCRIPTION

1. the action of forbidding something; banning, inhibiting or choosing not to do
2. condemnation or denunciation of something

PARTICIPATION

1. the action of exchanging gifts, skills and passions with others
2. the act of engaging with others in valued social roles and contributory civic efforts

LIBERATION

1. the action of setting someone free from imprisonment, slavery or oppression; release
2. freedom from limits on thought or behaviour

The proscription against doing harm is at the heart of medical ethics and is beautifully captured in the modern version of the Hippocratic Oath. Most clinicians quote the well-known dictum, 'First do no harm' (Latin: *Primum non nocere*). Interestingly, those words do not appear in the original Greek text, although the phrase 'I will utterly reject harm and mischief' does. In effect, this is proscription.

My sense is that we really need our doctors to use their proscriptive power to engage in more mischief making, if not outright heresy, while at the same time doing no harm to the people and communities they serve.

Dr Robert Mendelsohn, a self-proclaimed medical heretic, was the very embodiment of an ethical doctor. As well as being honest to a fault, he believed that his primary role was to ensure that he did nothing to displace the health-producing capacities of people and their indigenous communities. In other words, he was more engaged in medical proscription than in prescription. He writes,

In the late 1960s, my patients began to return to me with the diseases that I had previously created. The first group of patients were the ones with cancer of the thyroid gland, because, when I was trained at Michael Reese Hospital as a pediatric resident, I learned that the proper treatment for tonsillitis was X-ray therapy. Together with hundreds of other doctors, I prescribed X-rays for the tonsils. This led to an epidemic of tens of thousands of cases of thyroid cancer.

(Mendelsohn, et al., 1985)

He goes on to list other ailments caused by medical treatments of the 1960s and concludes that today's doctors have learned little from the past and continue to cause illness.

The Role of Gapper

Beyond distinguishing prescription and proscription, Mendelsohn also teaches us about a third role: the 'gapper'. Society is composed of two distinct domains: the institutional domain, governed by legal, contractual and administrative norms (bureaucracy); and the community domain, where citizens associate for their own purposes in more covenantal than contractual terms. While these two domains occupy the same space, they are fundamentally different and perform different functions when it comes to learning, justice, safety and wellbeing. Some social policies and the institutions that implement them respect these differences and work to keep the two domains in the right relationship with each other and assign each their appropriate functions. Most institutional advocates, however, do not respect the integrity of the community domain, their primary agenda being to treat perceived problems with institutional solutions, not to defend community capacities. In the process, communities lose the capacity to perform the functions that were and still are, in principle, their birthright.

Within this frame, the role of the ethical professional is to occupy the gap between these two domains and to challenge any colonial/imperial impulses of bureaucracies, hence opening more space for communities to grow and become more powerful and health creating. The role of the doctor is critical to community and individual wellbeing, and the doctor's impact can stretch well beyond the surgery.

The Problem With the Term *Social Prescribing*

Medicine is currently going through a great transition, from the science of treating sickness to the science and art of health creation (see Chapter 11). Increasingly savvy doctors, allied health professionals and VCSE organisations are recognising that they cannot unilaterally produce health, that in fact health is not a product to be dispensed by professionals and consumed by 'the sick'.

In the UK, social prescribing is being put forward as evidence of this transition. However, we must ask, is social prescribing the correct term to use to describe health creation? More specifically, does this term properly describe and value the process by which doctors enable their patients to make the journey towards interdependence that is at the heart of community life? To answer these questions, I give three reasons that I believe the term *social prescribing* is a misnomer:

1. The word *prescribe* does not accurately describe what impactful doctors, with the support of community development workers, are doing to broker people back into interdependent relationships or to support them in maintaining existing bonds.
2. In some instances, the practices of social prescribing have become too oriented towards referral and signposting, partly because prescribing is programmatic, insufficiently relational and largely devoid of longer-term community development efforts.
3. The doctor has authority over the medicine cabinet but no real authority over associational life in modern communities, and hence needs the support of allies. That said, they have much in the way of tacit influence among community members.

To summarise, the word *prescribe* does not describe what impactful doctors do.

Freirean Critique of *Prescription*

In his book *Pedagogy of the Oppressed* (1970), thinker and educator Paulo Freire gives his critique of education, describing it as a 'banking' concept in which students are treated as containers into which educators

put knowledge rather than enabled to discover their own knowledge. As banking is to pupils, social prescribing is in danger of being to patients. Building on the banking critique, Friere asserts that prescription is one of the basic levers of power between the oppressor and the oppressed. The alternative to prescription or banking is *liberation,* which situates the doctor in the role of 'alongsider', which is to say, a proscriber and heckler extraordinaire of the imperial impulses of their medical systems, in favour of more community-led responses, wherever possible.

The Problem With Prescription Referrals

The fact that this approach to care is called social prescribing is revealing. The term is, it seems, a political concession made by well-intentioned reformers in the hope that those who resist going beyond the medical model will feel better about doing so because the term *prescribing* is appended to a word that supposedly gives them cause for concern: *social.* I am not convinced that, in the long term, this tactic will adequately address the resistance at the heart of why so many non-sick people have been medicalised in the past and why so many others who have sought community alternatives have been drawn back into 'Serviceland' again and again.

Referring people to social activities within a community simply addresses the symptoms of a social 'disease'. Referring people to community activities should not be confused with a process that genuinely creates pathways towards satisfying and enriching life experiences or adequately addresses poverty and social justice issues, which are often the root cause of many maladies.

People will never belong when they are just dropping in. People who are socially isolated are deficient not in social activities per se but in opportunities to contribute their gifts and to receive the gifts of others outside of contract or even necessarily the exchange of money. They are missing reciprocal connections that create a sense of belonging, power and belief in their own gifts, agency and passions.

Doctors know better than most people that when individuals are devalued it has life-altering consequences for their wellbeing:

- They become seen as their condition. Which is to say, they become 'unseen' in the existential sense.

- This leads to a deficit orientation in which other people cannot see the capacities or the potential of the person. They become bereft of any valued social role.
- When people focus solely on a person's deficits, they assume that person needs to be in 'special' places with other 'special' people who possess similar deficits and supported by 'qualified' people who can look after them. In effect, they become labelled people and aggregate with other labelled people.
- In this way, labelled people often end up being rejected by and ejected from mainstream society and segregated into such places where the opportunity to experience roles that are socially valued in society at large is foreclosed on.
- The net effect of this rejection is being distanced from neighbours, neighbourhoods and community life, being set apart and sometimes put away, either physically or socially, in what some have aptly called 'Serviceland' and others have called 'Apartheid'.
- People get cast into negative roles, such as being considered not fully human or alien, being treated as objects or being viewed as objects of pity or burdens.
- People may literally lose their identity by being referred to not by name but as clients or service users. People become defined by what they are in relation to the service system, not by who they are in themselves or how they relate to family, friends and their community.
- Worse still, people who are assigned limited role expectations are regularly subjected to all kinds of discrimination and abuse.

Challenging Dominant Narratives

I believe it is time to state clearly that specific situations and circumstances are 'sickening', rather than that people themselves are sick. The symptoms which modern medicine attempts to treat often have little to do with the condition of our bodies; they are, rather, signals pointing to the disorders and presumptions of modern ways of working, playing and living.

(Illich, 1975)

Mary walks into a doctor's surgery with her partner, Richard, who is her full-time carer. They are seeking support in figuring out how to live well together now that Mary has been diagnosed with dementia. They are already well on their way in that they are determined to be seen for their capacities, not for Mary's diagnosis. They've asked for help to 'live well, given that dementia is a feature of our lives' instead of asking for help as 'dementia sufferers'.

The sad fact is that Mary and Richard are seeking support within a dominant narrative that characterises them and their lives as follows:

1. These folks have problems/deficits that need to be fixed, needs that need to be addressed.
2. These needs are best addressed by qualified people in a service/programmatic context.

Until we address the culture that underpins such narratives, no matter how progressive a new initiative may be, it will not get past go. To use an old saying, culture eats innovation for breakfast.

Table 16.1 summarises my tips for how health and care practitioners can move from a medical model to a social and asset-based model of social prescribing.

A Village Problem, Not a Health Problem

To engage in systems reform without facilitating community building at the neighbourhood level would be analogous to monocropping. The seeds would be metaphors for the people referred to communities by general practitioners or other professionals, and the land would be a metaphor for the communities that are losing their carrying capacities (their connectability) and their ability to be health producing while having ever-increasing numbers of people, many with complex support needs, referred to them.

I see that system leaders are changing the language from an individual focus to a village or population focus, but practitioners often still concentrate on the person with needs. It is a mistake to bypass the process of facilitating citizen-led discovery, connecting, and mobilisation—what I refer to as community building. But we are seeing many commissioners pay third-sector organisations (whom they treat as the 'community' or as a proxy for the community) to accept referrals from clinicians and then claim this approach to be asset-based community development. It is not.

TABLE 16.1 Effective Clinical Practice in Social Prescribing

Deficit Model	Asset Model	Enablers for Effective Practice
'Dementia sufferer;	Living well with dementia	A conversation that explores the couple's existing connections as well as their support needs in sustaining these connections and building up new ones.
Individual patient focus	Citizens with contributions to make to the wellbeing of their community	See past the label *dementia*. Shift the conversation from diagnosis or deficit towards Mary's and Richard's gifts (which they were born with), skills (which they know well enough to teach another) and passions (what they care about enough to act on). Work alongside a connecting practitioner (community builder) who sees those gifts and knows what part of the community they can best fit into.
Referrals directing people to activities	Referrals that link people to meaningful roles and reciprocal relationships	Ask: What is the community alternative to my clinical intervention? Use system leadership to genuinely engage in social change and community development.
Institutional systems leadership with antibodies against innovation	VCSE leadership that encourages disruptive thinking and social innovation	Create a dome of protection around community inventiveness rather than displace community invention by becoming the primary inventors.
		Go small and local, resource well, relocate authority, then get out of the way. The best route out of institutionalisation is re-communalisation. Ask: What matters to you that you'd like to join with others in doing? and What are the assets/resources/capacities and wants that exist near the person's doorstep that would help them to make that contribution?
Needs assessments that break down trust, reinforce labels and lead to prescription of the very services provided by those who analyse the person	Conversations that build trust and create a narrative and biography of the person and possibilities towards connections	Ask: What does a good day look like for you? What would I need to know to live well in your community/your life? Co-create a therapeutic, advocacy and community development vision of a good life.
Focus on how the social prescribing service will work	Focus on why social prescribing will help	Balance biomedical education (for both the professionals and the couple, Mary and Richard) with education about what makes people well (see Chapter 3), which may be summarised as somewhere to live, someone to love and something meaningful to do. An abundant community offers all of this.
Employ salaried strangers as link workers	Work alongside allies who have a deep, ongoing relationship with the local community. Tap into local community development practitioners and local resident connectors	Seek to discover what's already there. Identify and support small community associations and social enterprises that are rooted in the community.
		A connecting practitioner will be careful not to displace the capacities of local resident connectors and can support them and extend their capacity and reach.

Making the Case for a Community-Building Approach

If we do not directly invest in our communities—in 'a place and all its creatures' (Berry, 2002), and I would add its economy, ecology and cultures—we may one day find there is no longer a community at all. We cannot expect to engage with and refer to communities unless we first support them to be built from the inside out.

The Creation of a Culture of Care

We need to create a new culture, where we say, 'Where have you been all this time? You matter to us, we cannot do this without you, we need you and we need your gifts. Don't worry about your fallibilities; we all have them. We'll work with you as you are, so you can participate in your own unique way and contribute your gifts on your terms. Let's go!'

This is the other side of the 'What matters to you?' conversation. In practice, I can only truly answer the 'What matters to me?' question when I know I matter to others.

Conclusion

Supporting people to create pathways towards a good life is not about prescriptions or referrals. It is about walking alongside people in their life's journey. System leaders such as doctors can't do that alone, but they can advocate for greater participation to ensure that social issues are not medicalised and community efforts are not devalued.

Citizens need opportunities to be identified and to be supported in using their gifts so that they feel they belong and build their self-belief. People can then feel able to find their own solutions rather than, to paraphrase Freire, be filled up with prescribed care. This approach is in contrast to 'othering' people, which may limit their expectations or even alienate them.

Illich's (1975) observation that society is sick reminds us of Sir Michael Marmot's (2015) insight that it is the social determinants of people's lives that make people sick. Our strategic focus should not be on fixing 'sick' people and returning them to the same conditions that made them sick. Until we address the root causes, social prescribing runs the risk of becoming the ambulance at the bottom of the cliff, driven by well-meaning but beleaguered volunteers.

It is time to awaken to the fact that we don't have a health problem, or a social care problem, or a youth problem, or even a safety problem. We have a village problem. The neighbourhood becomes our primary unit of analysis and change. This path could lead to genuine place-based working, pooled budgets and the release of resources to work upstream and stem the subsidence of our social fabric, which is causing people to fall into the river quicker than we can pull them out.

. Communities have a huge reservoir of assets to offer each other, but we must first support local laypeople to discover, connect and then mobilise these assets. We cannot hope to engage with the community until we first support local residents in building community. If social prescribing continues in the absence of effective community building at the street and associational levels, it will carry on like an app without a smartphone, and eventually it will die from the very afflictions it wishes to address.

Postscript: This chapter is a summary of a series of blogs written by the author. Ideas can be investigated in greater detail by visiting https://www.nurturedevelopment.org/blog/abcd-approach/social-prescribing-panacea-another-top-programme-part-1/ *(Accessed 3 January 2024).*

REFERENCES

Berry, W., 2002. The Art of the Commonplace: The Agrarian Essays. Counterpoint, Washington, DC.

Freire, P., 1970. Pedagogy of the Oppressed. Continuum Books, New York.

Illich, I., 1975. Limits to Medicine: Medical Nemesis—The Expropriation of Health. Calder & Boyars, London.

McKnight, J., 2012. You can't command care. Abundant Community. Available from: http://www.abundantcommunity.com/home/videos/you_cant_command_care.html (Accessed 24 November 2022).

Marmot, M., 2015. The Health Gap: The Challenge of an Unequal World. Bloomsbury, London.

Mendelsohn, R., Crile, G., Epsein, S., et al., 1985. Dissent in Medicine: Nine Doctors Speak Out. Contemporary Books, Chicago.

Chapter 17

The NHS Foundation Trust as Catalyst for Change

Salma Yasmeen, Sue Barton, and Phil Walters

Introduction

South West Yorkshire Partnership Foundation Trust (SWYPFT) is a specialist NHS Foundation Trust that provides community, mental health and learning disability services to 1.2 million people across Barnsley, Calderdale, Kirklees and Wakefield. We provide some medium secure (forensic) services to the whole of Yorkshire and the Humber. We are also part of two Integrated Care Systems, West Yorkshire and South Yorkshire.

Our daily mission is to help people reach their potential and live well in their communities. We employ over 4800 staff, in both clinical and non-clinical support services, who work hard daily to make a difference in the lives of service users, families and carers. How we work is as important to us as what we do—we pride ourselves on being a values-led organisation.

As an NHS Trust, we interpret social prescribing as being about genuine co-production with the communities we serve, working with the strengths of each person and those of their carers and wider community. Our ambition is to invest in and develop services and approaches that are focused on principles of recovery, including place-based recovery colleges that are led by volunteers and people with lived experience.

We have over 200 volunteers that are a valuable and integral part of our workforce and a growing number of peer support workers that are part of our teams. We work in partnership with the voluntary sector to deliver the Live Well Wakefield service (www.livewell-wakefield.nhs.uk), which provides social prescribing services to the people of Wakefield. In 2021, Live Well Wakefield won the award for the best larger social prescribing project in the social prescribing network awards for the partnership approach.

Our Journey

The Trust began by developing the right conditions for our approach to flourish, starting with open conversations with over 2500 service users, carers and staff. Consistent themes emerged, leading to the shared agreement of the mission statement: 'Enable people to reach their potential and to live well in their community' and our underpinning values:

- We put the person first and in the centre.
- We know that families and carers matter.
- We are respectful, honest, open and transparent.
- We improve and aim to be outstanding.
- We are relevant today and ready for tomorrow.

Many of our developments have happened during a time of austerity and within a financially challenging context in the NHS. During this time, we have also seen increasing policy emphasis on the development of the national social prescribing approach as part of personalised care within which creativity and the arts in health care can flourish.

We decided that we were not purely a provider of care and treatment and that we should also consider how we enabled people to live a full and rewarding life. In this work, we were conscious of getting the right balance between governance and innovation. At the time, we articulated the need to be brave and to amplify the assets that already existed across our places. We used evidence and examples from asset-based community development work, including the pioneering work by Cormac Russell (Chapter 16), and underpinned it with the work of Michael Marmot (Chapter 5) to address the wider determinants of health and health inequalities if we were to deliver our mission.

Increasingly, service users, carers and staff are reporting favourably on their experiences, in terms of finding a greater meaning in their lives by including creative and spiritual approaches. We received feedback such as 'I started seeing things differently…, my whole life changed, my purpose in life changed, I started acting differently, it [creativity] gave me a different perspective and that's what I needed.'

An Anchor Institution for Community Development

SWYPFT hosts a national organisation, Altogether Better (www.altogetherbetter.org.uk). This is an example of how we have invested in, nurture and develop approaches that enable health-producing communities that stimulate creative and cultural activities to enable people to connect and find purpose, meaning and hope through shared interests.

Altogether Better

Altogether Better works with commissioners, services, leaders, clinicians and citizens around the UK to offer solutions to the challenges the NHS is currently facing. Their model is one of 'Collaborative Practice', inviting local people to gift their time to their GP practice or health service in a new, collaborative relationship (see the prologue of this book, written by David Ashton, as an early example). As a result, the practice changes how it works—people become 'champions' and stimulate and lead new groups and activities. Much of the work is in primary care where Altogether Better has helped over 350 GP practices to develop the skills, mindset and culture needed to create a general practice fit for the future. Their work complements and amplifies the role of social prescribing link workers by increasing capacity and reducing demand. They support the practice to use their data to connect patients into a plethora of new offers and activities that respond to the problems that medicine alone cannot fix.

Creative Minds

This is one of three charities linked to the main SWYPFT charity EyUp! It is the bridge between the NHS and the communities it serves through community development principles and asset-based approaches. It operates as a social movement, which empowers local communities to be part of decision-making and development. It brings NHS and community funding together to pool resources and extend our offer and cement our partnership with communities.

Launched in 2012, Creative Minds develops and supports the delivery of creative projects that improve health and wellbeing. It has over 120 creative community partnerships and strong pathways to people who are in the greatest need through staff champions in SWYPFT services.

These co-produce and deliver creative arts, sports, recreation and leisure activities. This includes activities such as horticulture and the use of green and blue spaces.

The main issue that we tackle is the loneliness and social isolation that people experience when they have mental and physical health issues. This can affect their personal resilience and lead to negative outcomes including loss of confidence, poor self-esteem and feelings of negativity. Service users and carers told us that engagement in creative activity needs to start with a safe, supportive environment. Creative engagement was seen as an opportunity for people to work as equals by shifting power and creating personal autonomy. This then allows people to challenge themselves constructively, imagine a different life for themselves and make plans to move their lives forwards.

Under Creative Minds, project groups are micro commissioned to focus on the activity. Participants share ground rules and develop social norms. They offer a safe environment where participants can test out relationship-building skills and establish supportive social networks. Our match-funding model brings NHS and community funding together to develop projects with broader scope and offer opportunities for more people.

Creative Minds can get alongside individuals who use services and support them to connect with meaningful activities in their communities and neighbourhoods that help individuals to regain hope, meaning and fulfil their potential. Peer-led projects are a priority area of development for Creative Minds, where participants from an existing programme who develop a passion for a particular activity can go on to develop their own groups.

Spirit in Mind

This is also a linked charity to EyUp! and focuses on the development of partnerships with locally based faith and humanist organisations. This enhances the range and diversity of support available to people who use our services and promotes a deeper understanding of the role of spirituality in health care. Spirit in Mind fosters synergetic patterns of collaborative working around bringing together and drawing upon the resources and wisdom of both faith-based organisations and the NHS.

Community Reporting, Research and Evaluation

Over the last 10 years, Creative Minds has been working with others to develop ways to research and evaluate creative activities in an empowered way that supports individuals and communities to play an active role in the process. We have developed a variety of participatory research approaches that have involved participants in designing and delivering the evaluation approach. This has included training a peer-led network of Community Reporters to collect stories from project participants to evaluate creative activities and provide new insights into why they feel creativity is important to health and wellbeing. Community Reporting is a storytelling movement that uses digital tools such as portable and pocket technologies (tablets, smartphones) to support people to tell their own stories in their own ways. Central to the approach is the belief that people telling authentic stories about their own lived experience offers a valuable understanding of their lives.

Systematising Creative Wellbeing

From the foundation of Creative Minds, health, local authority and community partners came together to develop a system-wide plan to make Calderdale a leader in using arts and culture to support people's health and wellbeing (Calderdale CCG, 2019). This followed the publication of the seminal report published by the All-Party Parliamentary Group (APPG) on arts, health and wellbeing, *Creative Health: The Arts for Health and Wellbeing* (2017). This concluded that the arts can help to:

- Keep us well, aid our recovery and support longer lives better lived
- Meet major challenges facing health and social care: ageing, long-term conditions, loneliness and mental health
- Save money in the health service and in social care through building health producing and better-connected communities

The National Centre for Creative Health (NCCH) was set up in response to recommendation one of the APPG report. The NCCH is working in partnership with NHS England to develop Creative Health Hubs within four Integrated Care Systems of which West Yorkshire Integrated Care System (WYICS) is one. West Yorkshire is an area where creativity and health work is already embedded, building on the successes of Creative Minds' work over the past 10 years.

The Mental Health Museum is a linked charity to EyUp! It is a progressive museum located at Fieldhead Hospital, Wakefield that holds a collection of unique and compelling artefacts that tell the story of mental health care. Museums and libraries are strong contributors to social prescribing approaches locally, and many are partners of Creative Minds locally. The Mental Health Museum made a conscious decision to work together with people who access services, carers, friends and family, and staff and visitors to develop a social prescribing type offer. This includes hosting information sessions, reading groups and creative activities for people.

During COVID, the museum team made outreach a priority, moving online and working remotely to co-curate exhibitions and content with our community and service user-led groups, securing funding to distribute over 2500 children's wellbeing craft packs to food banks across the district, encouraging discussions about mental health in families living in poverty, and receiving feedback such as 'It was great to see him have a quiet few moments of reflection, quite a contrast to the chaos and carnage of usual life!' The exhibitions and work of the museum develop around themes such as a recent one on sustainability, nature and the environment and how this links to wellbeing. The Green Year initiative included a grow-along with our community and a wildlife club that meets to explore the rich natural environment around the hospital, resulting in qualitative feedback such as 'I went into our back yard on the Saturday afternoon feeling tired and not much interested in anything … Spending an hour sorting out pots and mulch lifted my spirits considerably.'

Conclusion

We believe that a Foundation Trust can play a key role in developing and delivering asset-based approaches that promote recovery through a range of social prescribing approaches. We have found a way to do this which recognises and supports the strengths which are present in our communities and health and care system. This involves investing in the community where we work, making connections and building strong relationships. As a large NHS organisation, we play a key role as an anchor institution rooted in the areas we serve. Our role is to influence and act as a catalyst for change in our communities and places through convening, enabling and connecting. The recent development of integrated care systems provides a real opportunity to address the big issues of inequality and physical and mental health through innovative approaches which connect to and align with the priorities of people we provide support to or communities we are a part of.

Our experience tells us that there are some key ingredients to making this work. These include:

- **Committed Leadership at Board level**—recognising the value of creative health approaches and making this an integral part of strategic direction not just an add on
- **Investing in innovation**—investing in individuals and capacity to support and nurture innovations
- **Community powered priorities**—connecting with and creating the conditions for people and groups to develop the priorities that are important to them in their everyday lives
- **Developing good governance**—that enables and supports change and innovation
- **Diverse talent and skills**—recruiting and valuing a diverse workforce to support creative health approaches, creative practitioners, people with lived experience and community connectors as integrated members of teams
- **Creating the right conditions for change and integration**—enabling conversations between communities, the creative and cultural sector and health and social care practitioners and teams to co-produce approaches and systems that reflect the diversity of people in communities
- **Investing in system-wide partnerships**—developing shared priorities and plans for sustainable investment to address inequalities

We know this work is an important catalyst for transformational change. It focuses on the things which matter to people and can impact on wellbeing and healthier communities that are more connected, cohesive and productive. We are part of a growing evidence base that provides ways that we can help to address the inequalities which exist, and it results in stories which demonstrate how people can reach their potential and live well in their communities.

REFERENCES

All-Party Parliamentary Group on arts, health and wellbeing, 2017. Creative health: the arts for health and wellbeing. Available from: https://www.culturehealthandwellbeing.org.uk/appg-inquiry/Publications/Creative_Health_Inquiry_Report_2017_-_Second_Edition.pdf (Accessed 10 February 2023).

Calderdale, CCG., 2019. Living a larger life using creative activities to help people live well in Calderdale. Available from: https://www.calderdale.gov.uk/nweb/COUNCIL.minutes_pkg.view_doc?p_Type=AR&p_ID=69687 (Accessed 10 February 2023).

Chapter 18

The View From the VCSE Sector

Kate Jopling

Introduction

As the leading coalition of health and social care charities in England, National Voices brings together over 200 organisations working across a diverse range of health conditions and communities. The practical, social and emotional support provided by our members connects us with millions of people and to communities across the country.

The core insight underlying so many voluntary, community and social enterprise (VCSE) sector approaches to health is that our ability to live well isn't just about what goes on in our bodies but is also a product of the wider context of our lives—the places we live, the work we do, the money we have, our sense of our place in the world and the relationships we share with people around us.

Connector Services

At the heart of what the NHS calls 'community-centred approaches for health and wellbeing' is work by VCSE organisations to build people up and strengthen their communities (South, 2015). While diverse VCSE approaches have evolved in different places and for different people, many share common features. One such 'family' of approaches are the 'connector services' which boil down to connecting an individual to a trained supporter (who may be a paid professional or a volunteer) who gets alongside them and helps them to work through the issues and challenges that are getting in the way of a good life for them. Social prescribing services are among this wider family of connector services which encompasses community connectors and navigators, local area coordinators and more—as set out in Fig. 18.1 (Jopling and Howells, 2018).

'Social prescribing' tends to describe connector services that are linked to the statutory health system, usually primary care, and which offer support to connect to community-based support alongside, or as an alternative to, health services. Connectors within social prescribing services are commonly known as link workers. However, there remains a wide diversity of social prescribing schemes and approaches, and terminology differs from one area to the next (Buck and Ewbank, 2020).

Development

Social prescribing schemes were first developed as part of wider work to bring support in the community closer to the health system. They were built on a mutual recognition of the benefits of working together: for VCSE organisations, working in health settings was an important way to connect with people who need support; for health system leaders, linking to the VCSE sector provided a route to the wide range of non-medical support that people using primary care needed.

Schemes were established on the back of wider work to build relationships between VCSE sector organisations and forward-thinking health system leaders (sometimes individual primary care practitioners, sometimes commissioners within Clinical Commissioning Groups (CCGs), local authorities etc.). Often these relationships also encompassed commissioning and funding arrangements through which funds flowed from health and care budgets to the VCSE sector to provide services and activities. Many social prescribing schemes were piloted with support from innovation funders, trusts and

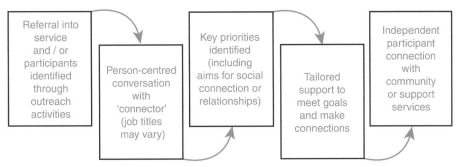

Fig. 18.1 Key features of connector services. From Jopling, K., Howells, A., 2018. Connecting communities to tackle loneliness and social isolation: learning report, British Red Cross.

foundations. In some—such as the Rotherham Social Prescribing Scheme—the scheme encompassed funding for link worker roles employed within the local VCSE sector umbrella body *and* the wider activities into which individuals could be referred (Dayson and Damm, 2020); in others—such as the Bromley by Bow centre—social prescribing approaches were part of a wider shared endeavour between the community and the NHS (Islam, 2019). The social prescribing link worker role was therefore born, and flourished, in contexts of wider support for community capacity building.

VCSE Capabilities and Flexibilities

Social prescribing works because link workers start with a conversation about the person rather than a presenting issue. Often the issues people face are complex—a tangled web of challenges with money, housing, health and care needs and personal relationships. Link workers have the flexibility to talk across these issues from the perspective of what matters to the individual, to help people prioritise and work out what to do next, drawing on the strengths and assets of the individual and their wider community, as well as formal services.

This greater comfort with walking alongside people in messy situations is one of the capabilities the VCSE sector brings to a health system which has historically been reluctant to uncover needs for which it has no solution. The other capability the VCSE sector brings is its ability to bring together support across messy systems. Community organisations have long experience of catching people who fall through the cracks in statutory support and in building new solutions where none exist. Thus creativity and flexibility are at the core of effective social prescribing approaches.

The importance of social prescribing was brought into sharp relief during the COVID-19 pandemic. In many areas the VCSE sector played a central role in immediate relief. Social prescribing schemes, particularly those that were more established when the pandemic hit, reoriented themselves to support people who were shielding, providing online or telephone services, and stepping in where existing community services were no longer able to operate. VCSE sector organisations told us they saw the cultural barriers to collaboration coming down as the close connection between health and non-medical needs came into clear focus.

The pandemic also demonstrated the value of social prescribing approaches in having the flexibility to respond to a rapidly changing and complex situation, and to coordinate, or support, a community response that made sure people got the help they need. At the same time it also increased the complexity and acuity of needs being dealt with by social prescribing link workers and increased demand on the wider statutory and voluntary sector safety net. Levels of needs have not abated since the pandemic. Indeed, with the cost-of-living crisis and the impact of NHS backlogs biting, the demands on link workers and the strains on the wider social prescribing systems are only growing.

Social Prescribing and the NHS

While interest in social prescribing had been growing over recent decades, NHS England's decision to invest in link workers, through the Alternative Roles Reimbursement Scheme (ARRS; NHS England, online) in general practice, represented a significant leap of faith in the direction of the power of the community to support people's everyday health and wellbeing and has enormously accelerated the rollout of social prescribing across England (NHS England and NHS Improvement, 2019). For many within the NHS, social prescribing is a relatively new model of care, understood primarily as a means of reducing demand for statutory services including health services, and particularly reducing pressure on GPs. However, strategically it sits at the heart of a wider shift.

National Voices has been working with NHS leaders over many years to support a faithful few—now thankfully growing in number and influence—to put people and communities at the centre of the health system. Both the NHS Five Year Forward View and the NHS Long Term Plan reflected this aspiration with significant commitments around personalised care and community-based support (NHS England, 2014, 2019). Our priority now is to ensure this results in real change for people who use health and care.

Social prescribing is one of a number of schemes that bring the NHS's theoretical commitments to life. The investment in social prescribing represents a significant shift *towards* recognising the expertise of people and communities, and the VCSE sector in keeping people well, and *away* from a merely medical model. It both aligns with, and expresses, the wider strategic shift the NHS is trying to make, as demonstrated in Fig. 18.2.

Challenges

However, the rollout of social prescribing has not been without its challenges. Many organisations sounded an alarm about the pace and scale of rollout in the context of a stretched VCSE sector. There were also voices within the sector who argued that the NHS investment in social prescribing represented a 'co-option' of something which previously was *of* the VCSE sector, and that this risked undermining the model.

For National Voices the priority has always been to ensure as many people as possible can access the support they need. So we worked to support the NHS rollout, in a spirit of realism that even the best-laid plans hit bumps in the road. Our role has been to act as a conduit between the real experiences of VCSE sector organisations and the people who use health services, and NHS leaders, and to help find a way to iron out those bumps.

In 2020, with support from NHS England, we set out to explore the perspectives and experiences of the VCSE sector of the NHS rollout of social prescribing which was, at that time, centred around an offer of funding for one link worker per Primary Care Network (PCN) in England under the ARRS. As our work to hear from organisations around the country continued, the COVID-19 pandemic hit. This not only changed our plans but also had a major impact on health systems and the social prescribing schemes and link workers that were operating within them. Nevertheless, we heard from over 300 VCSE organisations through a series of interviews, workshops and online engagements between December 2019 and June 2020 (Cole et al., 2020).

Overwhelmingly we found that the VCSE sector was supportive of social prescribing and keen to work constructively with the health system. Far from the polarised debates that sometimes occur on social media, our engagement with charities, large and small, national and local, health focused and not, showed that the sector shares the NHS's ambition to break down the boundaries between NHS services and non-medical support. The concerns we surfaced were not about whether to roll out social prescribing, but how.

The issue was that in practice, in some communities, social prescribing had been experienced as a top-down intervention from within the NHS, which had cut across rather than bolster existing work to bring sectors together. There were also concerns about strain on an already stretched VCSE sector and fears the VCSE was being asked to fill gaps in statutory services.

What the NHS funds through the ARRS is one part of the wider ecosystem that makes social prescribing tick. As noted above, the original social prescribing schemes were built in the context of wider collaboration across health system and community. Yet in some areas new link worker roles were created by the NHS

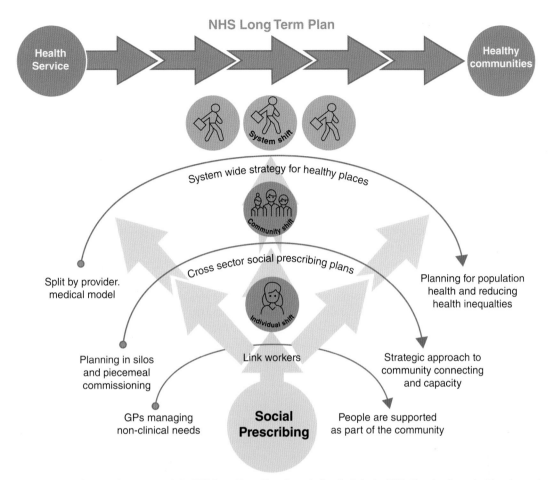

Fig. 18.2 Social prescribing in the context of the NHS Long Term Plan. From Jopling, K., Cole, A., 2022. Changing lives, changing places, changing systems: making progress on social prescribing, National Voices.

without proper consideration of the wider context of the local community—including other work linking the health system and VCSE sector. As such, the injection of new capacity didn't always land smoothly.

In some places there were gaps in communication. In others the pace of the rollout had a destabilising effect on existing connector schemes, and not enough was done to build on and invest in what was already in place. In other places, link workers were appointed without building links with the wider sector into which they wanted to make referrals. This left VCSE sector colleagues feeling excluded and undervalued.

However, there were also examples of successful integration of NHS-funded link workers into existing social prescribing schemes, primarily in places where

there were already strong relationships between the sector and statutory partners. For example, in Gateshead NHS-funded link workers were brought into the existing scheme run by Edberts House, benefitting from their networks, management structures and other programmes.

On the back of our consultations, we identified a range of areas for action to smooth the future rollout process. Some of the challenges we identified could be addressed directly by NHS England, including:

- The funding and management arrangements, role descriptions and performance expectations for new link workers
- The measures used to assess the outcomes of social prescribing

However, not all of the challenges we identified could be resolved by NHS England. These included:

- The need for funding to help the VCSE sector meet increased demand
- The need to ensure that social prescribing actively tackles inequality
- The need to invest in relationships and support ongoing collaboration and partnership

Funding

Perhaps unsurprisingly, securing sufficient, stable funding for services and activities the VCSE sector provides remains a paramount concern for our sector.

Social prescribing relies on the capacity of the community to respond and support people to stay well. It capitalises on the strength of the VCSE sector to connect up local services and support around a person. As an asset-based approach, it enables individuals and communities to draw on what they already have to achieve goals that are meaningful to them. However, community capacity is neither endlessly elastic nor free. While some community groups can welcome new members without increased cost, other more 'hard-edged' services, such as advice on debt or housing, come with a unit cost: additional demand translates directly into additional cost. Furthermore, not all communities have equal access to social infrastructure (All Party Parliamentary Group; APPG Left Behind Neighbourhoods, 2020). Investing in community capacity is therefore vital. Without it, social prescribing cannot succeed.

It is not just activity that needs funding. Money to provide groups and services is vital, but there is also a need to fund VCSE infrastructure bodies including councils for the voluntary sector etc. These organisations play a critical role in coordination and information sharing around social prescribing. Many of these organisations have long been underfunded, having borne the brunt of cuts in recent years, and are now under additional pressure as a result of the COVID-19 pandemic (Haslam, 2022).

The NHS has always made clear, in its formal communications, that the funding provided to support link workers is a *contribution* to local social prescribing ecosystems (NHS England and NHS Improvement, 2020). Despite this, in some areas new schemes have been launched without any additional funding for the wider activities that surround link workers, placing demand on already stretched services. In areas where the social infrastructure is weak this is a serious problem.

Social prescribing will only work as a mechanism for addressing health inequality if additional investment flows to more deprived areas. Without investment to meet the costs of tackling disadvantage, social prescribing could exacerbate inequality, as generalist link workers may lack the specialist skills to reach more marginalised communities and would face fewer services to meet the needs they encounter in more deprived communities—further exacerbating the inverse care law.

National Voices has always been clear that it is not the sole responsibility of the NHS to fund social infrastructure. However, our research showed a clear consensus that as social prescribing identifies unmet needs and drives new demand to the VCSE sector, funding needs to flow to meet it; and where the VCSE sector helps to deliver outcomes for the NHS, funding should flow from budgets allocated to their achievement. The challenge for NHS England is that those leading the social prescribing agenda cannot direct local NHS bodies to adhere to their guidance around funding provision, and they lack influence over the other funders of VCSE sector provision.

Galvanising Wider Action

Addressing the gaps in funding—and securing the strategic commitment to social prescribing needed to attract funding—is not something NHS England or the VCSE sector can resolve alone. A much wider range of organisations need to come together in support of the vision behind social prescribing.

In 2021, in partnership with New Philanthropy Capital and supported by NHS England, we convened a series of further discussions with stakeholders including Integrated Care System (ICS) leaders, local government representatives, funders and charities providing services at a national level, and national government representatives. We wanted to understand what would unlock progress on creating more stable cross-sector funding and collaboration in support of social prescribing (Jopling and Cole, 2022).

Funding for the VCSE sector in communities already comes from a wide range of sources—both national and local, statutory, corporate and voluntary. But the ecosystem around social prescribing does not begin and end with the VCSE sector. It also encompasses provision from statutory bodies and other national organisations—including the Department for Work and Pensions, Department for Levelling Up, Housing and Communities and others. Ideally all of these stakeholders would come together to plan for the future.

In relation to VCSE capacity, leaders across NHS England, and in the National Academy for Social Prescribing, have advocated for the creation of shared funding pots to support social prescribing activity. Bringing together funding across sectors—from statutory, charitable and corporate funders—to support work to achieve agreed outcomes has significant potential to deliver better results and avoid duplication and high procurement costs for all involved. However, given the variety of contexts for collaboration between the NHS and VCSE in different areas—ranging from virtually non-existent to well established—and the wide range of ways in which capacity is already being funded, it is going to be important that any new mechanisms and structures build on where the energy is and avoid reinventing the wheel.

Opportunities for Collaboration

The creation of integrated care systems (ICSs) offers an opportunity to get the right systems in place for collaboration on strategy, and funding for, social prescribing. However, ICSs already have a lot on their plates, and it is not clear that conversations about social prescribing will be prioritised. Furthermore, different ICSs are at radically different stages in terms of their wider obligations to establish links with VCSE sector.

Changes in NHS structures have made relationships across sectors challenging, not least because the new NHS footprints do not match those of VCSE organisations or other parts of the public sector. Primary care networks (PCNs) are significantly smaller than the CCG/local authority scale at which many medium-sized charities operate; meanwhile, ICSs cover far larger areas than most local VCSE sector organisations but are too numerous for national organisations to engage with individually. Work is now underway to develop ICS level VCSE alliances to bridge this divide, but these structures are still emerging and already look different in different places.

Function is more important than form when it comes to cross-sector collaboration. Social prescribing planning could be led by ICS-level forums in some areas, but in most areas it will be more appropriate for plans to be developed at place level, with the ICS taking an oversight role. The key will be to build on existing relationships wherever possible, not least because capacity for partnership working within the VCSE sector is already at significant stretch. NHS England will also need to do more to align the asks being made of the VCSE sector across its programmes on health inequalities, population health management, anchor institutions, voluntary sector partnerships and more, as all of these draw on the same capabilities and strengths.

Engaging Beyond Health

Collaboration will need to go beyond ICSs, though, to bring in national bodies, funders and others. Their capacity and approach will have a material impact on whether social prescribing is effective, and their work may be impacted by link workers' activity, for example, through increased referrals as needs are uncovered. However, as yet, their voices are rarely heard in discussions about social prescribing, and many do not see social prescribing as a priority.

In our discussions with these stakeholders, we found general support for the underlying principles of social prescribing. They saw the potential of personalised, holistic, targeted, community-based and preventative support that enables people to live well in the community. They recognised that this was urgently needed in the context of the impact of the pandemic on communities, the strains on health and care services, with more than 7 million people now on NHS waiting lists (NHS England, 2022) and the compounding impact of the cost-of-living crisis. However, this has not yet translated into engagement with the social prescribing movement.

Hearts and Minds

Social prescribing still has a 'PR problem'—people are enthusiastic about the end goal, but the concept is not always well known, and there are a range of unhelpful preconceptions about it. Some colleagues in the VCSE sector see social prescribing as an NHS-led endeavour, as an attempt to recast social needs within a medical model and antithetical to asset-based ways of working. Some in local government sometimes see social prescribing as the NHS 'reinventing' connector services that they have been driving forward for decades. Some colleagues in funding bodies perceive social prescribing as 'niche'—a new model of care, among many, which will go in or out of fashion.

Greater clarity and honesty around where the NHS's involvement in social prescribing begins and ends could help to address these issues. The NHS's leap of faith in investing in social prescribing link workers, while significant, remains only a contribution to the systems that can keep people healthy in the community. The success (and failure) of social prescribing must be owned collectively.

Recognising the diversity of models that fit under the 'social prescribing' umbrella will also be important, as will generous recognition that other models of connecting and linking can be just as effective. More explicitly stating the link of social prescribing to broader programmes of NHS reform is also necessary.

However, what funders and commissioners most need to hear is how social prescribing links to *their* core agenda—ICSs need to know how social prescribing can help to improve population health, tackle inequalities and deliver value for money; local authorities need to understand its relevance to addressing health inequalities and tackling wellbeing; central government departments need to understand how effective social prescribing schemes can be in identifying need and linking people to support around priority issues such as debt, housing and employment; charitable funders need to see where social prescribing schemes deliver on objectives that they are interested in, for example, addressing mental health, increasing physical activity, building community capacity, addressing youth exclusion, tackling loneliness etc.

Being clear about links between social prescribing and other agenda is the only way to ensure that social prescribing comes out of its niche and is recognised as cross-sector endeavour in support of a generational shift in our approach to health. Only when this is recognised will it be possible to secure the cross-sector leadership and funding needed for the future.

Conclusion

Social prescribing was 'invented' by leaders in the VCSE sector and the health system who mutually recognised that:

- More of the things that keep us well exist outside the medical system than within it; and
- for many people the NHS is the first port of call when things go wrong—sometimes because needs escalate to the point of making people unwell, and sometimes simply because the GP's office is accessible and recognised.

The insights that informed this approach remain true, and the potential of social prescribing is enormous. But for it to achieve its potential we must be smart, generous and flexible in how we implement it. We need to exemplify the approach that sits at the heart of such asset-based approaches—to build on what's strong.

REFERENCES

APPG Left Behind Neighbourhoods, 2020. Communities of trust: why we must invest in the social infrastructure of 'left behind' neighbourhoods, Local Trust. Available from: https://www.appg-leftbehindneighbourhoods.org.uk/publication/communities-of-trust-why-we-must-invest-in-the-infrastructure-of-left-behind-neighbourhoods/ (Accessed 14 February 2023).

Buck, D., Ewbank, L., 2020. What is social prescribing? The King's fund. Available from: https://www.kingsfund.org.uk/publications/social-prescribing (Accessed 14 February 2023).

Cole, A., Jones, D., Jopling, K., 2020. Rolling out social prescribing: understanding the experience of the voluntary, community and social enterprise sector, national voices. Available from: https://www.nationalvoices.org.uk/publications/our-publications/rolling-out-social-prescribing (Accessed 14 February 2023).

Dayson, C., Damm, C., 2020. Evaluation of the Rotherham Social Prescribing Service for Long Term Conditions: a review of data for 2016/17–2017/18, CRESR, Sheffield Hallam University. Available from: https://www.shu.ac.uk/centre-regional-economic-social-research/publications/evaluation-of-the-rotherham-social-prescribing-service-for-long-term-conditions (Accessed 14 February 2023).

Haslam, D., 2022. A focus on funding: the role of voluntary sector local infrastructure organisations during the COVID-19 pandemic in England, Open University. Available from: https://www.open.ac.uk/centres/voluntary-sector-leadership/blog/focus-funding-role-voluntary-sector-local-infrastructure-organisations-during-covid-19-pandemic (Accessed 14 February 2023).

Islam, N., 2019. Social Prescribing Service Bromley by Bow Centre Annual Report: April 2018–March 2019, Bromley by Bow Centre. Available from: https://www.bbbc.org.uk/wp-content/uploads/2019/09/BBBC-Social-Prescribing-Annual-Report-April-2018-March-2019-FINAL.pdf (Accessed 14 February 2023).

Jopling, K., Cole, A., 2022. Changing lives, changing places, changing systems: making progress on social prescribing, national voices. Available from: https://nationalvoices.org.uk/publications/our-publications/changing-lives-changing-places-changing-systems (Accessed 14 February 2023).

Jopling, K., Howells, A., 2018. Connecting communities to tackle loneliness and social isolation: Learning report, British Red Cross. https://r.search.yahoo.com/_ylt=AwrIedr4C.JlwyYXXN-93Bwx.;_ylu=Y29sbwMEcG9zAzIEdnRpZAMEc2VjA3Ny/RV=2/RE=1709341817/RO=10/RU=https%3a%2f%2fwww.redcross.org.uk%2f-%2fmedia%2fdocuments%2fabout-us%2fresearch-publications%2fhealth-and-social-care%2fconnecting-communities-learning-report.pdf/RK=2/RS=j4Ho.vujo0DYY1L4kLhu-Vc2P4K0- (Accessed 1 March 2024).

NHS England and NHS Improvement, 2019. Network Contract Directed Enhanced Service: Additional Roles Reimbursement Scheme Guidance December 2019. NHS England and NHS Improvement. https://www.england.nhs.uk/wp-content/uploads/2019/12/network-contract-des-additional-roles-reimbursement-scheme-guidance-december2019.pdf (Accessed 3 January 2024).

NHS England and NHS Improvement, 2020. Social prescribing and community-based support: Summary guide: updated: June 2020. NHS England and NHS Improvement. https://www.england.nhs.uk/wp-content/uploads/2020/06/social-prescribing-summary-guide-updated-june-20.pdf (Accessed 20 March 2024).

NHS England, 2014. Five Year Forward View. https://www.england.nhs.uk/wp-content/uploads/2014/10/5yfv-web.pdf (Accessed 20 March 2024).

NHS England, 2019. NHS long term plan. Available from: https://www.longtermplan.nhs.uk/ (Accessed 13 February 2023).

NHS England, 2022. Consultant-led referral to treatment waiting times data 2022–23, NHS. Accessed from: https://www.england.nhs.uk/statistics/statistical-work-areas/rtt-waiting-times/ (Accessed 13 February 2023).

NHS England. Expanding our workforce. Available from: https://www.england.nhs.uk/gp/expanding-our-workforce/ (Accessed 13 February 2023).

South, J., 2015. Health and wellbeing: a guide to community-centred approaches. Public Health England. Available from: https://www.gov.uk/government/publications/health-and-wellbeing-a-guide-to-community-centred-approaches (Accessed 13 February 2023).

Chapter 19

Workforce Transformation

Michelle Howarth and Jacqueline Leigh

Introduction

Social prescribing has emerged to reflect changes in society that have been brought into sharp relief by the recent coronavirus pandemic and associated widening health inequalites. Educators in health and care are shifting to prepare the future workforce to not only address the strategic priorities of personalised and holistic health and care but also consider how strengthen the communities they serve by working alongside them.

The post-war welfare state emerged predominately to 'care for' people and 'fix' them with innovations such as antibiotics, immunisations and improved sanitation. But lately we are concluding that we need to understand better how people live their lives, what makes for a good life and the root causes of their problems. Educators increasingly appreciate how to balance this pathogenic paradigm of fixing people to prevent or cure illness with a salutogenic or health-creating one that understands what makes people healthy and enhances citizen capabilities by focusing on their strengths. This chapter will present a case study from Greater Manchester exploring the use of non-clinical placement opportunities in community organisations that promote not only personalised approaches, but ways of integrated working and coproduction across a range of sectors.

Preparing the Workforce: Changing the Dialogue

The World Health Organization (WHO) Sustainable Development Goal (SDG) 3 encourages workforce development programmes that focus on maximising access to services that can promote wellbeing (Akachi et al., 2016).

That SDG goal, in conjunction with clinical services, has highlighted the need for non-medical strategies to tackle the wider determinants of health that underpin inequality.

More recently in England, the NHS Long Term Plan (2019) promotes a personalised model, typified by the phrase 'what matters to me' rather than 'what's the matter with me'. The plan explains that more of the same is not enough and workforce development requires a change to educational outcomes.

The post-pandemic era has subsequently *'highlighted the significant role of the community and social support'*, leading to debate about the workforce development needed to support healthy communities (Czabanowska & Kuhlmann, 2021). Given this picture, the workforce development challenge lies in how we prepare a workforce that can combat the health legacy of COVID-19, address backlogged NHS services and tackle wider health disparities such as housing and poverty, when health and care curricula are predominantly focused on a pathogenic paradigm.

Notable nursing academics such as McCormack and Titchen (2014) use Aristotelian thinking to go further, suggesting that health and care workers could and should maximise citizens' strengths by creating the conditions for them to flourish (rather than just heal) by pushing people's boundaries in various ways, using, for example, social and artistic approaches. Shades of this thinking are seen in disciplines such as learning disability and mental health services but are yet to be reflected in mainstream education standards.

Lord Nigel Crisp's quote of the African proverb *'health is made at home, hospitals are for repairs'*

(2020) helps to contextualise what makes people well, rather than just help them when they are ill. Yet despite the move in the debate from health and health care to wellbeing, little has changed in education.

Leigh et al. (2022) suggest that to achieve a salutogenic focus, nurse education must rapidly change, which in turn will influence students' attitudes and perceptions to what they prioritise, learn and internalise. One way to do this, Leigh argues, is to expose undergraduates to non-clinical settings such as those in the independent, voluntary, community and social enterprise (VCSE) sectors. Historically, nursing models have supported this with, for example, Beattie's model of health promotion (1977) rooted in the understanding of social and cultural practices.

The focus on 'fixing' a person, as opposed to understanding what's important to them, appears to be at the forefront of the nursing education paradigm. Helpfully, in the UK, the current undergraduate nursing curriculum is predicated on the Nursing & Midwifery Council standards for pre-registration education (NMC, 2018), which includes nurses' ability to understand social influences, health literacy and individual circumstances on lifestyle choices and relate these to mental, physical and behavioural health outcomes. However, the promotion of clinical skills by the NMC and other professional regulatory bodies has created challenges in the ability for students to learn in non-clinical placements, where proficiencies such as the insertion, management and removal of oral/nasal/gastric tubes (NMC, 2018: 5.6: 34) are not always attainable. Despite this, nurse educators have begun to use non-clinical social and community placements to help students understand what makes us well: belonging, relationships, purpose, control and enough money to live.

Similarly, Rakel and colleagues (2008) argues that complementary alternative medicines (CAM) education is predicated on a pathogenic model and that a shift in medical education towards 'what is needed for the creation of health (salutogenesis) can bring balance to a curriculum that is currently weighted in teaching about the creation of disease (pathogenesis)'. A comparable move was recently adopted by the College of Medicine's (2022). Beyond Pills programme, which has lobbied the Government to 'immediately address the nation's unsustainable prescription service through re-prescribing and social prescribing'. This paradigm shift is encouraging doctors and non-medical prescribers to recognise that they need to review and reduce their prescribing and incorporate social and complementary approaches. The College, NHS England and the National Social Prescribing Network have also launched a movement within medical, Allied Health Professionals (AHPs) and nursing student groups through the National Social Prescribing Student Champion Scheme to champion social prescribing (College of Medicine, 2017).

Case Study

In response, Health Education England (HEE, 2017) has collaborated with several higher education institutions to understand how to best prepare an undergraduate nursing workforce using non-clinical settings. We present a case study funded through the HEE Medical Outreach Programme in Greater Manchester to develop innovative non-clinical placements for student nurses.

A total of 10 pre-registration nurses from across the fields of practice—mental health, adult, children & young people—participated in the project. An NHS primary care placement acted as the primary placement and then arranged 'spoke' placements' of 3 weeks with local third-sector organisations supporting people from a range of backgrounds in a variety of ways. These organisations were well regarded and stable and had an existing relationship with the university that enabled collaborative negotiations to take place. This is important because one of the challenges of third-sector placements is their fragility and thus their dependability. The three organisations that took part provided a range of non-clinical interventions: an outreach 'Tech and Tea' for seniors wanting to improve their knowledge of technology; a forest school (free play outdoors to assist with learning and behaviour) for children and families; and an arts-based service, for people with mental health problems.

The student nurse learning outcomes were mapped to the undergraduate curriculum to ensure that the experience aligned with the professional education standards (see Table 19.1).

The students were allocated a placement in one of the three organisations, depending on the branch of nursing

Continued on following page

Case Study—(Continued)

that they were studying; for example, children & young people's student nurses were allocated to the forest school, students from a mental health branch were allocated to the arts-based service, and students on the adult branch looked at Tech and Tea. This allowed exposure to a different learning environment where what mattered to a person took precedence. The pilot enabled insight into the experiences from both the student and organisational perspective and revealed the benefit of these placements from a university, student, third-sector and the primary care organisational perspective. The feedback was overwhelmingly positive and highlighted the learning that enabled students to see the person, not just the patient.

TABLE 19.1   Learning Outcomes

1. Identify and discuss the needs and strengths of the client population in the VCSE sector. Evaluate any existing social prescribing connections between the clinical hub and the VCSE sector using a SWOT analysis.
2. Apply concepts and principles from the 'All Our Health' framework (Public Health England, 2015) and analyse how community-centred approaches may benefit the current patient/client population within the VCSE sector.
3. Effectively communicate findings considering appropriate and creative methods of dissemination for both client/public/patient (non-health and social care specialist) and practice audiences (specialist).

Student (Learner) Feedback

The students were initially apprehensive about learning in a non-traditional placement—in particular, they were concerned that they would not be able to achieve their proficiencies. However, once the placement had commenced, the students were able to learn about the wider influences on wellbeing and understand how social determinants affected them psychologically, physically, economically and socially. For example, one of the students attended art therapy sessions which included people from a diverse range of backgrounds, ages and populations. The student described how the group collaborated and supported each other, enabling them to bond, build friendships and thus improve their confidence. Other students described how they supported those with mental health difficulties and learning disabilities to take part in courses that enabled individuals to work towards employability, through certified courses. One student experienced a 'job club' and learned how staff empowered people to seek and apply for appropriate jobs, practice interview skills and build confidence. Overall, students expressed that it was a valuable opportunity to understand how non-clinical, strengths-based and health-creating approaches can support people (see Box 19.1).

The following quotes highlight how working in this way had supported learning:

'It is a great experience, in terms of us seeing alternatives to non-clinical interventions, in the sense that you could see that this is a kind of therapeutic way to help the health and wellbeing of people with mental health'.

(Student nurse C)

'It really helped me to learn so much about other ways to care for … to meet the needs of this group of people'.

(Student nurse F)

Other students reflected on learning and highlighted how the experience had benefited nursing philosophy:

'It is a great way in improving patients' wellbeing without the need of clinical intervention. I have really enjoyed my time …. and believe it has been beneficial to my personal philosophy of nursing'.

(Student nurse A)

Overall, the students valued the learning experience and benefitted from working with staff and service users. Significantly, they learned how the wider social determinants influenced the individual's physical and

BOX 19.1 'TECH AND TEA' LEARNING OUTCOMES

Tech and Tea is a 5-week basic IT course for older people, delivered by a charity called Inspiring Communities Together, funded jointly by Salford City Council and the NHS. It is delivered in the community, with the social part being just as important as the learning. Thirty-five percent of people have reported a decrease in loneliness while taking part in the course.

Student learners observe that:
- People feel more connected
  - People stay in contact with family and friends
  - People meet new people on the course
  - People make new friendships, which continue outside of the group
  - People feel more included in society
  - Some participants progress to other volunteering opportunities
- People are enabled to access learning more easily
  - Training is available at local community venues that people already use
  - Participants are recruited to the course by the people that work in the venues
  - Family members are supported to enable older people to participate
  - Older people are specifically targeted, meeting their specific needs
- Wellbeing is improved
  - Mood and cognition are improved by staying in touch with others, listening to music, talking about hobbies and reminiscing
  - Research shows that social connects improve immunity and reduce cardiovascular problems and depression

From Rimmer, V., 2017. Evaluation of the technology and tea project: executive summary and project report. MSc public health dissertation project. Available from: https://extranet.who.int/agefriendlyworld/wp-content/uploads/2018/04/Tech-and-Tea-Evaluation-Report-.pdf (Accessed 15 November 2022).

mental health and the impact on those from deprived populations in society.

Organisation Feedback

The organisations involved were asked to describe their experiences of the student placements. Like the students, the organisations expressed initial anxieties about hosting students. They were concerned that they would take up too much time and would need a lot of support. Following the placement, all the organisations provided positive feedback about the students, reporting that the students were assets, being able to help and support a wide range of individuals. They valued the student learning and how it had highlighted the work of the VCSE sector and the benefit of non-clinical approaches.

'They learnt a great deal about the holistic approach, because although they're taught about it, it's not always something they can actually put into practice. Because when you go into a very regimented NHS place with wards that only deal with a certain condition or whatever, you're not seeing the whole person, you're not seeing the social aspects and the whole range of different issues that person is experiencing'.

(Organisation 1)

Critical to the success of this pilot was the need to ensure that both the organisations and students were supported. Typically, NHS placements are facilitated through an array of roles such as Practice Education Facilitators, Academic Assessors, Practice Assessors and Practice Supervisors, supporting students and mentors in clinical areas. However, many third-sector organisations do not have appropriately 'qualified' staff in place to comply with the NMC Assessor and Supervisor guidance, which clearly advocates for a registered nurse to be in the learning environments. This can cause challenges and has promoted a response from some universities to explore how models could be adapted in community organisations. Despite the challenges, there was a significant paradigm shift amongst nurse educators because of the pilot.

Discussion

A culture of learning is possible through the adoption of strategies of challenge, openness and debate (Ward and McCormack, 2020). This case study and others across the country demonstrate the challenge of building new relationships to deliver truly integrated and person-centred care. To do so successfully, the relationship between statutory, education and voluntary services must change, power and resources must be exchanged, and solutions must be co-designed and produced (Crimlisk, 2019; Hunt, 2019). Resources for the VCSE sector require stabilising to enable the sector to thrive, and pedagogic frameworks and regulatory frameworks must be updated. As with all systems leadership, change will take place at the speed of trust. The strengths-based approach that applies to citizen growth will equally need to be applied to the partners, who each have different resources and different requirements to thrive.

Conclusion

Social prescribing has been driven to the fore by increases in health inequality and societal change, not least due to the coronavirus pandemic which exacerbated existing health and wellbeing disparities (Druss, 2020). A social movement for change within a medically driven health paradigm has gained significant momentum within medicine, nursing and other allied professions. Future health and care workforce development relies on the ability to shape the education of the workforce within higher education contexts to meet the challenges of a changing society. Barriers to such changes in education include bias towards the importance of secondary care, the pressures on and instability of the VCSE sector and the mindsets of those defining the competencies and supporting placements.

REFERENCES

Akachi, Y., Tarp, F., Kelley, E., Addison, T., Kruk, M.E., 2016. Measuring quality-of-care in the context of sustainable development goal 3: A call for papers. Bull. World Health Organ. 94 (3), 160.

Beattie, A., 1977. Making a curriculum work. In: Allan, P., Jolley, M. (Eds.), The Curriculum in Nursing Education. Croom Helm, London, pp. 55–71.

Crimlisk, K., 2019. Blog: Educational partnerships with the third sector: a model to address NHS workforce challenges? Health Foundation. Available from: https://www.health.org.uk/news-and-comment/blogs/educational-partnerships-with-the-third-sector-a-model-to-address-nhs (Accessed 15 November 2022).

Crisp, N., 2020. Health is made at home, hospitals are for repairs. SALUS Global Knowledge Exchange, Billericay.

College of Medicine, 2022. Beyond Pills campaign. Available from: https://collegeofmedicine.org.uk/beyond-pills/ (Accessed 15 November 2022).

College of Medicine, 2017. National Social Prescribing Student Champion Scheme. Available from: https://collegeofmedicine.org.uk/national-prescribing-student-champion-scheme/ (Accessed 15 November 2022).

Czabanowska, K., Kuhlmann, E., 2021. Public health competences through the lens of the COVID-19 pandemic: What matters for health workforce preparedness for global health emergencies. Int. J. Health Plann. Manage. 36 (S1), 14–19. doi:10.1002/hpm.3131.

Druss, BG., 2020. Addressing the COVID-19 pandemic in populations with serious mental illness. JAMA Psychiatry Crossref, Medline, Google Scholar.

England, N.H.S., 2019. Universal personalised care: Implementing the comprehensive model. NHS England, London.

Goldman, M.L., Druss, B.G., Horvitz-Lennon, M., Norquist, G.S., Kroeger Ptakowski, K., Brinkley, A., Greiner, M., Hayes, H., Hepburn, B., Jorgensen, S., Swartz, M.S., 2020. Mental health policy in the era of COVID-19. Psychiatr. Serv. 71 (11), 1158–1162.

Health Education England, 2017. Facing the facts, shaping the future—a draft health and care workforce strategy for England to 2027. Health Education England. Available from: https://www.hee.nhs.uk/sites/default/files/documents/Facing%20the%20Facts%2C%20Shaping%20the%20Future%20%E2%80%93%20a%20draft%20health%20and%20care%20workforce%20strategy%20for%20England%20to%202027.pdf.

Hunt, L.A., 2019. Developing a 'core of steel': The key attributes of effective practice assessors. Br. J. Nurs. 28 (22), 1478–1484.

Leigh, et al., 2022. Has the pandemic response to covid 19 further entrenched a pathogenic emphasis in nurse education? BJN, In press.

McCormack, B., Titchen, A., 2014. No beginning, no end: An ecology of human flourishing. Int. Pract. Dev. J. 4 (2). Foundation of Nursing Studies.

NMC, 2018. Future nurse: standards of proficiency for registered nurses, NMC, London.

Public Health England (2015) All Our Health: personalised care and population health. https://www.gov.uk/government/collections/all-our-health-personalised-care-and-population-health (Accessed 20 March 2024)

Rakel, D.P., Guerrera, M.P., Bayles, B.P., Desai, G.J., Ferrara, E., 2008. CAM education: Promoting a salutogenic focus in health care. J. Altern. Complement. Med. 14 (1), 87–93.

Ward, C., McCormack, B., 2000. Creating an adult learning culture through practice development. Nurse Educ. Today. 20 (4), 259–266.

Chapter 20

Summary Section 3 Perspectives

Heather Henry

We can look at the health and care 'pivot' towards wellbeing with the introduction of social prescribing from many angles. In this section we have seen views not only on the whole idea but also on how it is being interpreted and delivered too.

Top Down, Bottom up and Co-produced

Griffith's ethnographic perspective (Chapter 15) sees primary care grappling with an NHS policy that, although co-designed with primary care entrepreneurs originally (Chapter 2), has suffered from a lack of engagement with the wider primary care community as it has been rolled out. Overall, GP surgeries appreciate that the primary determinants of wellbeing lie outside of health and care. Yet, in supporting it, individuals understand and 'sell' the concept differently, some as a transactional 'service' and others as a relational, holistic model. Other confusions come from the nature of general practice itself, where complex circumstances mean that practitioners have difficulties interpreting whether patients need a more passive *care* or a more proactive *choice* approach.

Jopling (Chapter 18) describes a voluntary, community and social enterprise sector that likewise is supportive of social prescribing and has been heavily involved at all levels in its development. However, both she and Russell (Chapter 16) can sometimes identify more of a co-option of the VCSE into social prescribing, rather than a co-production.

Both Mitchell and Jarvis-Beesley (Chapter 14) and Yasmeen, Barton and Walters (Chapter 17) present a more co-produced model of social prescribing. In 2020, NHS England & NHS Improvement (NHSE&I) commissioned the Social Prescribing

Youth Network, led by StreetGames (streetgames. org), an organisation that uses the power of sport to help young people, to develop a proposal for 'youth social prescribing'. It's clear from the description of the social prescribing youth network (SPYN) on the StreetGames website that leaders feel that social prescribing should be developed and owned by the community, in partnership with the statutory sector. SPYN is developing as a social movement, being a network that is free to join. It has developed resources that have been co-produced with members, based on a test-and-learn approach that is reminiscent of Cottam's design approach in the previous section (Chapter 12).

NHS Trusts are also finding that co-production is getting results: NHS South West Yorkshire Partnership Foundation Trust leaders clearly feel that using an asset-based community development approach is the way to support the recovery of their patients and strengthen the local communities that they serve at the same time.

In both South West Yorkshire and with Street-Games, the model is one of shifting power to communities and enabling change rather than 'delivering a service'.

Co-ordination

Throughout the previous chapters, it is clear that the desire is there for health and care leaders to create the conditions for community assets to thrive (Selbie and Stevens, in South, 2015), yet the coordination structures aren't always there and the skills to coordinate social prescribing appear to be variable.

Jopling points to the mismatch in organisational footprints that is hampering the coordination of social prescribing: primary care networks that are too small to match VCSE networks, and integrated care systems that are too large. Organisations representing the wider determinants of health, like housing and policing, may find it difficult to contribute their strengths (see Chapters 25 and 26) and end up working in parallel.

Workforce Development

And at the front line, how is the workforce adapting to a social model of health? Although social prescribing is now part of the GP contract, community pharmacy, as a highly accessible primary care contracted service, is also keen to embrace it. An International Social Prescribing Pharmacy Association (ISPPA; https://www.socialprescribing.health/) has been established and offers education and support to community pharmacists, including undergraduates, across the world. The benefit here is that as well as being on most high streets, they are regularly visited and are trusted. The model for social prescribing here is more around assessing people and signposting them towards a social prescribing link worker rather than more active community engagement. This makes sense because the pharmacist needs to be in their premises during dispensing hours.

Russell (Chapter 16) describes the role of the doctor in various ways—although this could be expanded to nurse, pharmacist, paramedic etc. He wants doctors to be people who 'walk alongside' communities, who develop the skills of 'gappers' to keep the institutional domain and the community domain delivering their appropriate functions. There is an excellent parable by James Mackie (2012) about this, based on the ideas of Edgar Cahn, founder of time-banking.

Yet it must be a huge behavioural change for health professionals to become, as Russell describes it, 'proscribers'—people who should look out for communities and 'heckle imperial impulses'—rather than prescribers. This unlearning of a medical model may be difficult because making people better makes you feel good and because people look to clinicians as professionals who have the answers. This change is described in detail by GP Mark Spencer in Chapter 27, where, having realised that medicalising people no longer works in complex situations, he makes this journey to becoming a proscriber by walking alongside the people of Fleetwood. That means a reinvention of his GP role from leader to cheerleader.

Spencer came to the realisation himself that GPs are not the solution to complex challenges in people's lives, but we must consider how future workers are prepared for a changed vision of health and care where undergraduate doctors, nurses, allied health professionals and more need to learn how to create the enabling conditions for people to heal. Howarth and Leigh (Chapter 19) then look to see how the introduction of social prescribing is reflected in changes to undergraduate nurse education. They present a challenging picture, because student nurse learning outcomes are still invested in a biomedical model, and this may be the same for other disciplines. Health Education England, which supported Howarth and Leigh's work in Greater Manchester, are certainly aware of this conundrum, but awareness and action are now needed by professional regulators too.

One of the new roles that is now being recognised in health and care are what are called 'system convenors' (NHS England, online). This is different to what Russell calls 'gappers'—people who maintain and respect the gap between the institutional domain and the community domain. The founders of systems convening, Bev and Etienne Wenger-Trainor, describe it thus:

You may not have heard about them; what they do is rarely in their job description. You may not even be aware of what they do; they tend to act as enablers rather than taking credit or seeking the spotlight. But they are here— working on sustainable change, across challenging silos, in complex social landscapes, amid changing circumstances. We call them systems conveners.

(Wenger-Trainor, 2021)

Systems convenors have the important role of looking across the landscape of a complex problem (such as how to further develop social prescribing) and draw together people across boundaries to create new conversations and opportunities for learning. The NHS is now adopting this idea and incorporating it into work around spreading and adopting innovation (NHS England, online). Perhaps the role of the systems convenor in social prescribing is to make the 'gifts' that communities have to offer more visible and then connect them to helpful resources, without the institutional creep that Russell warns us against. Certainly, Jopling (Chapter 18) sees VCSE support organisations as having that role, and it could be argued that clinicians such as Dixon (Chapter 2), Spencer (Chapter 27) and Monteith (Chapter 25) could also claim the role of convenor. There are also those convenors that lie outside health and care, representing, for example, criminal justice (Shrivastava and Christmas, Chapter 25) and housing (Sharpe, Chapter 26), and we shall turn to what they see and contribute in the next sections on social prescribing in practice.

Resources

Contributors such as Russell (Chapter 16) and Yasmeen, Barton and Walters (Chapter 17) encourage us to see the full potential of civic society in supporting wellbeing. This is summarised by Fell:

VCS [voluntary and community services] aren't services, they are a whole range of things including community safe spaces, advocates, peers, health creators, confidence builders, connectors. That's the value that is gained from having embedded organisations. We need to recognise that multiple role in investment terms. Organisations need places and people to run them as well as the people that provide services. We need holistic investment, if we want to fully realise community benefits.

(Fell, 2022)

When we invest in the third sector, we are investing in an ecosystem that has emerged to address the wellbeing needs of local people, not just a range of services. If the rhetoric becomes how social prescribing is just another range of services to help manage NHS demand, then there is a danger that community resources will be perceived as being exploited. As Cottam (Chapter 12) explains, the question should always be about how we can enable people, families and communities to flourish rather than how to harness social prescribing to address the problems within the system.

On top of this is the problem highlighted by National Voices in their national surveys and focus groups, that while ongoing funding in the GP contract is available for social prescribing link workers, funding to enable community building is a real issue (Chapter 18). This then leads to the commonly heard cry of 'too many travel agents and not enough holidays'. An under-resourced

third sector is often living from one grant to another, which hampers their sustainability, and many, often smaller VCSE organisations fold as a result. This dents the confidence of statutory organisations that are signposting people towards community organisations. This can then become a vicious cycle of underfunding, instability and lack of confidence.

Community-Enhanced Social Prescribing

Behind the language in the preceding chapters, therefore, is a need both to develop the social prescribing model and to enable the community to connect and create for themselves the right sort of solutions for their community. This is the focus of more recent work, called 'community-enhanced social prescribing' (CESP; Morris et al., 2020). The authors comment that:

The NHS Long Term Plan (NHS England, online) is arguably too narrowly focused on individual outcomes and new social prescribing schemes will need to engage with, and orientate themselves more towards, local communities. [...] Key paradigms of community capacity building and connecting individuals to community currently run in parallel rather than being part of an integrated whole.

(Morris et al., 2020, p. 180)

At the time of this writing (2023), joint research by the University of York, the University of Central Lancashire, London School of Economics and Bluesci Trafford (a community interest company), funded by the National Institute for Health Research, is in progress to test the feasibility of CESP. Reporting in 2024, the team will test out bringing together the models of Connecting People (Webber et al., 2016) and Connected Communities (Parsfield et al., 2015) in CESP as shown in Fig. 20.1.

Essentially, CESP combines a model of community capacity building with a model of connecting an individual into that community.

'Connected Communities' Model

The community-building element of CESP starts with bringing a panel of interested local citizens together to map the community assets. This not only leads to

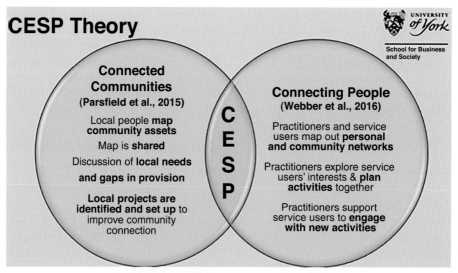

Fig. 20.1 CESP theory. From The University of York.

a discussion about whether there are gaps in community support but also seeks to build and strengthen connections between parts of the community that may have not been connected before. This in turn leads to ideas about how the assets in a community may link together differently to support needs.

The asset map is then shared by the citizen panel with residents, social prescribers and a partners panel consisting of organisational stakeholders such as members of the local authority, health and care, VCSE, business and housing representatives. The partners panel can then help to develop citizen-led ideas and build capacity. An example of this might be that the community panel identifies loneliness as an issue, and the partners panel may help citizens to connect with assets to, for example, create a befriending scheme.

Connecting People Model

Meanwhile, the connecting people model is the part aligned to social prescribing, where the link workers support individuals in identifying their own personal and community support networks, exploring interests and developing a person-centred plan.

CESP is built on community power that is supported, but not led by, organisational stakeholders, to increase community capabilities (Chapter 12).

Combining social prescribing and community building may offer synergy, as one feeds into the other and back again. CESP then has potential to offer a holistic *approach* to deliver holistic *support,* and it will be interesting to see how the research progresses.

This is familiar to those who practice asset-based community development, who know to ask questions in the right order so that we do not usurp community power:

- What can you (the community) do on your own?
- What can you do with our help?
- What are you asking us (statutory workers) to do?

From Perspectives to Practice

We turn next to how social prescribing operates in practice. Again, the contributors invited to write in this section could not possibly cover every aspect of social prescribing. What I hope is that they represent the more 'unusual suspects' who can offer food for thought.

REFERENCES

Fell, G., 2022. The voluntary and community sector: from 'integrated care' to 'social prescribing' and into social value & social capital. Available from: https://gregfellpublichealth.wordpress.com/2022/06/15/the-voluntary-and-community-sector-the-secret-weapon-for-joining-up-care-for-people/ (Accessed 1 September 2023).

Mackie, J., 2012. Video: the parable of the blobs and squares. Available from: https://vimeo.com/42332617 (Accessed 5 September 2023).

Morris, D., Thomas, P., Ridley, J., Webber, M., 2022. Community enhanced social prescribing: Integrating community in policy and practice. Int. J. Community Wellbeing. 5 (1), 179–195. https://doi.org/10.1007/s42413-020-00080-9.

NHS England, online. Systems convening. Available from: https://www.england.nhs.uk/spread-and-adoption/systems-convening/ (Accessed 25 July 2023).

Parsfield, M., Morris, D., Mokuolu, B., Knapp, M., Park, A-La., Yoshioka, M., Marcus, G., 2015. Community Capital. The Value of Connected Communities. Royal Society of Arts, London.

South, J., 2015. A guide to community-cantred approaches for health and wellbeing. Project Report. Public Health England/ NHS England.

Webber, M., Reidy, H., Ansari, D., Stevens, M., Morris, D., 2016. Developing and modeling complex social interventions: Introducing the connecting people intervention. Res. Soc. Work Prac. 26 (1), 14–19. https://doi.org/10.1177/1049731515578687.

Wenger-Trainor, E., Wenger-Trainor, B., 2021. Systems convening: A crucial form of leadership for the 21st century. Social Learning Lab. Available from: https://www.wenger-trayner.com/systems-convening-book/ (Accessed 25 July 2023).

Practice

Chapter 21

Connecting Community

Gay Palmer

Introduction

Social prescribing is about empowering a person by focussing on them and what's important to them. It's said that social prescribing is about community and feeling connected to others. If I consider these thoughts, then for me, social prescribing has been around for many years.

When I talk about my role as a social prescriber in South Southwark in London and what I do, people say that I am passionate and inspiring—they are correct in that thinking. This work comes naturally to me, and I credit that to the community I was raised in.

Community, Faith, History and Values

My parents were amongst many other elders from the Caribbean who came to England in the late 1950s and 1960s Windrush era. They came thinking that they would be welcomed and it would be a life of new beginnings and opportunities. It was a new life, but one filled with anger and hatred. They came and were treated like they were of no value.

They took the decision to show resilience and fend for themselves. They took themselves to churches, but were rejected, so many started their own. Over time, they built their own community as they wanted a sense of place, somewhere to feel valued and to feel that they belonged. This new community reflected on what from 'back home' made them feel safe and happy: being together, good music, good food and good vibes amongst people who understood the unspoken pain and understood the verbalised anger but could also share in the victories. For many the anger, hatred and rejection led to more damaging responses that impacted on physical and mental health.

Church and faith groups were important to many, so they formed churches as places where they were welcomed and valued and could share their faith and love of God together. For many, this helped to prevent feelings of loneliness and isolation. My parents have a strong faith in God which has helped them to keep going in both the good and the hardest of times. I was raised by the elders, who were those of my parent's age. Many had to work two to three jobs to make ends meet, whilst sisters within the church (female members) would act as childminders for two to three families. Children would come home upset, distressed, crying and bruised because of the treatment meted out by other children and teachers.

The churches started their own 'Saturday schools' where the educators from within our community would take their time to teach local children in a place of safety, where they could become empowered and encouraged instead of being dehumanised daily. A place where they were told '*you can do and be whoever you want to be*' instead of '*those jobs are not for people like you*'.

The church also realised that there were many within their local communities who were feeling the same emotions of being isolated, lonely, having no sense of belonging and needing a place of safety. So day centres, food banks and many other activities emerged, accessible to anyone locally. The church that I was raised in, the New Testament Church of God (https://ntcg.org.uk/), has many sites across the UK that are continuing to make a difference in local communities. Many elders manage allotments, allowing others to appreciate their handiwork throughout the year when the vegetables arrived on our table, with the size of the potatoes and pumpkins being something to behold. These activities have come from their own experiences of not being heard, valued and isolated so that ultimately their mental health becomes affected. They taught me how to value and respect a person and how the depth of difficulties they face may never be clear. But having a community, a place and a people that you feel connected to would make each day a little easier to face.

Professional Aspiration

If someone needed a plumber, electrician, a handy person, they could all be found within the church community. As many grew older, they left the local church and at times the local area to develop their own communities, but they didn't lose their sense of community and always gave back. They would join churches in their new areas or develop their own initiatives. Church sisters could boldly say that they were there when I was born, as many were qualified midwives. The church was—and is—full of many qualified professionals who would offer their skills and knowledge many times to help others. This example has led to us, the current working generation, becoming the people that we aspired to be like.

This spurred me on into a career in nursing and to working within the community. All my roles have been within community settings because it allows me to really understand what matters to a person and also then to be able to be their voice and empower them to make changes for themselves. I have been privileged to work in environments where people are vulnerable for various reasons and need someone to talk to, connect with, support them to access the right services, help them to feel seen, valued and heard—something I had seen my parents, elders and community do for many years, and still do now.

Art as Healing

I have grown up around communities whose voices were not always being heard by those who should have been there to listen. So, they looked within themselves, and their voices became louder. There was a collective sense of frustration, so they supported each other to make changes happen. There was heartache, loss. Singing became a collective way to express their feelings and emotions, a community who understood each other's hearts but with a common purpose: to use singing as their voice of hope, friendship, better mental health and improved breathing ability. Creative arts, music, drumming and poetry all became their outlets.

Alienation

For many, the answers do not lie in the health service. The lack of regard for communities whose families and ancestors have been repeatedly looked down on has had grave consequences. Historically they bore the brunt of being tested and tried on in relation to new services or treatment that professionals hoped would help. This has led to people finding their own way of managing their health and wellbeing. The lack of trust in a system means they either go without support or look to others for help or only get help when they are in dire straits.

For many the answers do not lie in the education system. Many are not who they had the potential to be because educators killed their dream daily by telling them they can't, downgraded high marks so they would not succeed, did not write honest references and gave incorrect diagnoses that would impact them for life. Many were diagnosed with learning difficulties and sent to special needs schools only to find that later on in their life the diagnoses were incorrect.

In our communities, services mean mistreatment to some: from within mental health systems where so many people are locked up, drugged up and become a shadow of themselves. One can see hurt and distress in their eyes—but numbed, with little or no energy to fight anymore. Other systems beyond health, like social care and policing, have stripped so much of their identity, their self-worth: forever being on the alert and unsure how to respond, as it can be misunderstood. Many families are living with the grief and loss of loved ones who were mistreated and sadly are not here to tell their story.

Factors such as increasing stress, financial implications and the breakdown of family and community as it was known have affected mental health. People have become disenfranchised—they stop engaging. They say, 'What's the point? No one else is listening to us'.

Social Prescribing

Social prescribing is giving a person time to talk and to share what matters to them—a space where decisions are made by them, with support. It is helping them to consider options and how to move forward with that. For some it gives them the connections to enable them to continue to move forward. For so many others it's about unpicking lives that have become increasingly complex and appear to be impossible, because their past experience of meeting previous blockages leaves them feeling that nothing can be achieved.

I work with them over a few sessions to look at what they want to focus on, and we work on that together, which may include offering them options. They research, and we attend something together. For others it's about accessing the right information, guidance and support services and preparing them for what they will need to bring for their appointments. For some people that has required me to be there to act as an advocate—to get clarity about a process or to get their needs conveyed in a way that can be understood.

Seeing the Benefit Is Its Own Reward

It's hard not to feel a sense of happiness when a 34-year-old mother with four children who has been living in an overcrowded accommodation and bidding to her social landlord for several years to get a bigger place, who is beyond frustrated and not getting anywhere, comes to you to help get clarity and the correct advice. A few months later she emails to say, *'Thank you, with your help I have been rehoused in a 4 bedroom with a garden … couldn't have done it without you … may heaven bless you'*.

Or you get an unexpected text from a 29-year-old who has a history of throat cancer. A year later after giving support they share that they are in a new accommodation, their mental health has really improved, life is getting better, and they are expecting a baby and now looking forward to a life filled with joy and new hope.

When you support someone and you watch them experience the frustration of trying to access a system and see the impact it has on their ability to cope with daily life, you feel it too. Or where a community of people suffer hardship as they have given up trying to share their needs only to have them dismissed—you feel that as well.

Conclusion

As a social prescriber, I am able to influence systems by sharing the gaps in the system with stakeholders and to look at how things can be done differently to improve the outcomes of communities that I know and understand.

I often say that those who are actually in need are the ones who have not completed the reports, because the systems that are trying to reach them don't know how to. So I am able to share with health colleagues the real health needs of a community, not what is being shared by reports or statistics, by repeating the voices and words that I hear. I find that being from a community that has faced hardships and difficulties, I am able to articulate their needs in a way that others don't have the privilege to. The facial expression, the sigh, the body language, the one-liner tells a whole story that other professionals are unable to understand. The smile, the wink, the *'yes you get it'* statement makes it all worthwhile. Positive outcomes help me to get up every day. Being able to share with system leaders the impact of a community not being heard and valued and how things need to change and the willingness of system leaders and communities to be open to change is satisfying. It's a joy to see an increase in activities and groups and witness others being able to see and share in the richness of a community and its culture. Watching generations share their wealth of wisdom and knowledge is of a greater value than words in a book that can't convey the pleasure in watching the next generation being bolder, more expressive and making a great impact.

I stand on the shoulders of a great community, and I am beyond proud of who they are and how they have come to this country and, despite all odds, have made a significant contribution. I am now able to give back to the community that has helped to shape me and to ensure that even as the elders fade, their voices will be heard by those of us left behind. I love my Caribbean heritage—you can't beat the sense of community and the sense of belonging that social prescribing brings.

Chapter 22

The DeStress-II Project: Enhancing Primary Care Responses to Poverty-Related Mental Distress

Felicity Thomas, Kathryn Berzins, Ilse Lee, Jane Horrell, Susanne Hughes, and Katrina Wyatt

Introduction

Often a first port of call in times of need, primary health care is in a unique position to deliver mental health support—indeed, 90% of people with mental health problems in the UK are cared for entirely within primary health care services (Royal College of General Practitioners (RCGP), 2017). Many primary health care teams in England now include social prescribers who can connect patients to local community and statutory services for practical and emotional support (Husk et al., 2019). Whilst there is some evidence to suggest that social prescribing can lead to positive health and wellbeing outcomes (Buck and Ewbank, 2020), little is known about how this process is operationalised within primary mental health care or the mechanisms that support or inhibit patient enrolment into this type of support.

This chapter draws on data from an ongoing study (DeStress-II) on the use of mental health treatments by patients from low-income households. Our research suggests that current primary care options to support patients in England experiencing poverty-related mental distress are over-medicalised and can be experienced as unsatisfactory by both patients and GPs. Mental health strategies now advocate more integrated social solutions that look beyond medication and talking therapies and encompass social prescribing. However, little is known about how this shift in working is being operationalised in practice or the factors that may inhibit this. Drawing on focus groups with people from low-income communities and reflective discussions with primary health practitioners, we identify how continued pressures to prescribe antidepressants and a lack of coordination within primary health care teams inhibit the effective use of social prescribing.

Context of the DeStress-II Study

Until recent years, mental health strategies and clinical guidelines in England have drawn heavily on a psychiatric diagnosis system which frames mental distress as an individual psychological problem rather than as an understandable response to wider social and economic problems (Byng et al., 2019). This in turn has meant that patients have been encouraged to understand their distress as a disease, with available support being dominated by medical or psychological interventions that aim to 'fix' the person, rather than interventions that seek to address (at individual or community level) what are often broader social and structural stressors associated with circumstantial factors: for example, poor housing, low pay, unemployment and social isolation.

Empirical data show that low-income populations experience high levels of mental distress yet frequently struggle to ask for and receive appropriate mental health support (Thomas et al., 2019, 2020). While the importance that patients attach to a trusted relationship with health care providers is high (Thompson and McCabe, 2012), evidence suggests that existing primary care responses to poverty-related mental distress—primarily antidepressant prescribing and talking therapies—are often deemed to be disempowering and inappropriate by people from low-income backgrounds. Patients in qualitative studies have reported feeling de-legitimised and 'fobbed off' with current treatment options and have recounted instances in which they felt judged by health professionals because of their low-income status (Thomas et al., 2019, 2020). At the same time, GPs have reported feeling conflicted and confused on how best to support these patients, as well as considerable frustration over the limited options and resourcing available to them to do so (Thomas et al., 2020).

Recognition that mental distress underpinned by poverty and intersecting inequalities is likely to require social solutions beyond medication and therapy has gained considerable traction in recent years (Skivington et al., 2018) and is now implicit within several core mental health strategy and guidance documents. The NHS Community Mental Health Framework (CMHF) for Adults and Older Adults (2019), for example, emphasises the need to facilitate more integrated, placed-based, primary and community care which looks beyond biomedical treatment (NHS England et al., 2019), whilst the recent NICE Guidelines on Depression in Adults (2022) mark a significant shift in thinking through promoting the use of a range of non-medical treatment options, specifically recommending that antidepressants are *not* routinely offered as a first-line treatment for less severe depression unless this is the patient's preference. More broadly, the NHS England Long Term Plan and the associated drive towards Universal Personalised Care have seen the rollout of social prescribing link workers, with a target of 900,000 people being referred to community-based activities and support by 2023/24 (NHS England, 2021).

Such shifts in thinking, particularly when backed up with appropriate resourcing to implement on-the-ground change, have the potential to play a significant role in reducing what can be unnecessary over-prescribing of antidepressants, as well as supporting patients, better and reducing the workload burden on GPs. However, little is currently known about how social prescribing is utilised within primary mental health care practice alongside other treatment options, or the factors that might inhibit its effective uptake.

Methodology

Focus groups were undertaken with people (n = 53) from low-income backgrounds to understand their experiences of seeking help for mental distress from primary care services. Focus groups took place across three areas of England (North West, South West, London) and were undertaken in person or online depending on participant preference and COVID-19 restrictions. Findings from the focus groups were supplemented with the insights of a team of low-income community partners from the three regions (n = 15) and fed into the co-development of a training intervention for primary health care professionals. Training was co-delivered by teams comprising a GP, a low-income community partner and a researcher in 47 GP practices across the three regions, purposively sampled for high antidepressant prescribing and high socio-economic disadvantage. Training aimed to provide a framework for health professionals to address social causes of distress in a person-centred way; to offer a set of micro-therapeutic practices to build trust, identify patient strengths and discuss alternatives to antidepressants (including social prescribing); and to give GPs confidence and legitimacy to know when to act as 'supporters' rather than 'fixers'. The training included reflective discussion on current practice working and the factors acting as barriers and facilitators to practice change. Ethics permission was granted by the Frenchay research ethics committee (IRAS303179).

Findings

HIGH USE OF ANTIDEPRESSANT MEDICATIONS

Despite shifts in policy-level thinking, antidepressant prescribing rates have increased markedly in recent years (Iacobucci, 2019) and remain a first-line response within many primary care consultations. Prescribing rates are known to be especially high in low-income areas, with medication use reported over long (and growing) periods of time (Public Health England, 2019). A perceived over-reliance on antidepressant prescribing for low-income patients was a commonly raised theme during focus group discussions, with participants such as Julia and Lucie describing being prescribed antidepressants inappropriately when they felt that this treatment was not likely to help them.

Every single time I've been [to the doctor], that's been the first port of call, it's been antidepressants [...] I just don't like how it makes me feel and it's true, it's just masking the problem, it's not fixing it.

(Julia, South West)

It's very much business, business, business, like, 'What do you want? Right, I can't help you', bosh, or 'Here's a prescription'. And reaching for the pad all the time and just giving people prescriptions, and then nothing really happens so you're still doing that five years later, saying, 'Have some more antidepressants' or whatever and nothing's changed.

(Lucie, London)

For many focus group participants, the rapidity of the prescribing process was felt to be problematic, with people feeling that medications were prescribed before the doctor had got to know them or understand the issues underlying their poor mental health. Yet participants also acknowledged the very high pressures facing primary care and surmised that doctors who no longer had the time to listen and build a relationship with their patients would commonly prescribe antidepressants as a practical response.

Although there is this huge value in the doctor–patient relationship and that continuity, you get to know someone, you understand—but that takes time. And often there isn't that realisation, there isn't that capacity, and quite often, dare I say it, I don't think GPs now want to get that involved [...] But actually, it's easier to write a prescription than it is to sit down, button up and not say anything and listen.

(Nina, South West)

Such findings concur with research which suggests that some doctors are reluctant to explore psycho-social issues in case they open up a multitude of complex issues that they do not feel they have the skills or resources to address effectively (Dew et al., 2005). Indeed, the lack of time for listening and relationship building within primary care was considered by both focus group

participants and GPs as a major negative shift in primary care practice, and one which both undermined trust and exacerbated reliance on medications.

A range of additional reasons for high antidepressant prescribing were discussed during the training sessions with primary care teams. These included the desire to do something to help a patient relatively quickly; a perceived lack of alternative options; a belief that antidepressants could be helpful in getting patients into a space where they could then take action to help themselves; and pressure for medications from patients themselves, which was often exacerbated when patients were required to evidence welfare entitlements.

There was a general lack of awareness amongst both primary care teams and focus group participants around the relatively limited effectiveness of antidepressants for people with low- to medium-level mental distress. In line with a recent Public Health England (2019) review of dependence and withdrawal associated with prescribed drugs (including antidepressants), it was widely agreed that better information and understanding were important in shifting current decision-making around mental health treatment within primary care. GPs explained that feeling confident in imparting reliable information to their patients on the limitations of antidepressants and the potential benefits of non-medical options (where evidence existed) would enable more honest discussion and informed joint decision-making around treatment and support options and would help them to justify referrals into social prescribing. Discussions with the DeStress community partners also evidenced a strong willingness to be informed about alternative treatment options and a recognition that wider public education would help to initiate a cultural shift in patient expectations along the same lines as that seen in antibiotic prescribing.

PRACTICE TEAM WORKING

Recent mental health policies have influenced substantive shifts in the composition of primary care teams, with most practices in the three regions involved in this study now drawing on GPs, social prescribing link workers, mental health nurses and other allied health professionals to deliver a more holistic bio-psycho-social approach to mental health care. It was evident within the training sessions that the conceptualisation of these teams and the ways that they functioned varied widely, with diverse implications for both staff and patient experience. Focus group participants such as Ted, for example, felt that some GPs were now more inclined to refer people on to other practice staff rather than attempting to deal with an issue themselves:

They are the initial point of hearing about distress, hearing about anxieties and maybe what people are experiencing mentally, but they tend not to want to deal with it as such, they will just pass it on.

(Ted, London)

It was recognised that this could be an effective use of time and that the support from non-medical practice staff could have positive outcomes; however, focus group participants stressed that because GPs still played a key role as the initial point of contact, 'feeling heard' rather than 'dismissed' remained paramount to building trusting patient–health care provider relations. At the same time, and as Husk et al. (2019) have highlighted, effective health team working around social prescribing relies on a series of relationships, *all* of which need to function together if they are to successfully meet patient need. Yet, we found that practice staff did not always have full oversight of the roles and remits of other team members. Despite referring patients on to the social prescribers within the practice, for example, some GPs disclosed that they did not always know who they were, what they did or how relevant the onward-referral options might be for their patients. Some GPs also did not realise that social prescribers could themselves have long waiting lists despite this having negative implications for the support available to their patients. There was also little evidence to suggest that GPs followed up with patients once they had referred them on to the social prescriber, or that social prescribers routinely fed this information back to GPs.

Research within primary care has found that weak endorsement by health professionals can make patients feel undermined and disincentivised and can result in low uptake and adherence to recommended treatments (Ford et al., 2019). Research also suggests that patients are more likely to enrol in social prescribing if they believe it will be of benefit, if the referral is presented in a way that matches their needs and expectations, and if any concerns they might have are adequately addressed by the referrer (Husk et al., 2019). The data from our study indicate that GPs do not always understand when social prescribing might be relevant to their patients and may not therefore endorse this as an option that people feel encouraged to take up. As the following quotes demonstrate, focus group participants also felt that a lack of awareness amongst GPs as to the social prescribing opportunities available meant they did not routinely offer it to patients when discussing treatment and support options.

I've recently found out about social prescribing which, again, has been kept quiet from me forever. I only found it out, it feels like a little secret, that actually, there's some funding through my GP surgery to access sporting things, so swimming and stuff like that.

(Julia, South West)

I think that there are a lot of resources in the UK that are not NHS, and unfortunately they don't put them together and say, 'We could refer here, here or here', there are lots of places that can offer people talking support that don't charge, but you don't hear GPs talking about them at all.

(Bella, London)

If you don't know and the GP never refers you, you don't know what is there.

(Tina, London)

For the minority of focus group participants who had been referred into social prescribing, the diverse nature and quality of the activities and support on offer were highlighted. One person, for example, explained how social prescribing had done little that they could not have done for themselves.

It's not a great positive support, it depends on who is the social prescriber. Some people there are able to support you in putting together an application for PIP (personal independence payment), for example, or any other benefit, but others of them, they just give you the information—you can even Google this information if you are really in need of something, maybe sometimes it's even quicker.

(Bella, London)

However, other participants stressed the value of the support received in enabling them to make positive changes to their health and wellbeing:

I was overweight, 14 stone, and I went to my doctor, and he said would you be interested to go to the gym, and he gave me a letter to take to the gym [...] So I started going the gym and started losing the weight, and I lost a couple of stone and I carried on going for a good few years, and that was a really good thing because if the doctor hadn't said to me do you want to go to the gym, you know, coz I was overweight, I wouldn't have lost that weight and I wouldn't have gone.

(Peter, North West Coast)

You come here and you forget everything. And [organisation name] as well, I did a course there, it's brilliant. They need to do more social prescribing. You can sit down and chill out, and we're all working to one purpose, you learn something new every day.

(Ada, North West Coast)

Some of the most valued mental health support amongst focus group participants came from the social support they had received through involvement in local community groups. Here, people praised the sustained, non-judgemental, one-to-one mentoring and support that they had received from their peers. However, with only a few exceptions, the participants concerned had accessed this support through word-of-mouth rather than via a referral from primary care.

Conclusion

Social prescribing is gaining in prominence in the UK, yet little is known about the factors that inhibit take-up within primary care. Work undertaken during the DeStress-II project identified core challenges that inhibit (effective) referral into social prescribing. Time and resource pressures within primary care, as well as patient demand and the need for patients to evidence welfare entitlements, mean that reducing antidepressant prescribing in favour of alternative support options remains far from straightforward. Awareness raising amongst both health care practitioners and patients around the relative limitations of antidepressants and the merits of non-medical options was agreed by participants to be an important area where further research is needed to inform shifts within public expectation and health care practice.

Primary care practice teams have undergone considerable shifts in recent years, with a range of allied staff now in place to support patients with their health and wellbeing. However, the study found that team-based working was not always well coordinated, and that doctors were not always fully informed about what they were referring patients into, or how effective or appropriate this might be for the patient's needs. This has significant implications for the likely enrolment and engagement of patients with social prescribing opportunities, as well as with the relationship and trust they hold with their GP. Further work is therefore needed to understand how primary care teams can more effectively work together to ensure that patient need can be met.

REFERENCES

Buck, D., Ewbank, L., 2020. What is social prescribing? Accessed from: https://www.kingsfund.org.uk/publications/social-prescribing. The King's Fund (Accessed 15 February 2023).

Byng, R., Groos, N., Dowrick, C., 2019. From mental disorder to shared understanding: A non-categorical approach to support individuals with distress in primary care. Br. J. Gen. Pract. 69 (680), 110–111.

Dew, K., Dowell, A., McLeod, D., Collings, S., Bushnell, J., 2005. 'This glorious twilight zone of uncertainty': Mental health consultations in general practice in New Zealand. Soc. Sci. Med. 61 (6), 1189–1200.

Ford, J., Thomas, F., Byng, R., McCabe, R., 2019. Exploring how patients respond to GP recommendations for mental health treatment: An analysis of communication in primary care consultations. BJGP Open. 3 (4).

Husk, K., Blockley, K., Lovell, R., Bethel, A., Lang, I., Byng, R., Garside, R., 2019. What approaches to social prescribing work, for whom, and in what circumstances? A realist review. Health Soc. Care. 28 (2), 309–324.

Iacobucci, G., 2019. NHS prescribed record number of antidepressants last year. Br. Med. J. 364, l1508.

NHS England and NHS Improvement and the National Collaborating Centre for Mental Health, 2019. The Community Mental Health Framework for Adults and Older Adults. Accessed from: https://www.england.nhs.uk/wp-content/uploads/2019/09/community-mental-health-framework-for-adults-and-older-adults.pdf (Accessed 15 February 2023).

NHS England, 2021. NICE guidelines on depression in adults. Accessed from: https://www.nice.org.uk/guidance/gid-cgwave0725/documents/draft-guideline-4 (Accessed 15 February 2023).

Public Health England, 2019. Dependence and withdrawal associated with some prescribed medicines: an evidence review. Accessed from: https://assets.publishing.service.gov.uk/government/uploads/system/uploads/attachment_data/file/940255/PHE_PMR_report_Dec2020.pdf (Accessed 10 September 2022).

RCGP, 2017. Mental health in primary care. Accessed from: https://www.rcgp.org.uk/representing-you/policy-areas/mental-health-in-primary-care (Accessed 15 February 2023).

Skivington, K., Smith, M., Chng, N.R., Mackenzie, M., Wyke, S., Mercer, S.W., 2018. Delivering a primary care-based social prescribing initiative: A qualitative study of the benefits and challenges. Br. J. Gen. Pract. 68 (672), e487–e494.

Thomas, F., Hansford, L., Ford, J., Wyatt, K., McCabe, R., Byng, R., 2019. How accessible and acceptable are current GP referral mechanisms for IAPT for low-income patients? Lay and primary care perspectives. J. Ment. Health. 29 (6), 706–711. doi:10.1080/096 38237.2019.1677876.

Thomas, F., Hansford, L., Wyatt, K., 2020. The violence of narrative: Embodying responsibility for poverty-related distress. Sociol. Health Illn. 42 (5), 1123–1138. https://doi.org/10.1111/1467-9566.13084.

Thompson, L., McCabe, R., 2012. The effect of clinician-patient alliance and communication on treatment adherence in mental health care: A systematic review. BMC Psychiatry. 12, 87.

Chapter 23

Learning From Buurtzorg in Community Nursing Services

Brendan Martin

Introduction

This is the story of what I experienced as a carer for my mother at the end of her life. With time and reflection on what happened, I set out to find ways to address the issues that I saw. I found something called 'Buurtzorg' which was founded by a Dutch nurse called Jos de Blok. It features self-managing neighbourhood community nursing teams that make connections and harness community power that resonates strongly with the concept of social prescribing.

How My Mum Put Me on the Road to Buurtzorg

On 17 April 2011, at 1:42 in the morning, my mother Betty Martin took her last breath as I held her hand in Lewisham Hospital, South East London. She had taken her first nearly 88 years earlier in Dunmanway, West Cork. I have devoted most of my time since that night trying with many others to ensure that, by the time it is my turn to go, Britain and Ireland have the kind of community health and social care I would have liked for my mum.

Around 16 hours before Betty died I had arrived at her house, the same one in which she and my dad brought up my four brothers and me, to spend the day with her, as I had done increasingly often towards the end of her life. As I drove across London that Saturday morning, her overnight care worker called me because Betty was not getting out of bed and seemed unwell. As soon as I arrived in her bedroom, I was quite sure she would not survive the weekend. But what did I know? I'm not a clinician, Betty was unable to express any wishes she might have had at that moment, and how would I explain it to my brothers had I not at least called her GP practice? So I did that, knowing that I was probably starting Betty down a pathway that could be far more traumatic than if she'd stay where she was. I knew and trusted her GP, but what I got was a locum who knew nothing about my mum or her circumstances. (In fact—in a stark illustration of what industrialisation of general practice had done—he had only flown in from Germany for the weekend to supplement his regular income.) What would you have done in his position? Would you have risked a conversation with me about what was most likely in her best interests, and how to make it happen? Or would you have taken the professionally safer route?

The ambulance arrived within an hour—the paramedics were lovely—and so we found ourselves in a cubicle of the busy accident and emergency department. I hope triage procedures have improved since then, even if the pressures on staff have increased, but as we waited, I saw Betty deteriorate in front of my eyes, suffering a stroke, perhaps a second one. I spent the rest of the day wheeling her around various departments, including X-ray. By early evening, the doctors concluded that only abdominal surgery could save her, but she was probably not strong enough to survive it. We agreed enough was enough and to let her go. As you can imagine—or perhaps know—this was a profound experience, about which I have thought a lot in the years since it happened. The conclusions I have reached were informed also by what I learnt in the preceding years as her care needs increased.

By the time she died, Betty needed someone under her roof every night, as well as two or three home care visits a day. This was costing about £75,000 a year, and, with power of attorney, I knew her liquid assets were close to exhaustion. Perhaps she knew it too. Yet the care workers who looked after my mum earned only minimum wage—and not even that for the time spent travelling between their clients' homes—and the quality of the care they provided was undermined by its fragmentation into timed tasks.

I knew we could do better because since 1990 I had worked internationally researching, developing and advocating approaches to public service reform based on enabling and supporting the intrinsic motivation and tacit knowledge of professionals. Drawing on experience in more than 70 countries, I had become convinced that self-managed teamwork was a vital ingredient of health and social care, and this now merged with my personal experience to inform my perspective about the future of home care.

The care workers who supported Betty were fine women but were stuck in a systemic and organisational environment that required them to focus on tasks rather than outcomes and inhibited their ability to really get to know the person in their care. They did an adequate job—in one or two cases a very good one—of keeping Betty safe from the harms that might have caused an earlier death, but they could not enable and support her to live the best life possible—or to experience a better death—in her final years.

Why Successive Governments Have Failed to 'Fix' Social Care

This is the social care system successive British governments have promised to 'fix', but they never do. Why not? In my view, the fundamental reason is that it is unfixable. Just as we have reached—and passed—the environmentally sustainable limit of our global industrial development model, so our industrialised model of social care is no longer compatible with enabling and supporting people to live with as much meaning, autonomy and warm social interaction as their health and time of life could allow. To face up to that reality is not to counsel despair. On the contrary, just as my experience with Betty showed me how fragmented

and unsatisfactory our existing system could be, it also revealed some of the seeds of change that, if we nurture them well, can give us hope.

One of my mum's favourite carers helped me to understand both what is wrong with our system and how it can be rebuilt. Fatima (not her real name) was always finding ways to do what was needed when needed, whether or not it was on her task list. The company that employed her—given a top rating by the Care Quality Commission—was less responsive. One day I asked Fatima if there was a secret number on which to call her agency because no one ever answered at the number I had. She laughed and said, 'They never answer for us, either!' So I asked her how she coped when there was an emergency, and she pointed to her mobile and said, 'We call each other'. It was a lightbulb moment that cemented my growing belief that while the system was broken, the people who kept it going regardless were not. It made me think: What if, instead of requiring those professionals to find ways around a dysfunctional system, we built the system around their commitment and capability to make and nurture the kinds of relationships with their clients needed to enable both to thrive?

As well as allowing care workers to provide more creative and flexible support, this would also raise their status and, by using their time more efficiently, reduce costs so that their pay could be improved.

I was caring for my mum at a time when there was growing controversy about 15-minute care visits, but I felt that debate missed the point because some days she needed little or no support while on others she needed a lot. What she always needed was support that responded appropriately as her condition changed, and relationships that made the best of and tried to strengthen her remaining capacities, supporting the autonomy she craved to live her life in a way that had meaning for her. However, it was also clear that even a great care service could not achieve this on its own, and another lesson I drew from that time was that my mum had become far more detached from her local community than was good for her wellbeing. She and my dad (who died 15 years before she did) had become quite insular over the years after their kids left home, and I could see how easily that happens, and how isolation increases even more after one spouse is left behind.

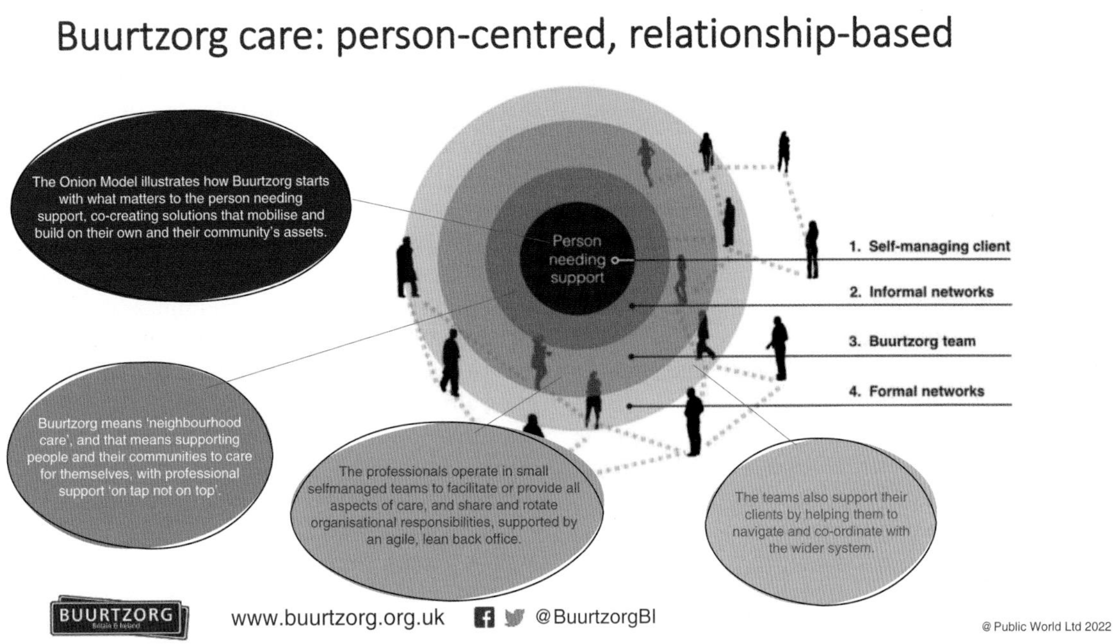

Buurtzorg care: person-centred, relationship-based

The Onion Model illustrates how Buurtzorg starts with what matters to the person needing support, co-creating solutions that mobilise and build on their own and their community's assets.

Person needing support

1. Self-managing client

2. Informal networks

3. Buurtzorg team

4. Formal networks

Buurtzorg means 'neighbourhood care', and that means supporting people and their communities to care for themselves, with professional support 'on tap not on top'.

The professionals operate in small selfmanaged teams to facilitate or provide all aspects of care, and share and rotate organisational responsibilities, supported by an agile, lean back office.

The teams also support their clients by helping them to navigate and co-ordinate with the wider system.

BUURTZORG
Britain & Ireland

www.buurtzorg.org.uk   @BuurtzorgBI

@ Public World Ltd 2022

Fig. 23.1 The Onion Model. From Buurtzorg Britain and Ireland and Public World Ltd.

I began to realise that the services we need could and should do much more than paper over the cracks in the fragmenting communities and families of modern industrial societies; they could and should also contribute to the creation of a new era of self-caring neighbourhoods. Drawing on my knowledge of community activism and work organisation in many countries, I went looking for inspiration and found Buurtzorg, which had been founded in 2007 by a group of friends around district nurse Jos de Blok.

Buurtzorg—Back to the Future

Buurtzorg's aim was to restore the neighbourhood nursing approach with which Jos had begun his career while mobilising the additional potential of modern information technology to enhance it.

'As a community nurse when I started in the 1980s I had responsibility for supporting the health and wellbeing of a neighbourhood and the freedom to decide how to take care of my patients', he has told me. 'We did what was needed when it was needed, without any management telling us how to do it.'

But in the 1990s, in a move similar to reforms in Britain and many other countries, the Dutch government established a Care Needs Assessment Centre (CNAC), which centralised assessments and the definition of tasks based on them. 'It led to a big change in how people talked about care', says Jos. 'We were told what to do and how much it should cost, and could no longer do what we thought necessary.'

Buurtzorg's approach was to start again from the perspective of the person needing care (Fig. 23.1) and to support people to manage their own as much as possible, building on their strengths and drawing on 'informal networks'—family, neighbours, community assets. Nurses would coordinate and complement these efforts as necessary.

In this approach, 'social prescribing' is not a novel addition to nursing practice but one of its fundamental characteristics, and is one of the reasons that Buurtzorg has reduced the average number of hours of care per client from 108 per year in 2014 to 70 in 2022, with ambition to reduce further in 2023.

Finding or creating non-clinical solutions to improve the health and wellbeing of clients operates not only at an individual level but also in the way the Buurtzorg teams engage with and help to develop the 'informal networks' layer of the onion model. An example of the creativity involved is the annual 'walker races' in which hundreds of older people in Buurtzorg's care, as well as many of their nurses, converge once a year on Amsterdam's Olympic Stadium for races of various distances with their walking frames. This started as an initiative of one of Buurtzorg's self-managed teams, stimulated by a conversation between a nurse and an older woman in her care, so that older people in their village could have fun, enjoy each other's company and maintain or improve their fitness. The team involved shared news of what they had done on the Buurtzorgweb—a digital tool that serves as a Facebook-like intranet—and others adopted the idea as well. Pretty soon it became not only a neighbourhood-level activity but also an annual national festival.

This not only resonated strongly with what I had imagined as an alternative to the system I had encountered with my mum. It also showed how it could succeed in practice, because Buurtzorg has not only greatly improved care and reduced costs but also become an international exemplar of good employment and organisational practice. So, as Jos had generously invited me to come and spend some time with him, a Buurtzorg team, a coach and back office staff, I took myself off to the Netherlands. It so happened that Public World was about to begin a programme of work to support change in community services in the London boroughs of Lambeth and Southwark, with Guy's and St Thomas's NHS Foundation Trust (GSTT). So we invited its then newly appointed head of community nursing, Cepta Hamm, to come with me.

Bringing Buurtzorg to Britain

Soon afterwards, we began a programme of support to GSTT in introducing a new model of neighbourhood nursing in Lambeth and Southwark, and Buurtzorg Britain & Ireland was born when Jos invited my social enterprise, Public World, to be its partner. (You can read some of the GSTT nurses' reflections in Kamara et al. [2022].) Since then, we have worked in more than 40 settings in the National Health Service and in social care and the hospice movement in Britain and Ireland, in each case co-creating solutions suited to their own context.

We have found that British nurses and care workers are just as able as Buurtzorg's to self-manage, and that their clients and communities are no less willing than in the Netherlands to be supported to care for themselves. However, an equally consistent lesson of our experience has been that if such an approach is to grow to scale successfully and sustainably, organisational and system leaders and administrative arrangements require radical change in culture, methods and mindset. Some of this learning has been derived from our participation in a project partly funded by the European Union's Interreg 2Seas Transforming Integrated Care in the Community (TICC) programme (https://www.interreg2seas.eu/en/ticc). We have been supporting Medway Community Health, Kent Community Health Foundation Trust and Kent County Council to experiment with applying Buurtzorg principles in their contexts. Similar trials took place in the Calais and Lille areas of France, through Soignons Humain, La Vie Active and VIVAT Service a la Personne.

Between them, the organisations involved in the TICC project reported more than 200 'barriers and challenges' to their efforts within their own organisational arrangements and systems. The details are available online at www.publicworld.org. Some of these were generic, such as change of any kind being a challenge, staff shortages and the global pandemic severely restricting space for trying new things. But most arose from tensions between how systems and organisations are designed and operate and what the model needs for success at scale. In particular, we found:

1. **Inconsistent goals throughout organisations** meant that teams were being funded and monitored according to a different set of outcomes from the outcomes they were trying to work towards within the Buurtzorg model.
2. **Lack of integration of services at all levels** meant that teams were trying to work in a holistic, patient-centred way but dealing with regulatory and monitoring systems that did not support this. Funders and regulators divided up work according to type of care (health or social)

and geographical boundaries that did not match the neighbourhoods served.

3. **Hierarchy and competition** within institutions had the effect of undermining the autonomy of the teams, obstructing their work and making it harder for teams to operate in a nonhierarchical and collaborative way internally.

4. **Systems-led working** meant that teams were often required to adapt their work to fit inflexible institutional systems, rather than having systems designed to support the purposes of the frontline work.

These obstacles have not prevented the TICC neighbourhood nursing and home care teams, as well as many others we have supported in several places, demonstrating their ability and willingness to take similar initiatives as those of the Buurtzorg teams in the Netherlands. On the contrary, there are some inspiring examples. For instance, one of the neighbourhood nursing teams employed by Guy's and St Thomas's NHS Foundation Trust helped a client with worsening leg ulcers to reverse a decline into immobility and isolation by finding a way to motivate her to leave the house and become more active. The nurse did this by suggesting an outing inspired by the information she had gathered about what mattered to her client, information that only a relationship built over time could yield. The result was that her ulcers cleared up and her mental health improved. The nurses in the team had the satisfaction of helping their client to solve her problems rather than simply addressing their effects, and the NHS was able to discharge a patient who had previously seemed likely to need community nurse visits for the rest of her life.

In Medway Community Health, nurses had a similar success by supporting a patient to resume her enjoyment of spending time with her beloved horse, initially by taking her out themselves while they tried to find others in her community who could help her on a voluntary basis. Such examples will remain atypical whilst nurses and care workers are under so much pressure that all they have time to do is the tasks that are needed to keep people alive rather than enabling and supporting them to live with purpose and a balance of personal control and community interdependence.

Conclusion

Reflecting on his own early career in district nursing and the practices developed by Buurtzorg nurses—now some 9000 of them in around 900 self-managed teams—Jos de Blok told me that they operate not only as clinicians but also as community organisers.

But to do that consistently they need manageable caseloads and the authority and support to do whatever they agree (within reasonable budgetary constraints) with their clients as needed, individually and as a team. In the Netherlands, they have shown that this need be neither a pipedream nor unaffordable. On the contrary, being enabled and supported to work in this way has allowed Buurtzorg to reduce costs by improving outcomes while halving the average number of hours of professional input per client.

The growth of social prescribing initiatives of various kinds in the British system demonstrates the value of building social connections and community power to not only complement clinical interventions but also, sometimes, prevent their necessity. But if we are to make the radical shift that is needed to take social prescribing from the margins of NHS and social care practice to being a routine aspect of nursing and care worker practice, we must make the radical organisational and systemic changes to support it.

In the Netherlands, Buurtzorg is part of the national collective bargaining agreement for nurses but pays above its required levels. By improving the job roles, pay and status of community nursing and home care we will also be better able to overcome the recruitment and retention issues that undermine them. By working in this way we might also find that the term *social prescribing* itself becomes redundant as we build stronger and healthier communities better able to care for themselves. After all, the English translation of Buurtzorg is 'neighbourhood care'.

REFERENCE

Kamara, Y., Rodriguez, C., Moyo, N., 2022. District nursing using neighbourhood care principles in practice: Reflecting on our experience. Br. J. Community Nurs. 27 (11), 552–556. https://bit.ly/BuurtzorgatGSTT.

Chapter 24

The Contribution of Allied Health Professionals

Linda Hindle

Introduction

This chapter gives an overview of the different professions collectively described as allied health professions (AHPs). It then outlines why and how many AHPs are already engaged in social prescribing and the spectrum of engagement across and within the professions. It concludes with some recommendations to further the social prescribing contribution of AHPs.

Introducing the Allied Health Professionals

In 2012, International Chief Allied Health Professions Officers came together to create a definition of the term AHPs, which states; 'Allied Health Professionals are a distinct group of health professionals who apply their expertise to prevent disease transmission, diagnose, treat and rehabilitate people of all ages and all specialties. Together with a range of technical and support staff they may deliver direct patient care, rehabilitation, treatment, diagnostics and health improvement interventions to restore and maintain optimal physical, sensory, psychological, cognitive and social functions.'

There is no international consistency about which professions are included in the AHP grouping. In England there are 14 professions represented by the Chief Allied Health Professions Officer, all of which are regulated and professionally autonomous practitioners. Collectively, these 14 professions are the third largest clinical workforce in the NHS behind doctors and nurses (see Table 24.1).

Why Allied Health Professions Are Interested in Social Prescribing

ALIGNMENT TO THE WAYS AHPs WORK

Allied health professionals tend to use a biopsychosocial approach to care (Lehman et al., 2017), focussing their assessment and care on a holistic view of an individual or population. They have been early advocates of person-centred care and self-management, and some AHPs would describe social prescribing as an integral part of their practice.

Whilst there is a wide difference between the different professions, many of the allied health professions are in a privileged position to spend more time with the people they care for than some other health care professionals; they will usually see people over a period of time and therefore can develop a rapport and focus on what matters to the individual with a view to tailoring their care and support appropriately. An example of this is in occupational therapy where the aim of care is to support individuals to enable them to return to or optimise participation in all the things that people do such as working, learning, playing and interacting with others. They may work with people with learning disabilities or mental health conditions or with those who have lost an occupational ability due to a physical injury such as acquired brain injury. One of the models used in occupational therapy is the Person-Environment-Occupation-Performance (PEOP) model (Baum et al., 2015) which proposes that intrinsic (i.e. person), extrinsic (i.e. environmental) and occupation (i.e. task/role) factors interact to produce the person's occupational performance and participation. It is

TABLE 24.1	The 14 Allied Health Professions in England

Arts therapists—Art, music and drama therapists are three distinct professions although each uses the medium of art, music or drama as a form of psychotherapy to encourage clients to explore a variety of issues including emotional, behavioural or mental health problems; learning or physical disabilities; life-limiting conditions; neurological conditions; or physical illnesses.

Dietitians assess, diagnose and treat diet and nutritional problems at an individual level and work with communities and populations to support healthy eating as part of wider public health interventions.

Occupational therapists (OTs) support people with a range of interventions to enable them to return to or optimise participation in all the things that people do, such as caring for themselves and others, working, learning, playing and interacting with others.

Operating department practitioners work in operating departments and critical care units and support patients in the preparation for, during and immediately after an operation.

Orthoptists are experts in diagnosing and treating defects in eye movement and problems with how the eyes work together, called binocular vision. These can be caused by issues with the muscles around the eyes or defects in the nerves enabling the brain to communicate with the eyes.

Osteopaths take a holistic view of the structure and function of the body to diagnose and treat a wide variety of medical conditions. They work on the principle that the skeleton, muscles, ligaments and connective tissues of an individual need to function smoothly together so as to maintain wellbeing.

Prosthetists and orthotists provide gait analysis and engineering solutions to patients with problems of the neurological, muscular and skeletal systems, including limb loss.

Paramedics, whilst best known for their roles in the ambulance and emergency care services, are increasingly working in other parts of the health care system such as primary care.

Physiotherapists use physical approaches to promote, maintain and restore physical, psychological and social wellbeing, working through partnership and negotiation with individuals to optimise their functional ability and potential.

Podiatrists specialise in the foot, ankle and leg, aiming to improve the mobility, independence and quality of life for their patients.

There are two types of **Radiographers:** diagnostic and therapeutic.

Diagnostic radiographers use a range of techniques to produce high-quality images to diagnose an injury or disease. They are also integral to many screening programmes including breast screening as well as ultrasound monitoring of pregnancy.

Therapeutic radiographers play a vital role in the treatment of cancer. They plan and deliver radiotherapy and provide care and support for patients throughout their radiotherapy treatment.

Speech and language therapists (SLTs) in the UK work with children and adults to help them overcome or adapt to a vast array of disorders of speech, language, communication and swallowing.

Other professionals who may be considered allied health professionals in other countries and contexts include professions such as psychologists, audiologists, counsellors, environmental health officers and exercise physiologists.

clear to see how this model aligns with the principles of social prescribing which recognise that people's health is determined by economic and environmental factors. The PEOP model therefore seeks to address people's needs in a holistic way by enabling people to be referred to a range of local, non-clinical services with the aim of supporting them to take greater control of their own health.

ALIGNMENT TO WHERE AHPs WORK

Allied health professions tend to work as part of a multidisciplinary team not just within health and social care but across a broader system. Whilst the majority work in the National Health Service, AHPs also work in other sectors such as social care, the criminal justice system, private sector, voluntary sector, education and housing, and therefore they are ideally placed to work across boundaries and sectors. This breadth of perspectives enables AHPs to appreciate the strengths and assets within individuals and communities and use this understanding to help those they are working with to access the support they need via social prescribing. Some examples of how AHPs work in non-traditional health settings include:

- Dietitians leading or supporting community cooking groups which support social connections at the same time as teaching and experimenting with recipes, new foods and cooking skills.
- Speech and language therapists supporting young people in contact with the criminal justice system. Over 60% of young people in justice settings have speech, language and communication needs which lead to difficulties understanding spoken words and using language to communicate, difficulty listening and understanding and potentially difficulties expressing feelings and emotions in an appropriate way, which may result in aggressive behaviour. Speech and language therapists can support young people to develop conversation and social skills and express their emotions more effectively.
- Podiatrists working with charities supporting those who are homeless. Not only does this involve providing care to minimise and prevent painful feet conditions, it also involves listening, developing trust and signposting to other support offers.

ALIGNMENT TO STRATEGIC PRIORITIES FOR AHPs SUCH AS PREVENTION AND ENVIRONMENTAL SUSTAINABILITY

Social prescribing makes sense environmentally because it is about preventing and reducing the need for carbon-intensive heath care. The agendas around public health, prevention, self-management, personalised care, environmental sustainability and social justice are inextricably linked with social prescribing. Sustainable health care is predicated on preventing and reducing the need for intensive health care services; we do this by supporting individuals and communities to improve health and wellbeing. A model for sustainable clinical practice has been described by Frances Mortimer as the combination of four elements, all of which lead to reduced demand for high carbon use and intensive health care services (Mortimer, 2010). These include:

- **Prevention**—promoting health and preventing disease by tackling the causes of illnesses and health inequalities
- **Patient self-care**—empowering people to take a greater role in managing their own health and health care

- **Lean service delivery**—streamlining care systems to minimise wasteful activities; an example of this could be the Beyond Pills Campaign established by the College of Medicine (2022) in response to the Chief Pharmaceutical Officer's National Overprescribing Review (Department of Health and Social Care, 2021) that revealed that 10% of prescribed drugs (approximately 110 million items) are unnecessary and may cause harm
- **Low-carbon alternatives**—prioritising treatments and technologies with a lower environmental impact, including social prescribing

Over the past 8 years AHPs have been on a journey to increase their contribution and recognition as part of the wider public health workforce delivering health improvement and reductions in health inequalities. AHPs are also developing their role as part of the net zero ambition. The health and care system in England is responsible for an estimated 4% to 5% of the country's carbon footprint. *Delivering a Net Zero NHS* (NHS England, 2020a) sets out how we will reduce the elements of this that the NHS controls directly to net zero carbon by 2040, and those that the NHS can influence to net zero by 2045, in order to ensure that our health system contributes towards the national ambition to be carbon neutral by 2050.

Reaching our country's ambitions under the Paris Climate Change Agreement could see over 5700 lives saved every year from improved air quality, 38,000 lives saved every year from a more physically active population and over 100,000 lives saved every year from healthier diets (NHS England, 2020b).

Barriers to the Use of Social Prescribing by AHPs

Whilst allied health professionals see the opportunity to contribute to the social prescribing agenda and the value of doing so, there are of course barriers to involvement such as limitations of time, awareness of social prescribing resources and teams, and the relatively large geographical footprint that many AHPs work within. This is especially true for those who work in regional organisations such as Ambulance Trusts or Tertiary Care Centres.

Nevertheless, many of these barriers can also be translated as opportunities; for example, the pressures on workforce capacity demonstrate the increased importance of working in partnership with others as opposed to in silos. This is very relevant in relation to social prescribing. Equally, increasing demand on services highlights the importance of intervening early, getting care right the first time and identifying with clients the enablers to support them to self-manage or prevent deterioration of their condition; clearly this is a link to social prescribing.

The development of integrated care systems and primary care networks in England provides a mechanism to facilitate increased collaborations between all health care professionals including AHPs and social prescribing networks. An example of this could be through reciprocal training placements for AHPs and social prescribing link workers, supporting each other to understand the roles and work context of the other to facilitate improved collaboration.

How Do Allied Health Professionals Engage in Social Prescribing?

As previously discussed, there are wide differences in the roles of the allied health professions; some are more acute care focused whilst others have a longer-term therapeutic or preventative approach providing care closer to home. For this reason, it is not surprising that AHPs will be connected to social prescribing to a greater or lesser extent and in different ways.

In 2019, AHP leaders from Public Health and the NHS worked with the Royal Society for Public Health (RSPH) to develop a framework to explain the spectrum of involvement in social prescribing by AHPs (RSPH, 2019). This work started with a series of conversations, surveys and tweet chats with AHPs to explore their understanding of social prescribing and the different ways they were engaging.

AHPs described social prescribing as taking a holistic view of the health and wellbeing of an individual and connecting people to services that can help to support them. They highlighted the importance of social prescribing as a non-medical means of tackling specific health needs alongside the wider determinants of health. Participants were enthusiastic about the potential for social prescribing to support the needs

of the people who use their services and were keen to build their skills and knowledge. There was clearly a breadth of opportunities for involvement in social prescribing depending on roles and context and, encouragingly, enthusiasm to do more.

The AHP social prescribing framework was co-produced with AHPs and service users. It includes four levels of social prescribing related activity:

1. **Active signposting**
   Active signposting is a light-touch approach where AHPs in local agencies provide information and choice to signpost people to services using resource directories and local knowledge. Active signposting works best for people who are confident and skilled enough to find their own way to services after a brief 'making every contact count' conversation (MECC, NHS England, 2024).
   Example—A physiotherapist in a hospital discharge team often works with people who have fallen. The physiotherapist makes time to listen to what is important to each individual and helps them to identify strategies to increase their confidence and reduce the risk of falls. This often includes signposting to local groups and services.
2. **Referral to a social prescribing link worker**
   In cases where a person needs more support than active signposting can provide, AHPs may offer a referral to a social prescribing link worker whose role is to work with individuals to build trust, understand their needs and create a shared plan based on what matters to them, to help them take control of their health and wellbeing. The link worker will help individuals to navigate and access local groups and support networks.
   Example—A dietitian had been supporting a lady to lose weight. It became clear during conversations that the lady was isolated, lonely and lacking in confidence following the death of her husband; this was causing her to comfort eat. A referral to a social prescribing link worker helped the lady to connect with her community, reduce her social isolation, re-kindle past hobbies and re-build her confidence.
3. **Delivery of social prescribing**
   AHPs are likely to undertake social prescribing themselves when they are already providing long-term intensive support to a person as part

of their job role. AHP social prescribing is for individuals needing specialist assessment and intervention outside the competency of a link worker or when the social prescribing forms a natural part of the individual's therapy.

Social prescribing is much more time intensive than active signposting or referring to a link worker. It involves supporting people of all ages to work out which local groups and services would be beneficial to them and helping them to access them in a variety of ways. AHPs may need to work through multiple options with a client and accompany them on first visits.

Some AHPs are likely to do more social prescribing themselves than others because of the nature of their role. Occupational therapists, physiotherapists and speech and language therapists, for example, are more likely to carry out social prescribing activities than diagnostic radiographers who are likely to have short, one-off interactions with clients.

Example—A community occupational therapist in a mental health team often works with people over an extended period to help them re-develop a sense of purpose and confidence to manage their condition. This role involves exploring with an individual: what matters to them, what they need and what will (and won't) work for them. The therapy involves supporting people to make connections, try out solutions and find strategies to enable them to cope with their illness.

4. **Development of the social prescribing infrastructure**

AHPs can, and do, support the development of social prescribing across the health, social care and voluntary systems in several ways, including:

- Providing community groups and services that are socially prescribed by link workers and other health care professionals. Examples include community choirs run by speech and language therapists or music therapists for people with dementia or other difficulties communicating, or community cooking groups led by dietitians.
- Providing guidance, advice, supervision and training to link workers, including raising

awareness of referral routes to AHP support when a person's needs goes beyond link workers' level of competence.

Further Developments

Opportunities to further embed this approach into the routine practice of AHPs include:

- Increasing multi-professional education and practice to encourage collaboration and reduce the risk of professional protectiveness or working in professional bubbles.
- Ensuring that performance targets do not result in unintended consequences which negatively affect what is best for the patient in the longer term. For example, longer term intervention or easier routes for the public to engage with health care services when needed will in many cases result in a better outcomes and less intensive health care input than a one-size-fits-all, over-medicalised approach.
- Increased use of health coaching, behaviour change interventions and motivational interviewing to support identification of what really matters to individuals.
- Use of population health care to identify high-need populations and potential future demand with a view to intervening early. This approach will identify underlying causes of ill health and inequalities which are similar across different partner organisations and therefore highlight the benefits of working with partners and communities to plan and deliver services collaboratively.

Conclusion

This chapter has described a spectrum of engagement in social prescribing by AHPs and acknowledges the predictable differences in social prescribing–related activity across the AHP community owing to variations in the nature and duration of clinical interactions across professions and contexts. It is clear that social prescribing or increasing access to nonmedical support—whether by signposting, link workers or direct delivery—will be increasingly important to AHPs to improve the health and wellbeing of the population and ensure a sustainable health and care system.

REFERENCES

Baum, C.M., Christiansen, C.H., Bass, J.D., 2015. The person-environment-occupation-performance (PEOP) model. In: Christiansen, C.H., Baum, C.M., Bass, J.D. (Eds.), Occupational Therapy: Performance, Participation, and Well-Being, fourth ed, 49–56.

College of Medicine and Integrated Care, 2022. Beyond pills campaign. A beyond pills campaign fights to stop over-prescribing in the UK—college of medicine and integrated health. https://collegeofmedicine.org.uk/beyond-pills/ (Accessed 11 March 2024).

Department of Health and Social Care, 2021. National overprescribing review report. Available from: https://www.gov.uk/government/publications/national-overprescribing-review-report (Accessed 14 February 2023).

Lehman, Barbara, J., David, Diana, M., Gruber, Jennifer, A., 2017. Rethinking the biopsychosocial model of health: understanding health as a dynamic system. Soc. Personal. Psychol. Compass. 11 (8), e12328. http://dx.doi.org/10.1111/spc3.12328.

Mortimer, F., 2010. The sustainable physician. Clin. Med. 10 (2), 110–111.

NHS England, 2020a. Delivering a 'net zero' national health service. Available from: delivering-a-net-zero-national-health-service.pdf (england.nhs.uk) (Accessed 14 February 2023).

NHS England, 2020b. Being a greener AHP. https://www.england.nhs.uk/ahp/greener-ahp-hub/understanding-environmental-sustainability/being-a-green-ahp/ (Accessed 14 February 2023).

NHS England. 2024. Making every contact count. https://www.e-lfh.org.uk/making-every-contact-count-mecc-e-learning-programme-updated/ (Accessed 11 March 2024).

Royal Society for Public Health, NHS England and Public Health England (2017).

Chapter 25

The Role of Urgent and Emergency Services

Steve Vincent, chapter editor

Introduction

This chapter explores a snapshot of some of the work that emergency services are undertaking to support individuals and families with complex needs. The work will be seen by some as not the traditional or core activity of the respective agencies involved, and it would be fair to say that the terminology of social prescribing will not be common language in their day-to-day activities. However, as you will see when we look through the perspective lenses of urgent health care, policing and fire, their contributions are making a significant impact on the individuals and families involved. In essence, these case studies identify the 'upstream work' undertaken—much of this is preventative around the social determinants of health and delivers better results when delivered collectively.

The challenge is that in an era where results are measured against individual organisations, there are few targets that are a collective responsibility. This is reinforced through individual inspection regimes that can drive work in the wrong direction due to the performance results being over short-term periods.

Prevention is a long-term commitment that needs to be sustained using a whole system approach. Taking into account my own experience within the fire sector, the sustained investment in prevention activity over decades has paid dividends in relation to the reduction of fire deaths and accidental fires. This was championed throughout the sector with a few fire and rescue services (FRS) making the link to health inequalities and has been recognised for that work by Sir Michael Marmot.

If you can forgive the pun, many blue light services have long since recognised that 'firefighting' the drug misuse, the falls and the major fires is a fight too late. Instead, we have turned our attention to understanding the social causes and how we may intervene earlier. Here we showcase how we do it—our version of 'social prescribing' and how we might support it.

The High Intensity Use Programme—Urgent and Emergency Care Lens

Rhian Monteith

Introduction

The high intensity use (HIU) programme has been developed over the past 10 years. It works one-to-one with thousands of individuals who all have two things in common: they access health care more often, or differently, than expected; and they need an alternative form of support, support that involves grit, determination, persistence, patience and bucketloads of heart!

The revolving door of doing the same thing—whether that be going to hospital or the GP many times or calling 999 on a regular basis—is frustrating for both the individual in need (clients) and the organisation offering help. People who access health care more often, or differently, than expected have a bad name both inside and outside of the NHS. You've heard words like 'manipulative' and phrases like 'they get a kick out of what they're doing'. Most of all, there is sense of futility: 'if you "fix" one of "them", they will only be replaced by another, so what's the point'. It's easy to understand the frustration. Clinicians work hard to qualify in a medical role so that we can help those with medical needs. We're sympathetic when we hear someone's sad story the first time, but with high users of health care their story can lose impact. At the second, third or even tenth time of telling we can become numb to their tragedies. The budgetary constraints we are all under only compound the frustration felt.

Frequent Attenders: Why and How?

When behaviours and actions become routine, clients can end up sleepwalking their way through interactions with services or support offered. This can easily lead to unconscious, automatic responses instead of really being aware of what we as an individual think, what we feel, what we do and the impact it's having on us. This can be equally true of organisations involved in clients' care who feel frustrated and helpless because the support they have to offer never seems to be enough.

Frustrations with frequent attenders to A&E or callers to 999 may result in reactions such as punishment, deterrence and shaming. Threats of prison or antisocial behaviour orders (ASBOs) or official letters setting out how much someone has cost the system—and, by implication, how little they contribute to society—are the hallmarks of how some people 'manage' high-intensity users.

While this approach gives vent to frustration it misses two important facts: they are people, and it doesn't work. Not for anyone, and not long term.

Listening

The origins of the HIU Programme came from within an ambulance service in 2012 where, as a frontline advanced paramedic, I saw the frustrations first-hand.

I decided to take my medical head off, put my coaching head on, and find out what people presenting to A&E and calling 999 repeatedly really need. I spent the next 6 months listening and asking questions, more listening and more questions, until the answers and the approach needed became clear. This led to the next decade of coaching and mentoring clients and workers in this space to fine-tune the approach and ultimately help those who call out an ambulance, visit the GP or go to hospital more than expected.

Responding

The fundamental principles of this approach are not to criminalise people for being in crisis, not to medicalise everything coming through medical front doors, and to use a profoundly human approach. NHS England (2022) has now adopted the approach and is rolling it out across the country, with over 60% of emergency departments with access to an HIU Programme—a community-based, assertive outreach service that serves pressured environments like hospitals, ambulance services and GP practices. Interestingly, the vast majority of HIU programmes are not actually based within these pressurised settings but within the community, or hosted by voluntary sector organisations.

Who Are the Client Group?

The short answer is—anyone!

'When I grow up, I want to be dependent on alcohol and suicidal'.

Said nobody; ever

It sounds obvious but people accessing health care frequently weren't made that way. Something has happened in their lives to leave them in a place where regularly calling the emergency services, going to hospital or visiting their doctor seems attractive. This could have been divorce, bereavement, unemployment or crippling anxiety.

Left alone, some people understand that a medical complaint attracts an immediate human response in a way that a social complaint does not. Going to hospital or to the GP may be the only time they feel that somebody is listening to them, and thus their cycle of high contact is established. People—who shall remain anonymous—on the receiving end of the HIU Programme and who spring to mind include someone who worked in a mental health hospital for 22 years, another who brought up three wonderful children, and a teacher at a school for disabled people: all honest, hard-working, generous human beings.

We all need a leg up at some point in our lives. Whether we hide away for weeks on end, lash out at people we care about the most, go on benders, drink prosecco every night and look down on those who drink cider to numb the pain, or go to A&E seeking solace and for the pain of living to stop. It's all the same stuff. It's a way of expressing ourselves the best way we know how, at a precise moment in time.

HIU Role Essentials

Although HIU has aspects of social prescribing to it, the programme doesn't base itself on endless referrals to already saturated services because when someone is drowning, it's not the time to teach them how to swim. To truly connect with others, we use the art of storytelling because it is stories that connect us. Do we really expect clients to open up their bag of memories from 1957 and talk about what's closest to them to a stranger, just because they have a lanyard on, not knowing who *we* really are? Stories, told well, have the ability to bring us to life, to remove the mask of who we pretend to be and provide the human element to a conversation—what is most personal is most universal.

People undertaking HIU lead roles need a well-developed emotional intelligence and have excellent negotiation skills. The role demands people who think and feel differently in order to relate to those people who think and feel differently.

When I was growing up, my mum read one poem to me over and over again—'The Invitation', by storyteller Oriah Mountain Dreamer.

A standout line in the poem reads:

'It doesn't interest me who you know or how you came to be here. I want to know if you will stand in the centre of the fire with me and not shrink back'.

The biggest skill, therefore, in a client-facing role of this nature is someone who is there for the client no matter what and can naturally awaken other people—the technical stuff we can learn. Those who can demonstrate a different approach recognising and building on people's strengths, not character flaws, will go far. Working with people who have difficult lives has almost exclusively been about removing disabling conditions—a method that doesn't work in isolation. Instead, what really does work is to create enabling conditions in which people can flourish.

Knowing the mistakes people have made in life doesn't interest me. These things separate us, label us, isolate us from others. Instead, imagine if we highlighted what **connects us**, sharing who we really are—what we like and don't like, on a human level.

Imagine if a person's care plan was replaced with a 'Take Noticeboard'. This would be mine....

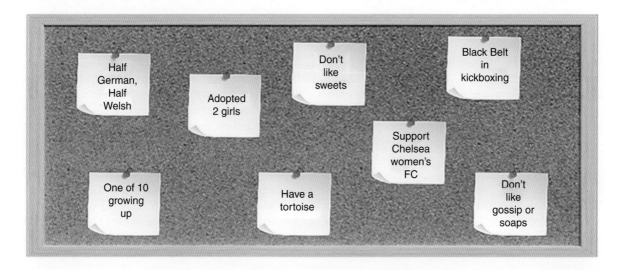

I'm sure you'd remember this more, long after you've finished this book.

So far, it may sound like I'm describing techniques used in motivational interviewing, and there are elements of that. However, people in crisis need something else. With others, I have developed a model that goes deeper and wider and teaches people *how* to change in a sustainable way, not just *what* to change, and to come off script when needed. It's called the Switch Model® (Think Outs, 2019; https://www.thinkouts.com/the-switch-model/).

It's not a group of 'them' and 'us'. There is only 'us and a crisis can happen to anyone, so the Switch Model® is designed for workers and clients alike.

Ten years on, the same tools and techniques—based on empathy, encouragement and compassion—have been used to sustainably reduce hospital attendances and admissions and 999 calls. In addition there have been reductions in GP contacts, mental health contacts and those made to overstretched call centres, both in the UK and abroad. The most important part is that people—often some of the most vulnerable in our society—have what they need to cope with life's twists and turns; worker burnout and overwhelm is staved off, keeping workers in position.

Conclusion

The HIU approach succeeds because it has kept its roots firmly in the ground while the information that informs it does so from the floor up. We haven't tried to figure this out from a distance. In this way it has the ability to constantly evolve in line with changing times and patterns of behaviour. The major strength of this approach is that it's not plagued by rigidity but based on some solid core principles that keep people moving forward so positive results are sustainable over time.

This way of connecting with people and affecting positive change is completely transferrable to environments and organisations where people 'do things more than or differently than expected (or needed)', including 999 frequent callers, complaints departments, GP practices and call centres.

REFERENCE

NHS England, 2022. High Intensity Use Programme. Available from https://www.england.nhs.uk/high-intensity-use-programme (Accessed 5 March 2023).

Policing Lens

Justin Srivastava and Helen Christmas

Introduction

Some of you may be asking: 'What is modern policing doing in a book about social prescribing? (And some of you may be officers and staff within policing itself.)' Our response to that is that there is more common ground than you may think.

Social prescribing is a holistic approach, recognising and seeking to meet a person's underlying need, rather than 'treating' a presenting problem. It recognises that the GP (or police officer…) a person is seeking help from might not be able to provide an answer within their own professional 'toolkit'—but they could look to ensure that a person can access an intervention or opportunity that's right for them.

Public health approaches in policing, or trauma-informed policing practice (The Scottish Institute for Policing Research, 2019), have a very similar focus starting with underlying causes not the outward-facing symptoms. Underpinning all of this is prevention.

Prevention

So, is prevention the policing hook? It does have a long policing history. In police training environments up and down the land you will hear talk about the Peelian Principles of Policing. Although these principles were adopted and first used in 1829, their timeless value continues today (Reith, 1956). But, most importantly, the first Peelian Principles of Policing were predicated on prevention, namely: 'To prevent crime and disorder, as an alternative to their repression by military force and severity of legal punishment' (Home Office, 2022). This prevention focus is as relevant today as it was then.

But prevention of what? Modern policing is complex (The Leadership Centre, 2022). It's not like some of the media portrayal of it, 'blue lights and pub fights'. National policing demand research has identified that over 80% of calls to the police are not directly about crime (College of Policing, 2015). Many of these are about complex social needs, vulnerability, mental health or social isolation. It is not uncommon for the police to receive emergency calls from community members who are socially isolated, maybe living alone with complex vulnerabilities, who are simply reaching out for someone to talk to. Whilst policing may attend such calls, it is often not the right response service with officers unable to offer appropriate resources to provide long-term support or problem solving.

There is clear evidence that noncrime demand is impacting on police resources; combined with cuts to other public services, this can result in unmet need and ultimately crisis situations. Her Majesty's Inspectorate of Constabulary and Fire and Rescue Services' report 'Policing of Mental Health: Picking up the Pieces' (HMICFRS, 2018) was direct in its language:

'. . .in our view, too many aspects of the broader mental health system are broken; the police are left to pick up the pieces. The fact that almost every police force now has its own mental health triage team indicates that there isn't nearly enough emphasis on early intervention and primary care to prevent the need for a crisis response'.

The report calls for collaboration across public services, for prevention and for early recognition of and response to people's holistic needs.

In a recent poll the public agreed and recognised that the police need to improve their ability to tackle the causes of demand (rather than managing the symptoms), which in turn requires the police to work more effectively as part of a wider system of public services (Crest Advisory, 2018). However, this is not common practice across policing (yet).

There are some excellent examples of pilot programmes involving integrated teams working together towards a common goal across the country. One such example is the Government investment of £28m in 2021 into Project Adder which is a new intensive approach to tackling drug misuse, combining targeted and tougher policing with enhanced treatment and recovery services. Project ADDER (which stands for Addiction, Diversion, Disruption, Enforcement and Recovery) will bring together partners including the police, local councils and health services (HM Government, 2022).

Causes of the Causes

Ask any police office or staff member, and whilst they may not mention public health approaches or social prescribing by name, they will talk about the need for society to tackle the underlying causes of the issues that they deal with every working day. This point was reinforced recently by the educationist Sir Michael Barber, when he reminded policing that the best way to reduce crime is to prevent it from happening in the first place (The Police Foundation, 2022). Thus, together as community and statutory partners we must address the societal needs of vulnerability, crime, people failing to thrive, poverty, violence, mental and physical health deterioration and the intergenerational cycle of trauma.

In recent years, policing has seen a growing drive to adopt a different approach—'a public heath approach' (College of Policing, 2022d). Importantly, this does not mean that policing is doing the job of public health, or vice versa. It is rather a way of combining different professional skills and perspectives to achieve better outcomes. By drawing on the strengths of other statutory agencies, the voluntary sector and, most importantly, communities, we can make our future generations stronger, safer and healthier (College of Policing, 2022c). This mirrors the NHS approach of 'Right Care, Right Place' (NHS England, 2022a) or, in common policing terminology, 'it's not all for us to do!'

Public health approaches, whilst different from traditional models of response policing which often focus on individuals and enforcement, build on police experiences of neighbourhood policing and problem-solving. Public health approaches in policing support the Policing Vision 2025, which talks about proactive preventative activity, working with partners to problem-solve, vulnerability, cohesive communities, improving data sharing, evidence-based practice and whole system approaches (Christmas and Srivastava, 2019).

The College of Policing recently developed a collection of Principles of a Public Health Approach to Policing (College of Policing, 2022b), and the first of these champions 'intervening early with at-risk groups to reduce the harm caused by the issue, including by promoting recovery and increasing resilience'. This sits comfortably alongside a social prescribing approach, a point well understood by Devon and Cornwall Police Domestic Abuse Behaviour Change Programme. This adopts a 'whole family' approach to reducing offending and harm by minimising the impact of adverse childhood experiences through early intervention and policing/health collaboration. Absolutely key is the multi-agency support that is put in place before criminal proceedings against the perpetrator begins. After a family is referred to the programme, the support involves deploying a children's resilience worker and a behaviour change independent domestic violence advocate, working with a perpetrator as part of the integrated offender management team (College of Policing, 2022).

There are many other fantastic examples of public health approaches in practice, most recently in the creation of violence reduction units (VRUs) which bring together police, local government, health and education professionals, community leaders and other key partners to ensure a multi-agency response to the identification of local drivers of serious violence and collaboration to take necessary action to tackle these (College of Policing, 2021; HM Government, 2020). This approach is strongly reinforced and promoted in the forthcoming Serious Violence Duty (HM Government, 2021). Again, these teams are bringing together different professional backgrounds and skills—recognising that no one sector can meet needs holistically.

Many of the same VRUs are often led by policing or the wider policing family (e.g., The Office of the Police and Crime Commissioner) and recognise, support and in some cases fund projects that fit within the social prescribing ethos, often with a strong focus on reachable and teachable moments across multiple settings. One such example is the A&E navigators who are now present in many UK hospitals, supporting patients with a violence-related injury by addressing changeable risk factors and promoting protective factors for violence involvement. The same navigators use techniques such as counselling, mentoring and/or referrals to community services to address psychosocial challenges, such as substance abuse or mental health concerns, and to support attitude and behaviour change (College of Policing, 2022a).

Police custody suites are arguably another setting where social prescribing methodology is utilised. This is a system well known to the 'DIVERT' coaches in Lancashire who are affiliated with local sports clubs and recognise that police custody can be a particularly low point in a young person's life. DIVERT coaches use this time as a teachable moment. They help to address the underlying social determinants and health inequalities prior to diverting young people into education, training and employment and have a genuine interest in each young adult they meet in an effort to start meaningful engagement and effective intervention (Lancashire Violence Reduction Network, 2020).

Challenges

Increased need and reduced capacity—whether in policing or primary care—make it harder to go the extra mile, to take the additional time to understand a person's story or to help them access the support they need to flourish. It's harder to evidence prevention and long-term outcomes than it is to evidence crisis response and a box ticked. There are worries that an overemphasis on enforcement at the expense of prevention and community engagement can be detrimental, a point made recently by The Police Foundation (2022) when it suggested that 'heavy-handed tactics and changes in policy … will inflict further damage on the relationship between the police and the community'. At the time of writing, the UK faces a long recession, public sector cuts and a significant increase in the number of people living in poverty. All of these may increase the pressure towards short-term crisis responses.

We cannot underestimate the potential for unintended consequences in our political and public desire for police to pursue enforcement—a point well made by the retired Chief Constable of Durham Constabulary Mike Barton (The Daily Express, 2022). In our policing efforts to do the bidding of the public through arrest and enforcement, we can create an environment where even more violent and cunning drug dealers replace the arrested ones. Thus, not only does society increase its ever-growing prison population, but it doesn't deal with the drivers of the drug market in the first place. As Mr Barton summised, we are never going to arrest our way out of the problem, and he called for a 'grown-up debate around drugs'. Taking this a step further, we would argue that this debate must and should include social prescribing and a true multi-agency public health approach to prevention by addressing the 'causes of the causes' of the drugs market.

Conclusion

So does policing have a role to play in social prescribing? The evidence would suggest 'absolutely', through the effective use of a public health approach seeing a shift to earlier intervention working collaboratively across the local system (National Police Chiefs Council, 2022). We need leadership at the front line in a way that traverses traditional service sectors. 'The 21st century public servant should be able to cross organisational boundaries' (Needham & Mangan, 2011). However, no one sector can do it alone. All agencies have a key responsibility to address the 'causes of the causes', and we need to design, adopt and deliver an effective national preventative strategy across all government departments and new police leadership models and adopt a public health approach across all of policing and its partner agencies. Recognition of shared values and approaches (NHS England, 2022b) such as the basic social prescribing premise of understanding and meeting someone's underlying needs—should enable us to collaborate to improve outcomes rather than try to shift 'demand' around the system. We cannot afford to work in organisational silos any more (NHS England, 2022b).

REFERENCES

Christmas, H., Srivastava, J., 2019. What is a Public Health Approach in Policing. College of Policing, London.

College of Policing, 2015. College of Policing analysis: Estimating Demand on the Police Service. College of Policing, London.

College of Policing, 2021. Policing and Health—Landscape Review 2021. College of Policing, London (Accessed 27 March 2024).

College of Policing, 2022a. Accident and emergency navigators. College of Policing. Available from: https://www.college.police.uk/research/crime-reduction-toolkit/accident-and-emergency-navigators (Accessed 25 April 2024).

College of Policing, 2022b. Principles of a Public Health Approach. Available from: https://assets.college.police.uk/s3fs-public/2021-02/principles-public-health-approach-to-policing.pdf#:~:text=A%20public%20health%20approach%20to%20policing%20uses%20the,approach%20involves%20

effective%20use%20of%20evidence%20and%20intelligence (Accessed 25 April 2024).

College of Policing, 2022c. Policing and health collaboration. College of Policing. Available from: https://assets.college.police.uk/s3fs-public/2021-09/policing-and-health-collaboration-landscape-review-2021.pdf (Accessed 25 April 2024).

College of Policing, 2022d. Our approach to public health. Available from: https://www.college.police.uk/about/public-health (Accessed 25 April 2024).

Crest Advisory, 2018. Rethinking Police Demand: A Review of Drivers, Capability and Capacity. Crest Advisory, London.

Her Majesty's Inspectorate of Constabulary and Fire and Rescue Services, 2018. Policing and Mental Health: Picking up the Pieces. https://assets-hmicfrs.justiceinspectorates.gov.uk/uploads/policing-and-mental-health-picking-up-the-pieces.pdf (Accessed 25 April 2024).

HM Government, 2021. Serious violence duty. Available from: https://www.gov.uk/government/consultations/serious-violence-duty (Accessed 25 April 2024).

HM Government, 2022. £148 million to cut drugs crime. Available from: https://www.gov.uk/government/news/148-million-to-cut-drugs-crime. (Gov.uk) (Accessed 25 April 2024).

HM Government, 2020. Violence reduction unit interim guidance. Available from: https://assets.publishing.service.gov.uk/government/uploads/system/uploads/attachment_data/file/876380/12VRU_Interim_Guidance_FINAL__003_2732020.pdf. (Gov.uk) (Accessed 25 April 2024).

Home Office, 2022. Definition of policing by consent. Available from: https://www.gov.uk/government/publications/policing-by-consent/definition-of-policing-by-consent. (Gov.uk) (Accessed 25 April 2024).

Lancashire Violence Reduction Network, 2020. Divert custody programme. What is Divert? Available from: https://assets.publishing.service.gov.uk/government/uploads/system/uploads/attachment_data/file/876380/12VRU_Interim_Guidance_FINAL__003_2732020.pdf (Accessed 25 April 2024).

National Police Chiefs Council, 2022. Police, health and social care consensus. Available from: https://news.npcc.police.uk/releases/policing-health-and-social-care-consensus (Accessed 25 April 2024).

Needham, C., Mangan, C., 2011. The 21st Century Public Servant. University of Birmingham, Birmingham.

NHS England, 2022a. Right care right place. Available from: https://www.nhsinform.scot/campaigns/right-care-right-place (Accessed 25 April 2024).

NHS England, 2022b. What is social prescribing? Available from: https://www.england.nhs.uk/personalisedcare/social-prescribing/ (Accessed 25 April 2024).

Reith, C., 1956. A New Study in Policing History. Oliver and Boyd, London.

The Daily Express, 2022. BBC QT: ex-chief constable makes heartbreaking confession on knife crime- 'Its my fault'. Available from: https://www.express.co.uk/news/uk/1232695/BBC-Question-Time-latest-news-knife-crime-london-murder-rate-updates-Brexit-mike-barton (Accessed 25 April 2024).

The Leadership Centre, 2022. Critical, tame, wicked problems. Messy and elegant solutions. Available from: https://www.leadershipcentre.org.uk/artofchangemaking/theory/critical-tame-and-wicked-problems/ (Accessed 25 April 2024).

The Police Foundation, 2022. Strategic review of policing. Police Foundation, London.

The Scottish Institute for Policing Research, 2019. Moving towards Trauma-Informed policing: an exploration of police officers attitudes and perceptions towards Adverse Childhood Experiences. SIPR, Edinburgh.

UK Fire Service Lens

Gerard Devereux

Introduction

Tackling fires and other emergencies will always be the primary focus of every Fire and Rescue Service (FRS), because unfortunate and unplanned things happen and we need a service that is capable and ready to respond when the fire station bell rings. That's what the fire service does. Thankfully, the number of fire call-outs has decreased over the years and remains relatively low, compared to other causes of premature death and serious injury. Nowadays, many FRSs attend more road traffic collisions than fires. In 2002, English FRSs attended 577,053 incidents, and of these incidents only 26% were fire related (Home Office, 2022a). Add to this the growing scope for a modern FRS to respond to an ever-increasing list of demands including climate events such as flooding, wildfires and extreme weather events, and you start to get the picture. FRSs do a lot more than putting out fires.

The Road to Prevention

At the heart of FRS prevention work is the practical advice and follow-up that services carry out in people's homes. This is where most fire fatalities occur, and it remains the primary focus for the sector's prevention efforts. The sector has a strong prevention story to tell, and it is rooted in the principles of social prescribing that place the individual at the centre of what we do to promote home fire safety, support independent living and promote the wider health and being of the individual.

During much of the 1980s, the focus of FRS prevention strategy in the home focussed largely on the premises themselves, and with good reason. In the late 1980s, half of the deaths caused by house fires occurred because people were already trapped by the time they realised there was a fire. In 1987, only 9% of homes in the United Kingdom had a smoke alarm (Department for Communities and Local Government, 2008). A new emphasis emerged recognising the need to act; government began to promote the use of smoke alarms in homes through a national campaign, which began in 1988. This new emphasis also coincided with advances in technology that made the alarms cheaper to produce and more affordable for people to buy. In 1991, the Smoke Detectors Act was passed, leading to all new homes being fitted with smoke detection systems. Now the emphasis shifted to a person-centred approach to promoting fire safety.

The pivotal moment in the change to a proactive prevention approach came with the publication of *In the Line of Fire* (Audit Commission, 1995). This report promoted a shift from cure toward prevention, recommending to Government that FRSs should be given statutory responsibility to promote fire safety, to educate the public about fire, its causes, its dangers and ways to combat it. The report also recommended removing the Government funding formula for FRSs that gave local fire authorities more funding based on the number of fires they dealt with. In practice, in the mid-1990s there was no financial incentive to carry out fire safety work. In fact, it was a disincentive, as they would receive less funding for reducing the number of fires in their community.

The direction of travel for FRSs was set, and the late 1990s saw an explosion of local prevention initiatives to promote fire safety in the home. However, approaches to prevention remained patchy across individual areas. Poorly evaluated, it lacked any national direction. It wasn't until 2002 and *The Future of the Fire Service: Reducing Risk, Saving Lives* report (Lyons et al., 2002) that the prevention aspect of FRSs became a recognised central function. This was formally adopted by Government as part of the Fire and Rescue Services Act 2004.

The immediate impact of the Fire and Rescue Services Act saw Government investing £25 million to support Home Fire Risk Visits (HFRVs). After 2 years of financial support, the Government's evaluation of HFRVs showed that this approach was effective and especially successful when FRSs partnered with other agencies, which was vital for reaching vulnerable people, supporting referrals and carrying out HFRVs.

In 2012, Sir Ken Knight, a former firefighter, was invited by the then Fire Minister the Rt Hon Brandon Lewis to review the progress FRSs had made and to consider future efficiencies and ways of working (Knight, 2013). The Facing the Future review found that many individual services had transformed themselves from organisations that primarily responded to emergencies into those that first looked to reduce risk. However, this came at a price, as there remained widespread duplication in the effort to design, commission, implement and evaluate FRS interventions such as HFSCs. The emergence of a new Inspectorate regime through His Majesty's Inspectorate for Constabulary and Fire and Rescue Services (HMICFRS) has further strengthened the drive to a standardised evidence-based approach to preventing fire in the home that has seen the emergence of the Person Centred Framework (PCF) for the HFSV, which has drawn heavily from a social prescribing model.

In 2015, the Chief Fire Officers Association (CFOA) signed a national consensus agreement with Public Health England (PHE), Age UK and the Local Government Association (LGA) to work together to encourage joint strategies for intelligence-led early intervention and prevention. This ensured that people with complex needs get the personalised, integrated care and support they need to live full lives, sustain their independence for longer and, in doing so, reduce preventable hospital admissions and avoidable winter pressures/deaths (Public Health England, 2015).

Yet—to the wider observer and indeed some in the sector—prevention still doesn't grab the headlines, even though in 2019 and 2020 the total number of Home Fire Safety Visits (HFSVs) conducted by FRSs and partners was 588,666 (Home Office, 2022b), and this was achieved as we emerged from COVID-19 restrictions.

The Person-Centred Framework has been developed by the National Fire Chiefs Council (NFCC) in consultation with UKFRS and has the support of the Home Office. The NFCC is the sector's membership body and supports individual FRSs to develop the services that are offered.

In the first State of Fire Report released in December 2019, Sir Thomas Windsor outlined the following scenario for FRSs:

'The long-term decrease in the number of fire incidents is due to many factors, including prevention work by services for which they deserve great credit. As a result of responding to fewer incidents, services have used their capacity in a range of different ways to support their local communities. This includes expanding the breadth of their prevention work'.

(His Majesty's Inspectorate for Constabulary and Fire and Rescue Services, 2019, p15)

Windsor also raises the prospect that the very image of the firefighter should be challenged. *'The role of the firefighter. Services have expanded the role into broader areas, in particular health and wellbeing'* (His Majesty's Inspectorate for Constabulary and Fire and Rescue Services, 2019, p 24). This reflects the changing nature of FRSs which have seen an ever-increasing realisation that prevention work should include risk reduction measures developed around the wider needs of the individual, not solely the type of premises in which they live. It also challenges the perceived role of the firefighter as simply responding to emergencies rather than an operational role that can prevent emergencies happening in the first place. This remains an area of some national and local debate, but increasingly operational staff are seen as being central to operating in partnership with other public sector bodies, voluntary and community sector groups and individuals to prevent emergencies occurring.

The Person-Centred Approach

At the heart of this approach is a strong link to social prescribing through partnership working to identify risk and practical onward referrals to further support for the individual whilst acknowledging their needs and wishes. Warm words about being patient or person centred need to be backed up by evidence-based advice and interventions that support the individual in meaningful ways that enrich their lives whilst keeping them safe. The evidence that we can derive from fire fatalities across the UK indicates that there are common and complex risk factors that cut across fire safety and wider health and wellbeing needs.

Health, wellbeing and care issues, when coupled with fires in the home, result in worse outcomes including a much higher likelihood of serious injuries and/or fatalities. An in-depth review of fire-related fatalities and severe casualties carried out incorporating data from 2010/11 to 2018/19 (Home Office, 2022c) found that the profile of fatal fires had remained consistent with previous research studies. These factors include multi-morbidity and frailty, cognitive impairment, smoking, drugs, alcohol, physical inactivity, obesity, loneliness and cold homes. Some of these factors, such as smoking, increase the likelihood of having a fire, and others, such as frailty, increase the likelihood of sustaining more serious injuries or fatalities as the ability to respond to a fire is limited.

The aim of the Home Fire Safety Visits is about responding to local risk profiling, including that of strategic partners, and then reducing risk and changing behaviour, not simply a checklist of questions to be asked.

'The Person Centred Home Fire Safety Visit should include risk reduction measures developed around the health, behaviour and wider needs of the individual; not solely the type of premises in which they reside. As it is these underlying causes that can increase an individual's exposure to fire and can also reduce the chances of them surviving a fire in the home'.

(*National Fire Chiefs Council Person Centred Framework Guidance, 2020*)

The NFCC believes that the adoption of an evidence-based person-centred approach which reflects the needs of our most vulnerable individuals and communities is the way to reduce incidents of fire and fire-related deaths in the home setting. This approach will ensure that the sector is targeting its prevention capability to benefit those individuals and communities that are most at risk of having a fire in their home.

This work is often undertaken in partnership with other agencies and has sometimes been confused as FRSs doing work on behalf of other agencies. However, at the core of all FRS prevention work is the explicit aim to reduce fire risk as a statutory function. This social model of prescribing often means that FRSs will work in tandem with health and social care services and other strategic partners. This will be jointly undertaken by the agencies/organisations involved, based on mutual risk profiling, and visits will be jointly undertaken to ensure that all aspects of an individual's needs are addressed. This is highlighted in this brief case study from Nottinghamshire FRS.

Nottinghamshire Fire Service Working With Occupational Therapists

A few FRSs directly employ an occupational therapist (OT) to work with them. Evidence has shown that the addition of the OT's knowledge of physical, sensory, cognitive and emotional difficulties in daily living provides a greater understanding of fire risk and allows complex cases to be managed more effectively. An evaluation of the impact demonstrates the financial savings accrued by employing an OT by Nottinghamshire FRS, estimated to be between £2.51 and £7.16 for every £1 invested (Fig. 25.1). This has led to a more integrated approach to multi-agency working and has introduced the professional approach of the OT and NHS concepts such as Making Every Contact Count (NHS England, 2016) to the wider FRS workforce.

From the FRS perspective, if services provide a person-centred HFSV, then the following characteristics should be evident:

- dignity, respect and compassion
- coordinated support
- personalised support

Individuals may have varying and increasing levels of fire risk based upon numerous and changing factors which can be categorised under three headings:

Person factors—which are integral to the person or people living in a property; things that are temporarily or permanently a part of them and cannot be changed, such as their level of mobility.

Behaviour factors—which are actions, activities or behaviours, things that people do (or don't do) such as smoking a cigarette, taking medication or substance use.

Home factors—which are factors that are integral to the home itself, or its contents (physical environment), or how the person interacts with others (social environment) such as the layout of the property and other people that occupy the property.

The Benefits...

Reduced number of fire service call outs

Reduced number of hospital admissions

Reduced number of referrals made to other services

Collaborative learning opportuinty

Stronger link between fire and health services

improve individual health and wellbeing

Reduced risk of death

Reduced risk of property damage

Improvement in public health: reduced risk of falls

Time saved looking for relevant information

Delay care home admissions

Reduced risk of emotional and physical suffering

NOTTINGHAMSHIRE
Fire & Rescue Service
Creating Safer Communities

Fig. 25.1 Nottinghamshire OT model. From Lauren Markham, 2018. Business case for continuing the employment of an occupational therapist within Nottingham Fire and Rescue Service. Unpublished Master's Thesis. Nottingham Trent University.

Fig. 25.2 illustrates how this approach may result in services, understanding which individuals represent a higher risk of having a fire in the home, and is the model that the NFCC adopted in 2018. The model also sets out strong inputs on risk stratification and referral and signposting to address the requirements of the individual.

Conclusion

As we face emergent challenges such as the recent pandemic or the current cost-of-living increases, we also need to re-evaluate how we can work in a collaborative manner to support individuals and local communities. The NFCC believes that at the core of FRS prevention work is the explicit aim to reduce fire risk, but to do this the individual or community must be at the centre of all that we do, and we must encourage FRSs to work in partnership with others to address the underlying causes of fire fatalities and injuries. It is this social prescribing model of care that will lead to increased fire safety and the promotion of the health and wellbeing of some of our most vulnerable individuals and communities.

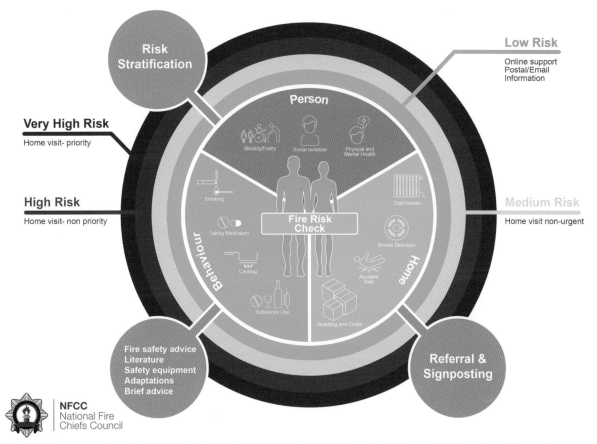

Fig. 25.2 The person-centred fire risk check. From National Fire Chiefs Council, 2020. Person Centred Framework Guidance. https://nfcc.org.uk/our-services/prevention/person-centred-framework/person-centred-framework-guidance/.

REFERENCES

Audit Commission, 1995. In the Line of Fire: Value for Money in the Fire Service—The National Picture.

Department for Communities and Local Government, 2008. Celebrating 20 years of fire prevention in the home. Available from: https://www.readkong.com/page/safer-houses-4029015 (Accessed 15 May 2024).

His Majesty's Inspectorate for Constabulary and Fire and Rescue Services, 2019. State of Fire and Rescue. The Annual Assessment of Fire and Rescue Services in England, p. 15, 24. Available from: https://hmicfrs.justiceinspectorates.gov.uk/publications/state-of-fire-and-rescue-annual-assessment-2019 (Accessed 20 March 2023).

Home Office, 2022a. Detailed analysis of fires attended by fire and rescue services in England, April 2021 to March 2022. Available from: https://www.gov.uk/government/statistics/detailed-analysis-of-fires-attended-by-fire-and-rescue-services-england-april-2021-to-march-2022/detailed-analysis-of-fires-attended-by-fire-and-rescue-services-england-april-2021-to-march-2022 (Accessed 10 March 2023).

Home Office, 2022b. Fire statistics data tables. Available from: https://www.gov.uk/government/statistical-data-sets/fire-statistics-data-tables (Accessed 20 March 2024).

Home Office, 2022c. An in-depth review of fire-related fatalities and severe casualties in England, 2010 –2018. Available from: https://www.gov.uk/government/publications/an-in-depth-review-of-fire-related-fatalities-and-severe-casualties-in-england-2010-to-201819 (Accessed 10 March 2023).

Knight, K., 2013. Facing the future; findings from the review of efficiencies and operations in fire and rescue authorities in England. Available from: https://assets.publishing.service.gov.uk/government/uploads/system/uploads/attachment_data/file/200092/FINAL_Facing_the_Future__3_md.pdf (Accessed 10 March 2023).

Lyons, M., Baines, G., & Young, A., 2002. The Bain Report: The Future of the Fire Service: reducing risk, saving lives. Office of the Deputy Prime Minister. https://webarchive.nationalarchives.gov.uk/ukgwa/20070506111045/http://www.communities.gov.uk/index.asp?id=1123804 (Accessed 15 May 2024).

National Fire Chiefs Council Person Centred Framework Guidance, 2020. Available from: https://nfcc.org.uk/our-services/prevention/person-centred-framework/person-centred-framework-guidance/ (Accessed 20 March 2024).

NHS England, 2016. Making ever contact count consensus statement. Available from: https://www.england.nhs.uk/publication/making-every-contact-count-mecc-consensus-statement/ (Accessed 10 March 2023).

Public Health England, 2015. Consensus statement on improving health and wellbeing. Available from: https://www.england.nhs.uk/wp-content/uploads/2015/09/joint-consens-statmnt.pdf (Accessed 10 March 2023).

Chapter 26

Housing, Health and Wellbeing: Perfect Partners

Noel Sharpe

'Our house, was our castle and our keep
Our house, in the middle of our street'
('Our House', Madness: November 1982)

Introduction

I suppose having a section on housing in the middle of a book on social prescribing and health may seem rather strange to some people. Really, what has housing got to do with health and wellbeing? Well, apparently a lot .... When Suggs and Madness sang about their house, in the middle of their street, they were locating their home within a wider community. A wider community (street) that was part of the sense of belonging somewhere, their house is place based, with the culture and idiosyncrasies of that particular community. This idea of housing families within communities underpins the key principles of modern-day social housing, recognising that health and wellbeing can often be improved by access to decent housing and thriving communities. Consequently, current housing providers (HPs) focus a significant amount of resources on the street/community/place within which social housing is located.

HPs recognised very early on that people rarely live in a vacuum. Whilst the house should provide shelter, warmth and security, it is also the place that people have a sense of belonging to something, their neighbourhood, community.

Housing Demand

There has always been demand for affordable rented housing, (House of Lords, 2022) and indeed altruistic philanthropists such as George Peabody and Joseph Rowntree began building social housing for workers in the Edwardian and Victorian period. These were some of the first Housing Associations and are still in existence today. However, social housing's first big breakthrough came in 1919 with Christopher Addison's Housing and Town Planning Act. The Addison Act made local councils responsible for assessing local housing needs and planning how to meet them. In response, councils began to build the first council housing (UK Parliament, online).

The Second World War brought devastation to many towns and cities across the UK. Consequently, the 1950s saw a marked increase in the amount of social housing being built, so much so that by the 1960s over a quarter of the UK's population lived in a council house (University of West England, 2008).

Investment, however, did not continue, and successive Housing Acts in 1980 and 1985 reduced house building by local authorities and decimated the numbers of social housing available to rent through schemes such as the Right to Buy (House of Lords Library, 2022).

Greater Manchester Housing Providers

Currently, housing providers across Greater Manchester provide over 264,000 homes for rent in the region, which equates to approximately 22% of housing stock in the region.

Greater Manchester Housing Providers (GMHP) is a unique partnership of 24 housing associations delivering housing and other services in the city region. One in every five households of GM live in a housing association home.

GMHP work collaboratively with GMHP, Greater Manchester Combined Authority and focus on housing as the key foundation to health creation and a good quality of life. The work of the GMHP is driven by the strategic commitments made in the Greater Manchester Tripartite Agreement (GMHP, 2021). The Agreement puts GMHP at the centre of long-term housing, health and placemaking strategy across the devolved city region.

Paul Dennett, Mayor of Salford and GMCA lead for housing, homelessness and infrastructure, states that the agreement

'will build on the unique involvement we have in Greater Manchester between our health and social care services, our housing providers and local government. … and now we will go further and faster in improving health, housing and quality of life'.

(GMHP, 2021)

More Than Just a Roof

Mayor Dennett's words illustrate how housing providers go beyond the usual landlord /tenant relationship to influence health and wellbeing (Box 26.1), including

- Sheltered housing for older tenants
- Support for people suffering mental health issues
- Supported tenancies for young people leaving care
- Support for women and girls experiencing domestic violence and perpetrators of violence
- Support and advice debt/benefits etc

BOX 26.1 ACHIEVEMENTS OF GMPH

In 2020/21 GMPH:
- Supported 7700 into employment and
- Supported customers to access an additional £22.3M in benefits and grants
- Created 594 new apprenticeships
- Provided advice and guidance to 4000 youths

From GMHP Online.

- Support to access employment and training.
- Support for people with addictions (alcohol/drug)
- Support to access Humanitarian Aid (food/energy/clothing etc)
- Community development to increase resilience within communities and develop peer support communities

Bolton—a Case in Point

Bolton at Home (BH) is a member of GMHP and exemplify the vital contribution to wellbeing and good health within their communities.

BH own, manage and maintain more than 18,000 homes across the Bolton borough. In terms of housing, they invest to improve the quality of properties for tenants and build new homes to give people the opportunity to live in a quality, affordable home.

However, the purpose goes far beyond bricks and mortar. BH tackle poverty with debt with money/benefits advice, support and deliver food and clothes initiatives and explore options to help people keep warm for less. BH also support tenants and residents into training and employment and deal with antisocial behaviour in Bolton's communities.

BH believe that if we want thriving and prosperous communities, then it is incumbent upon housing providers to invest in the tenants and residents living within those communities. BH currently invest just under £2M yearly to deliver thriving communities, including:

- community development support
- access to arts and cultural activities
- the provision of six Urban Care And Neighbourhood or UCAN centres, who provide advice and support in a wide variety of areas ranging from benefit/humanitarian support including pantries through to employment/unemployment support
- enabling local charities and grassroots groups to thrive through the provision of grants and funding and support through free use of community and UCAN centres
- access to employment and training opportunities

Together, we aim to build peer support networks that enable community and individual resilience. The difference we make is perhaps best seen via case studies (names changed).

Susan

Susan's story illustrates social prescribing in action via a partnership between BH and a GP practice. She first connected with the Arts on Prescription project when the social prescriber from her GP surgery made her aware of the lockdown craft packs from BH.

Pre-pandemic, health professionals at the surgery made referrals to the weekly Arts on Prescription group, supported by a BH Arts officer. During the pandemic, the home craft packs were a way to connect people through a common activity they could do safely at home alongside some online activities. Word of mouth and online engagement grew, and it is now an open access group for anyone with a health condition.

Susan suffered from mobility issues and her health deteriorated in 2019, leaving her unable to enjoy social activities. By the time lockdown restrictions ended, she had lost all her confidence and was completely isolated. It had been 3 years since she'd been out of the house; she felt like a prisoner in her own home. This led to her being incredibly anxious, and inactivity had badly affected her mobility.

When Susan received a call from Michelle, the Arts Officer overseeing the project, inviting her to the first in-person session, she panicked and told her she was housebound. Michelle arranged for her to receive some further art supplies and kept the relationship going by dropping them off for her. In a very caring and person-centred approach, as well as delivering bespoke craft packages, the officer offered to give Susan a lift to and from the session if she ever felt like she wanted to attend. Eventually Susan accepted the offer.

'Michelle picked me up and took me to the centre. Just having someone to walk in with and not facing it alone made a massive difference. The group were friendly and welcoming, and Laura (the group facilitator) was lovely. That little bit of extra support and encouragement was all I needed, and I've never looked back'.

Susan now attends weekly sessions of Arts on Prescription. Her confidence has grown so much that she

has started to access other community provision such as the luncheon club and the Wonder Women group, which is a group for women to come together, engage in activities and provide support for one another.

Susan is now a key member of many groups and provides support and encouragement for new members. She no longer feels lonely and isolated. Her mobility has improved and she feels far less anxious.

Bernadette the Peer Navigator

Peer navigators (PN) are salaried BH staff recruited from the neighbourhood they live in. They act to ensure members of their community can access local services and opportunities in a timely manner. They develop interest groups with local people; this not only offers individuals choice and ownership but also enables them to co-produce the opportunities. The support offer is wide ranging and goes beyond signposting and often includes:

- Ringing or messaging each week to remind and encourage individuals to attend a group
- Accompanying to a first appointment with a service
- Picking up or 'knocking on' on the way to a group session
- Signposting and referring but also encouraging and asking how things have gone
- Friendship, confidence building and positive encouragement
- Getting to know wider family including children
- Welcoming people who are new to the area

Bernadette, one of the first PN, described herself as being at an all-time low before starting her PN journey. She was unemployed, depressed, anxious and a regular 'Pantry' user, receiving weekly food parcels. Bernadette has lived in a Bolton at Home property all her life. She felt she knew everyone in her local community and was very aware of the local needs.

With some support from the Pantry staff, she applied for the 18-month PN post and was successful.

Throughout the role (fully supported by BH staff), Bernadette's confidence increased significantly.

'I built a great rapport and people wanted my help, as they knew I wouldn't judge, as I had experienced first-hand the problems we faced as a community'.

Bernadette became a role model for other residents. Her family and friends started attending activities and appointments and became far more active within their community in terms of attending and running groups of their own.

Local children and youths were more likely to attend community events and activities because they knew the people involved.

'My eldest boy would often tell me how proud he was of me'.

(Bernadette)

As a direct result of the peer navigator programme there was a significant increase in people having improved social networks, taking better care of themselves through healthy eating and regular exercise, being less anxious and generally feeling better about themselves. Through a women's group, the PN created a space where women could offload their worries and concerns, have a laugh and a cry. Bernadette's mum, who barely left the house due to severe depression, started attending regularly. At first she was coaxed into it but soon started to look forward to it and continued

to attend. Her mum even took on the ambassador role and brought others along after Bernadette's immediate support was no longer needed. She then went on to volunteer elsewhere independently. Others accessed courses after taster sessions organised by the PN, with some completing all three levels of a British Sign Language course.

Men in Sheds

Bill suffered with depression and was isolated, with no relatives living locally. After a redundancy leading to long-term unemployment, he became further isolated due to minimal contact with former colleagues. He started drinking heavily and was eventually admitted to hospital.

During his recovery Bill was engaged by a BH Community Development Officer and introduced to Willow Hey Men in Sheds (see Fig. 26.1). The Men in Sheds project is one of the many groups based at this thriving outdoor community growing site at the heart of a housing estate. The local community are supported to access a range of opportunities from woodworking, planting, crafting, cooking and eating together.

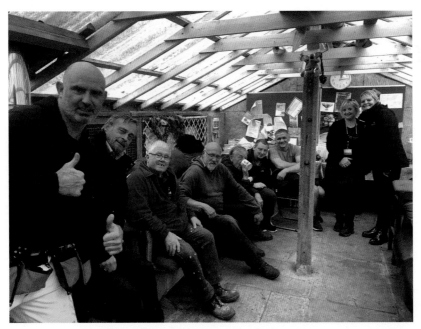

Fig. 26.1 Men in Sheds. (Image credit Bolton at Home.)

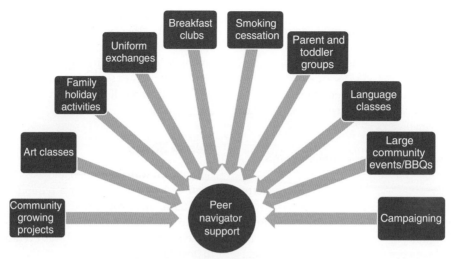

Fig. 26.2 Support offered via Bolton peer navigators.

The group gave Bill the space to share his endless creative and joinery skills with other project members. He has reconnected on both social and emotional/intellectual levels with other men, as in many instances men tend to communicate better about their feelings when working shoulder to shoulder. Bill now has a network of support. He helps to run the group as a committee member and treasurer, he has a trusted social network and he feels valued. He has since become a Bolton at Home 'Culture Champion' and delivers poetry sessions across the wider community.

Bill is one of the project advocates and actively promotes the benefits to other members of the community, especially men that are also isolated.

Bill's brother reflects that the project

'has probably saved his life by giving him purpose and a focus to his week—breaking up the monotony of daily life and reducing loneliness significantly'.

Outcomes

These brief case studies give only a limited impression of the impact of community-based activities delivered through housing associations. The improvement in health and wellbeing of participants is significant emotionally, psychologically and physically. Consequently, there is an overall improvement in quality of life.

The outcomes for first four PN recruited from one neighbourhood were extremely positive:

- One left to start a full-time post elsewhere.
- One applied for and was offered a post at Bolton at Home.
- One applied for and was offered a post with Bolton Council for Voluntary Services.
- One went on to do a full-time university degree in youth and community work.

Since beginning the PN programme, at least 2200 people have been offered practical support or signposted to a wide range of activities and services (Fig. 26.2).

Peer navigators work because they are local, activities are co-produced, they are trusted and they build and maintain resilience within communities and promote wellbeing and self-care.

Conclusion

Community-based activity, supported by our peer navigators, embodies the social prescribing approach. It encourages self-reliance, promotes joint endeavour, increases self-esteem and confidence and establishes community and individual resilience that can serve as a buffer against future crisis.

As Charlie Norman (CEO Mosscare St Vincent's Housing Provider and Chair of GM Housing Provider CEO Group) said,

'There is a very good reason why housing associations invest in people and communities. Not only is it the right thing to do, but it makes good and sound business sense too. By investing in customers, through health and wellbeing initiatives and supporting them to thrive within their communities, they are in turn more likely to be happier with their home, will keep and sustain their tenancy longer and contribute more to their wider neighbourhood. It is a win/win situation!'

Resources

Peabody Foundation. https://www.peabodygroup.org.uk/about-us/who-we-are/our-heritage/george-peabody.

Joseph Rowntree Foundation. https://www.jrf.org.uk/about-us/our-heritage.

REFERENCES

GMHP (Online). Our Impact. Available from: https://gmhousing.co.uk/about/our-impact/ (Accessed 21 March 2024).

Greater Manchester Housing Providers, 2021. Greater Manchester Tripartite Agreement. Available from: https://gmhousing.co.uk/tripartite-agreement/ (Accessed 17 January 2023).

House of Lords Built Environment Committee, 2022. Meeting Housing Demand. UK Parliament. https://committees.parliament.uk/publications/8354/documents/85292/default/ (Accessed 21 March 2024).

House of Lords Library, 2022. Right to buy: Past, present and future. Available from: https://lordslibrary.parliament.uk/right-to-buy-past-present-and-future/ (Accessed 17 January 2023).

Madness, 1982. Our House. https://www.madness.co.uk/songs/our-house/ (Accessed 21 March 2024).

UK Parliament (Online). Council housing. Available from: https://www.parliament.uk/about/living-heritage/transformingsociety/towncountry/towns/overview/councilhousing/ (Accessed 17 January 2023).

University of the West England, 2008. The history of council housing. Available from: https://fet.uwe.ac.uk/conweb/house_ages/council_housing/print.htm (Accessed 17 January 2023).

Chapter 27

Building Hope for a Better Future Fleetwood: A Small Town With a Big Heart

Mark Spencer

Introduction

Fleetwood, where I have practised as a GP for more than 30 years, is a small town of around 28,000 residents on the Lancashire coast, just to the north of Blackpool. As with many coastal communities across the country, Fleetwood faces significant challenges. What perhaps makes this town somewhat different, though, is how the community itself is being increasingly empowered to bring about positive changes through a programme called Healthier Fleetwood. Healthier Fleetwood's role is not to lead but to create an environment where residents can determine what's important to them, to ensure that somebody is listening and acting on their opinions and feedback, and to provide a forum for new ideas.

The programme is run by a partnership made up of organisations active in the Fleetwood community, including the NHS, local authorities, businesses, schools and the voluntary and faith sector. A 'spirit of a healthier Fleetwood' has seeped into the culture of the town as the way things are done.

In June 2022, Healthier Fleetwood was the proud recipient of the Queen's Award for Voluntary Service. Fleetwood is held up as an example of good practice in a report published in 2022 by the Institute of Health Equity (Marmot et al., 2022). The report states, 'Healthier Fleetwood is a ground-breaking approach and it is increasingly being recognised around the world for its willingness to listen and change practice, and for the difference these changes are making to the health and wellbeing of Fleetwood's residents'. One of the report's recommendations is to adopt the Fleetwood model to address the social determinants of health in primary care.

Why?

Fleetwood was a purpose-built new town dating back to the 1830s. Its purpose was to help construct the northern end of the west coast main railway line out of London. A newly built port would then ferry passengers further north by boat. A thriving fishing industry developed out of the port. Unfortunately, in the 1960s the railway station was closed and the line into Fleetwood decommissioned. During the 1960s and 1970s, the fishing industry was severely cut back as a consequence of the 'cod wars' between Iceland and the UK. The last deep-sea trawler left the town in 1982. The 'roll on, roll off' ferry service between Fleetwood and Northern Ireland ceased to operate in 2010, resulting in further significant loss of jobs. The nearby ICI chemical plant closed in the 1990s with thousands of further redundancies. All this left Fleetwood with not only poor transport links and high unemployment levels but also a complete loss of sense of purpose for the whole community. The town continued to decline over the next four decades, as did the health of the residents.

Fleetwood is now in the worst quintile nationally in terms of deprivation and poverty. Life expectancy and healthy life expectancy are significantly below the national average. There are very high prevalence rates for all long-term conditions, but especially mental illness, obesity and conditions associated with addiction.

The emotional health and wellbeing of children and youngsters are a particularly high priority for the town, not only because this is what the data tell us but also because this is what we hear from residents when ask, 'What matters to you?' Between April 2021 and March 2022, 147 Fleetwood children attended the paediatric A&E department of Blackpool Victoria Hospital due to significant risks associated with their mental health, including self-harm. There are similar statistics for adults with mental health and addiction issues.

Loneliness and isolation are often cited as important issues when we listen to adults and the elderly.

What's Hope Got To Do With It?

What I've noticed as a GP is what happens when people who are living chronically stressful lives begin to lose hope that things will ever get any better. People then start to take on habits that help them to get through yet another really bad day, but these habits are often harmful and self-destructive: alcohol, illicit and prescribed drugs, binge eating and smoking. Patients frequently say to me, 'Please don't tell me to stop smoking, it's the enjoyment I have in life'. The standard public health 'stop smoking' campaigns just don't work in these situations. Invariably people begin to isolate themselves, shutting themselves away in their own homes, not wanting to see anyone or do anything. People become less and less active, slowing down physically and mentally, becoming more sedentary, less and less motivated, day by day, month by month, year by year. In short, their physical and especially their mental health spirals downwards.

I vividly remember a consultation in 2015 which completely changed my own thinking about the importance of hope in people's lives. This was with a man in his mid-30s who had endured an abusive childhood. He'd begun drinking in his early teens in order to block out memories that he wanted to forget about but couldn't. As his drinking escalated, he developed severe alcohol-related liver disease. One day I said something to him that perhaps most doctors and nurses have said at one time or other: 'If you don't

stop drinking, it's going to kill you'. He replied, 'Doc, I know you're trying to help, but it's not the thought of dying that's stressing me out, it's the thought of living'. A few weeks after that he died.

A short while later I found myself sitting in a seminar at a conference listening to Hazel Stuteley, a retired health visitor who'd enabled residents to transform a downtrodden Cornish community. It was then that the 'how' started to become a little bit clearer.

Listen With an Open Mind, an Open Heart and an Open Will

Hazel had used her lived experience to work with colleagues at Exeter University to refine a community transformation approach called Connecting Communities (C2). In 2016, via my association with the Health Creation Alliance, formerly NHS Alliance, Hazel and the C2 team visited Fleetwood. They supported us through those early days of establishing Healthier Fleetwood, a resident-led social movement aimed at improving the health and wellbeing of each and every resident in the town.

At the heart of everything we do is actively listen to our residents. The email address listening@healthier-fleetwood.co.uk was chosen to reflect how we wanted residents to think of us. The main question is invariably 'What matters to you?' That conversation started 6 years ago and is ongoing. The very act of deeply listening will often create energy for change as local people start their own initiatives.

We hold a monthly 'residents connect meeting' led by residents, for residents. The topics discussed are the things that are important to residents, and everyone is encouraged to participate in their own time, within an environment of compassion and support. There are also informal drop-in sessions at places like the library and at our Healthier Fleetwood information session within the local shopping complex.

The main reason for health care professionals, local authority staff, housing association folk and others to attend the meetings is to actively listen in order to understand. This is really not as easy as it sounds. Clinicians listen all the time in the one-to-one situation in our consultation rooms. It's the very first thing that trainee GPs are taught. It's often cited as the main thing that strengthens the clinician/patient relationship:

'I trust my doctor/nurse because they listen to me'. However, put health care professionals and NHS managers in a room with residents, and the professionals will very quickly move into 'strategy' mode. They will start planning what 'the system' can do to fix the perceived problems in that community. Lots of very well-meaning organisations have come into Fleetwood in order to fix us. And you know what—nothing changes.

Connecting Our Community

'If Fleetwood were a giant dot to dot, then Healthier Fleetwood would be the pen'.

(Local resident)

Both C2 and the Health Creation Alliance (Chapter 11) say that to be well, people need three Cs: control, contact and confidence. If you visit Healthier Fleetwood or have a look at the website, you'll notice the strap line 'Connecting our community', one of the three Cs.

As social animals, we thrive when we're connected to other human beings, hence the health benefits, especially mentally. Connecting is ideally done in person by linking people into established groups or supporting the formation of new groups. We often notice that people will attend one group and then, becoming more self-confident, begin to attend other groups. They will then start contributing more at residents' meetings. One great example is an older gentleman whose wife passed away. He became more and more self-isolated. His only trip out was to walk to the corner shop to pick up his paper. Over time this walk took longer and longer as his walking pace became slower and slower. He described being hunched over, shuffling along. Eventually he stopped going out altogether and then spent all day, every day, on the sofa 'waiting to die', as he put it. His friend dragged him along to walking football. He spent the first few weeks as a spectator on the sideline, then he began kicking a ball about. Slowly he started joining in the games and a month or two later became team captain with a spring in his step and smile on his face. It was an absolute joy to see such a transformation.

This growing self-confidence will then result in increasing self-motivation and a desire to establish new groups of their own, or volunteer to help others setting up their group.

Healthier Fleetwood's role is to help create an environment where residents can take control of their health and wellbeing, as individuals and as a community. The support can vary but often starts with providing a forum to share ideas, seek support from others and deliver a valued project or group.

Tony had attended several of the monthly Healthier Fleetwood Open Meetings and had said he wanted to start a group for men to meet, chat and provide mutual support. Each time he spoke he was visibly growing in confidence until he announced he was starting a men's shed and invited others to join him. Two came to the first session, then five, then double figures, and the group quickly became a vital part of many men's lives, somewhere they could go for friendship without judgement and also signposting to other services and activities.

In these early weeks the Men's Shed Fleetwood was supported by several local organisations. Healthier Fleetwood assisted by holding funds they generated through donations until their bank account was open; we also designed and printed marketing material and acted as a sounding board for the group as they developed. Four years on, the Shedders are now a fully independent, registered charity led by a group of trustees all living and working in the town. They are an integral part of the local community.

The Men's Shed is now a registered charity, own their own premises and offer support to hundreds of men across the town. More recently women have become involved as well, and it continues to go from strength to strength. In my GP role, I now regularly encourage people who feel isolated, lonely, down and hopeless to call in at the Men's Shed.

Residents Debby, Victoria, Elaine and Diane came up with the idea for a community project called the Fleetwood Wellbeing Way, supported by Lancashire Mind. It's a walk along the promenade, marked at intervals with fun and interactive challenges based on the Five Ways to Wellbeing (Aked et al., 2008). They also attended Healthier Fleetwood's open meetings to share their vision and receive feedback from the community and get practical support until they were established. The group is now 2 years on, has a busy Facebook page, and we continue to work with them on themed campaigns to engage the community.

Fleetwood Beach Wheelchairs has been a fantastic success but also a great example of how sometimes it can be a slow and difficult path. Local resident Mick called into a Healthier Fleetwood drop-in as far back as October 2017. He wanted to bring a beach wheelchair service to the town and had the time and passion to lead the project but needed the support of others to drive it forward and make connections. We brought together the initial steering group and acted as accounts and marketing department until the group was ready to apply for charitable status, before launching with their first chair.

As we prepare to start the 2023 Summer Season, Fleetwood Beach Wheelchairs has their own premises, 10 specially designed chairs and a dedicated band of volunteers—an asset to the town both for local residents and visitors alike.

I can't overstate the importance of empowering people to do things for themselves rather than doing things for them or to them. It's simply being there to say, 'That's a great idea, go for it!' In helping to create this positive, connected environment for residents to take control of their lives and grow in confidence, Healthier Fleetwood works closely with the social prescribing team and allows them to focus on the one-to-one support of local residents.

So, What's All This Got To Do With Social Prescribing?

The NHS now formally supports social prescribing through the recently formed primary care networks and their employment of social prescribing link workers (SPLWs). Nationally, the role of the link worker is to take 'referrals' from health care professionals and then link 'patients' into social activities within their community. However, we seem to have medicalised a great idea and turned it into an NHS pathway whose activity in terms of 'patients' being 'put through' the pathway can be counted against targets. Somewhere along the line we seem to have missed some important fundamentals: listening, building trust and giving away control. That's where Healthier Fleetwood is different.

Some 'patients' are not ready to enter the 'social prescribing pathway'. Listening closely and building rapport and trust take some time and enable the listener to get an accurate understanding of what really matters to someone, not what *you* think matters. The whole process of knowing that they have been heard is empowering for people. This does not fit well with the rush to

get as many people as possible through social prescribing as quickly as possible. This undue haste can also be very de-motivating for the link worker themselves as 'patients' disengage from the process at an early stage.

Social prescribing reaches its true potential when professionals and system leaders feel out of, rather than in, control—one of the three Cs. Having actively listened, health care professionals, managers, local authority folk and others in leadership roles then need to work in equal partnership with residents to jointly deliver the changes that really make a difference.

Professional Wellbeing

Being an enthusiastic but small cog in a much larger Healthier Fleetwood Partnership has changed me as a human being and as a health care professional. Seven years ago, I was in my mid-50s and had been a GP for 25 years. Like many of my GP colleagues, I was completely burnt out and was ready to take early retirement. I was finding General Practice extremely stressful and had no hope that it was ever going to get any better. I'd reduced my clinical commitment to just 1 day per week and felt completely done. Seven years later, I'm thriving. I'm back up to full time, and even though General Practice is still extremely busy, I have the energy and motivation to continue to support my patients, the practice staff and the community as a whole.

Conclusion

When residents are actively listened to; when they are connected to each other and to those whose job it is to support them; when they have increasing self-confidence and are genuinely in control of their own health, their other own lives and their own community; then truly amazing things happen, both at an individual level and at a community level.

The Healthier Fleetwood approach is not only good for the health of residents; it's also good for the health and wellbeing of health care professionals. Given the difficulties that the NHS has in terms of recruitment and retention of doctors, nurses, therapists etc. at this time, perhaps not only listening to, and empowering, local communities but also listening to communities of professionals like me is one of the solutions for improved wellbeing to bear in mind.

Resources

Connecting Communities C2. Available from: https://www.c2connectingcommunities.co.uk/.

Healthier Fleetwood. Available from: https://www.healthierfleetwood.co.uk/partners.

REFERENCES

Aked, J., Marks, N., Cordon, C., Thompson, S., 2008. Five Ways to Well-being. New Economic Foundation, London. Available from: https://neweconomics.org/uploads/files/five-ways-to-wellbeing-1.pdf.

Marmot, M., Allen, J., Boyce, T., Goldblatt, P., Callaghan, O., 2022. A Hopeful Future: Equity and The Social Determinants of Health in Lancashire and Cumbria. Institute of Health Equity, London.

Chapter 28

London's Commitment to Social Prescribing

Tom Coffey

Introduction

I've been a GP in London for over 30 years, and in that time I've had to come to terms with an uncomfortable truth: medicine alone cannot solve every health problem.

In my time, I've seen medicine become more holistic. Health care is now about empowering patients to get more involved in their care while encouraging clinicians to treat the whole person and not just their symptoms. Social prescribing is part of that holistic approach to health. It recognises that many aspects of a person's life can affect their health and wellbeing—and things that can improve health are as likely to be found out in the community as they are in the doctor's surgery.

Case Studies

I've seen this with patients in my Tooting practice. Take Aisha, a 30-year-old primary school teacher who has been recently diagnosed with type 2 diabetes. She's on medication to manage her blood sugar, but her condition has also been helped by incorporating more exercise into her routine, having joined a community walking group. This is building her confidence to take a more active route to work. She's also joined a local cooking class to make changes to her diet, and the encouragement from people around her is keeping her on track.

Then there's 55-year-old Elias, who had been struggling with loneliness. The rising cost of living has meant he doesn't have much money for recreational activities, and visiting his family up north is nearly impossible these days. However, recently he linked up with a local creative group where he's made new friends, and he's also been connected to advice services for support with his finances. Elias and I are discussing reducing the dosage of his anxiety medication as his mood improves.

London's Commitment to Social Prescribing

Aisha's and Elias's experiences are echoed across the capital. They highlight the important role that social prescribing can play in improving lives and health. This is why we at City Hall have been eager to see social prescribing happening across London and being made available to all those who could benefit from it. And it's never been more important. With demand for health and social care services continuing to stretch our NHS and local government beyond capacity, we want to support and sustain approaches that help people to stay well. Here's how we're making it happen with social prescribing in London.

When Sadiq Khan became Mayor of London, he outlined his vision for a healthier, fairer city, in which all Londoners have the best opportunities to live a long life in good health. In my role as the Senior Health Advisor, I work closely with the mayor to identify our priorities for tackling London's stark health inequalities, and I've always felt that social prescribing could make a real difference. However, when I first joined City Hall, back in 2016, there was no national social prescribing programme. Despite some early adopters in London around that time, it was happening piecemeal across the city. This meant that far too many Londoners were missing out on an important opportunity to improve their health. Worryingly, these included some of our most vulnerable residents.

Unlocking Progress in London

Rather than wait for national action, the mayor set out to unlock progress in London. Working closely with the NHS's consultancy team, Healthy London Partnership[1], the mayor identified three keys: (1) establishing a strong London partnership with a shared commitment to social prescribing; (2) supporting and empowering the Voluntary, Community & Social Enterprise (VCSE) sector to play their vital role; and (3) taking a 'health in all policies' type approach to social prescribing—looking across all of the mayor's responsibilities and polices and thinking about where there were opportunities to support social prescribing, as a means of improving Londoner's health and tackling inequalities.

Let's start with the shared commitment. As I've already mentioned, the mayor is passionate about tackling unfairness and improving lives for all Londoners. London's Health Inequalities Strategy (Greater London Authority, 2018, updated 2021) is one of the most important tools the mayor has to address this. It outlines what he will do to tackle the social, financial and environmental barriers to good health in our city. It also provides a rallying call for collaborative working on some of London's greatest health inequalities challenges. Social prescribing is an important part of the mayor's strategy.

Five Principles

Delivering a social prescribing system that links Londoners into the wide range of support that can help them to live healthier lives requires close collaboration between different agencies and sectors. Therefore, it was crucial to bring a range of organisations around the table to develop our London approach. In 2018, the mayor and Healthy London Partnership convened the London Social Prescribing Advisory Group—bringing together the NHS, primary care, local authorities, public health

and, vitally, the VCSE—to design London's approach and set out our priorities. Together we published 'Next Steps for Social Prescribing' (Greater London Authority, Healthy London Partnership and The Social Prescribing Network, 2019), setting out five principles to underpin our work to build the best social prescribing system for the capital:

- Available for all—ensuring activities reflect the needs and priorities of communities
- Easy access—activities available through a range of channels
- A localised system—that allows collaboration between commissioners, the VCSE sector and Londoners
- A vibrant VCSE—that is regarded as an equal partner in the design and delivery of services, is adequately funded and has the necessary tools
- A supported workforce—ensuring that social prescribing link workers and volunteers receive the training and support that they need.

A Regional Approach to a National Plan

This groundwork meant that by 2019, when NHS England launched its ambitious Long Term Plan, we already had a regional approach to complement the national one. Under the Long Term Plan, social prescribing would be rolled out, establishing over 1000 trained social prescribing link workers across England by the end of 2020–2021. Working in partnership, we made sure that social prescribing was embedded in NHS London plans, and that social prescribing link workers—the glue that holds the system together—were being supported as their roles developed.

The national plan fitted well with our London approach, but something quite vital was missing— the VCSE. This was something our London Advisory Group, working closely with the wider VCSE sector, had identified; the sector was massively exposed to risk, and they needed our support. That's why coordinating and empowering the VCSE sector were the second key to unlocking social prescribing in London. Without a strong and vibrant VCSE, social prescribing simply does not work. The VCSE sector provides the community services, support and activities that link workers refer to, and people—like my patients, Aisha and Elias—depend on. They're also deeply connected

---

[1]Healthy London Partnership merged with health care consulting to become Transformation Partners in Heath and Care in 2023. HLP/TPHC is a joint citywide transformation unit that brings together a wide range of innovative partnerships to make progress on London's specific population health challenges to make London the healthiest global city.

to London's diverse communities, reaching people that public sector organisations often fail to.

Supporting the Voluntary and Community Sector

Therefore, in 2019 the mayor committed to funding a social prescribing network for VCSE organisations. London Plus was invited to run the network, building on their role as an umbrella organisation championing and supporting London's charities and community groups. The London network is unique in the UK. It raises awareness of the vital role of the VCSE in social prescribing and builds capacity in the sector, providing networking, peer support, training and learning opportunities for its 400 (and increasing) members. Crucially, by bringing together VCSE organisations, it helps to amplify their voices, and the voices of Londoners, in conversations about shaping and resourcing social prescribing.

This is important, as while the NHS is funded to deliver social prescribing and resource link workers, this resource does not extend to funding the services and activities provided in communities. With the cost-of-living crisis creating further pressures, sustainability of the sector remains an urgent concern for social prescribing. The way new integrated care systems work with the VCSE will provide both challenges and opportunities here.

Taking a 'Health in All Policies' Approach

The third key to unlocking social prescribing in London lies in the mayor's 'health in all policies' approach. London has so much going for it—world-class arts and culture, stunning green spaces and an excellent public transport system. All of these things can play a role in improving people's health. That's why the mayor has sought to identify where social prescribing might be able to help improve access to such opportunities.

Arts and culture can provide a route to happier, healthier and more fulfilling lives by helping us reconnect with our senses, body and mind. Over the past 3 years, the mayor has been exploring how to hardwire social prescribing of arts and culture in London. For example, in 2020 Merton and Southwark received funding from the mayor, Healthy London Partnership, and Arts Council England to pilot six art-based social prescribing programmes. The funding supported training for primary care and link workers, small group art sessions, drop-in drama groups and therapeutic creative writing sessions for people in south London. The pilot was a success in opening referral routes and building understanding between culture and health sectors. It supported over 150 Londoners across both boroughs, many of whom couldn't leave their homes due to COVID, and helped them to stay connected to others in their community.

Another example is improving access to social welfare and legal advice services. Many people struggle to do what's best for their health as they are battling other challenges in their life. While a GP has limited tools to support a patient who is grappling with financial or housing problems, social prescribing can provide avenues to support. The mayor has been investing in London's link workers by providing social welfare legal advice training, as well as further specialist National Vocational Qualification (NVQ) learning. This enables link workers to help Londoners with these issues. The mayor is also working to improve access to advice in other community settings, such as schools and community centres. Services like these have helped people, like my patient Elias, to navigate complex systems so that they can understand their rights and make informed decisions. This reduces financial strain and can increase a person's overall sense of security and wellbeing.

These are just some snapshots of the fantastic work that has been happening in London to build and strengthen social prescribing. And there is more to come. At the time of writing, London's five Integrated Care Systems are mapping out their approach to social prescribing for the future. Meanwhile the mayor continues to support the VCSE sector through the network, helping them to further enhance their collective voice, build capacity and take a lead role.

Conclusion

It really is amazing how much has changed in London since we first made the commitment to social prescribing in the 2018 London Health Inequalities Strategy. Things have certainly moved further and faster than I imagined when I spoke at a King's Fund event in 2018. Back then I said we would need 10 years to get going in London. Look what we accomplished in 5! With the continuing commitment and collaboration which has underpinned our work in London to date, I'm excited to think about what we can achieve together in the next 5 years.

REFERENCES

Greater London Authority, 2018. The London health inequalities strategy. Available from: https://www.london.gov.uk/sites/default/files/health_strategy_2018_low_res_fa1.pdf (Accessed 20 March 2023).

Greater London Authority, Healthy London Partnership and The Social Prescribing Network, 2019. Next steps for social prescribing in London. Available from: https://www.london.gov.uk/sites/default/files/social_prescribing_next_steps_document.pdf (Accessed 16 March 2023).

Greater London Authority, 2021. London's health inequalities strategy. Available from: https://www.london.gov.uk/programmes-strategies/health-and-wellbeing/health-inequalities/london-health-inequalities-strategy (Accessed 20 March 2023).

Chapter 29

Summary Section 4 Practice

Heather Henry

Despite extensive guidance developed by the NHS and the National Academy of Social Prescribing, the ways that social prescribing is now being delivered over the last few years in the UK and beyond are many and varied. Before we begin our analysis of the practice outlined from the contributors in this section, we perhaps need to examine the ways that social prescribing models may be designed.

Models of Social Prescribing

Perhaps the most well-quoted review of social prescribing models was by Kimberlee (2013) and focused on primary care and mental health predominantly. He identified three models and proposed that models became increasingly holistic over time.

Light
- Refer at-risk or vulnerable patients to a specific programme to address a specific need or to encourage a patient to reach a specific objective, e.g. exercise on prescription

Medium
- Health assessment by a facilitator and advice on lifestyle issues
- Advice on the promotion of self-care
- Signposts to voluntary organisations or self-help groups for a specific issue

Holistic
- A clear GP/primary care referral process
- Locally delivered with supporting organisations
- A jointly developed intervention which has been sustained over time
- A method to address beneficiary needs in a holistic way

- No limits to the amount of time a health facilitator/worker/officer spends with a referred beneficiary
- Addresses beneficiary wellbeing but anticipates that mental health needs may also be discovered

Oster et al. (2023) recently undertook a scoping review of the types of social prescribing models. They found significant variation in design and delivery and also commented that the articulation of specific models could be indistinct, making it difficult for decision-makers, keen to develop or refine a local model, to draw on. Instead, the authors drew out from the scoping review six key aspects to consider when designing a social prescribing model (Table 29.1) and options for delivery (Fig. 29.1).

A blind spot in Oster et al.'s scoping is that it stops at referrals to non-medical services and does not describe the community building that is necessary for this to succeed. So the development of any social prescribing model needs to consider and plan for this—something that we met in Chapter 20 with the community-enhanced social prescribing model.

A Continuum of Support

Oster et al. invites leaders to identify the generic/specific population and general/specific needs, but as we have seen from previous chapters, there is more to it than that: Primary care networks and integrated care system leaders also need to consider how they will progress from a purely biomedical model to one that recognises people and communities' agency and strengths and is more relational and builds community capability rather than foster dependency on services. As we have seen, this requires, on the one hand, traditional 'looking after' skills when this is required,

TABLE 29.1   Planning Stages and Decision-Making Options for Social Prescribing Model

1) which population(s) they will target
   a. general population: broad reach to capture all those potentially affected by non-medical needs
   b. specific population: e.g. relating to diagnosis, health behaviour (e.g. smoking, physical activity), or specific at-risk population with specific non-medical needs
2) which non-medical needs will be addressed
   a. general non-medical needs: encompassing the wide range of social determinants and behavioural health
   b. specific non-medical needs: e.g. sedentary lifestyle, homelessness, food insecurity, etc.
3) how supports and services will be identified
   a. personal knowledge (of link worker/other role)
   b. service mapping
4) where the program will be delivered
   a. health care
   b. community
   c. online
   d. mixed
5) how the program will be staffed
   a. existing staff (health/social services/community-based organisation)
   b. new link worker staff
   c. volunteer/student link workers
   d. training required:
      i. training to use the system
      ii. training deliver interventions, such as motivational interviewing
6) how it will be funded
   a. government funding
   b. charity
   c. other funding sources
   d. embed within existing services/funding

From Oster, C., Skelton, C., Leibbrandt, R., Hines, S., 2023. Models of social prescribing to address non-medical needs in adults: a scoping review. BMC Health Serv. Res. 23, 642. https://doi.org/10.1186/s12913-023-09650-x.

such as intervening with medications and treatments, and 'letting go' skills. This suggests a continuum of support from care and clinical intervention to wellbeing (Fig. 29.2). An empowered community can help leaders to join up care and even prevent care from being needed by creating social value that can support levelling up (Fell, 2022). A radical power shift, supported by confidence in citizens and investment of resources, is at the very heart of building individual and community capabilities.

Interpretations of Social Prescribing in Practice

So, what do our contributors offer to this analysis, based on their professional practice? Some services have a long history of identifying non-medical issues and connecting them to assets in the community as part of their work, although they may not refer to these activities as 'social prescribing' and may therefore not be identified in academic reviews. Let's look at some examples.

Community Nursing

Historically, community nurses, and especially health visitors, have taken an active role in both signposting and community building itself, perhaps acting as convenors: bringing together the assets of a community in new and useful ways. They have been mapping the local assets as part of their community profiles and connecting their patients to these assets for decades. A recent example of community building comes from district nursing and is reminiscent of the Buurtzorg self-managing teams model described by Brendan Martin in Chapter 23. Here Sarah Everett, a district nurse from Govan, Glasgow, identified that men's social isolation is an issue and has helped them to set up a men's shed—a space where they could come together to do practical activities (Allen, 2019). For this, Sarah was awarded the much-deserved title of 'nurse of the year'. But for seasoned observers, this is an example of what community nurses used to do before the levels of demand forced their practice to become more transactional. For example, two decades ago a district nurse called Ellie Lindsay established the Lindsay Leg Club® movement (Lindsay, 2004) where isolated people with leg ulcers come together in a social environment to have their wounds dressed and receive education and information. The model involves nurses, patients and local community collaborating as partners in the provision of holistic care. Branches of Lindsay Leg Club® have now proliferated across the UK and beyond.

Allied Health Professionals

Meanwhile, Linda Hindle (Chapter 24) helps us to expand our minds about how allied health professionals

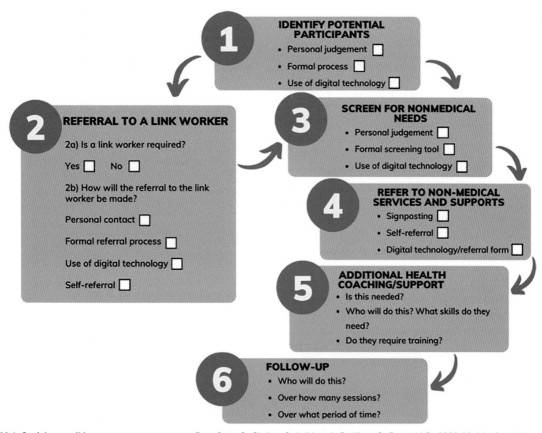

Fig. 29.1 Social prescribing programme processes. From Oster, C., Skelton, C., Leibbrandt, R., Hines, S., Bonevski, B., 2023. Models of social prescribing to address non-medical needs in adults: a scoping review. BMC Health Serv. Res. 23, 642.

Pathogenic practice:		Salutogenic practice
Medical model	⟷	Social model
Health	⟷	Wellbeing
Acute	⟷	Long term
Needs	⟷	Capabilities
Doing to	⟷	Doing with
Disease	⟷	Wellbeing
Directive	⟷	Distributive
Help	⟷	Ask for help
Deficit-based	⟷	Asset-based

Fig. 29.2 The continuum between an asset-based and deficit-based practice. From Henry, H., Howarth, M., 2018. An overview of using an asset-based approach to nursing. J. Gen. Pract. Nurs. 4 (4), 61–66.

are working. They not only offer holistic assessments and signpost people to community assets but also act as community assets in a holistic and multidisciplinary way, with dieticians helping with community cookery classes, for example.

Hindle also makes the important point about how social prescribing reduces the impact on the environment by reducing the need for carbon-intensive heath care: travel to appointments, heating and lighting, transport of goods etc.

Local Authorities and Social Work

Social work too has a jagged social prescribing history. The Barclay Report (Barclay, 1982) was a report on the roles and tasks of social workers in England and Wales. It was commissioned by the government and produced by a working party chaired by Sir Peter Barclay. The report recommended that social workers should focus more on community engagement and act as brokers of resources for people in need, rather than providing direct services. The Conservative government of the day, led by Margaret Thatcher, largely ignored the report because the policy was to reduce public spending and focus on individual responsibility.

Community-based social work, however, has received increasing focus in both central and local government with the introduction of local strategic partnerships and area agreements. Before the recent introduction of integrated care systems, it was local authorities who have been taking up the cudgels, by recognising and investing in enhancing 'community power' (Dabbs, Chapter 9). The 'Wigan Deal' is a classic example of this (Naylor and Wellings, 2019). Since 2011, Wigan Council has embarked on a major process of empowering communities through a citizen-led approach. This involves asset transfer to community groups and investment in community-led schemes. Over 1000 social work and other council staff have been retrained to offer a 'different conversation' with residents that focuses on identifying skills, interests and talents rather than problems and needs (Wigan Council, 2016). This echoes the NHS mantra of 'what matters to you' but goes further by empowering and investing in what matters to communities rather than just leaving community building to chance.

Political Mayors

Political mayors across the UK, such as in Greater Manchester, Birmingham and London, have also been quick to recognise the potential of social prescribing. GP Tom Coffey (Chapter 28) supported London's Mayor Sadiq Khan to instigate social prescribing long before the NHS Long Term Plan, as a way to help tackle health inequalities. This was no doubt bolstered by his contemporaries' success with initiatives like the well-known Bromley-by Bow centre (https://www.bbbc.org.uk/) where fellow GP Sam Everington and his partners work alongside other public services, voluntary organisations and local people to develop new initiatives to improve wellbeing.

Critically, London's City Hall instituted a 'health in all policies' approach. This sort of joined-up government has been championed by MP and former shadow health secretary Jonathon Ashworth, who, until recently, was shadow work and pensions secretary. From this position, Ashworth sees the value of health in employment strategy, such as providing young people with support for depression, stress and anxiety to help them into work, saying, 'If young people are not in education or training, and don't feel they can make a contribution because of mental health problems, we're at risk of writing off a whole generation' (Elgot, 2023).

Wider Determinants of Health

For leaders representing the social determinants of health, like housing, fire and rescue, and policing, social prescribing makes sound business sense (Sharpe, Chapter 26; Srivastava, Christmas and Devereux, Chapter 25).

Working alongside communities to improve their wellbeing will enable housing, policing and fire and rescue services to be more successful in, for example, helping people to maintain their tenancies or to reduce the risk of offending or fires. Some of these leaders may be well embedded within the local integrated care systems that are developing their social prescribing systems. Others may be working in parallel, or trying to find a way in.

Organisations such as The Health Creation Alliance, for example, in its previous guise as New NHS Alliance, have been promoting housing's contribution to wellbeing in the NHS for many years. One of the barriers to involving housing is the evidence that their contribution matters (Simpson et al., 2016a). The Alliance developed a guide for how the housing sector—or indeed other sectors—could set out its business case to persuade the NHS to view them as equal partners in wellbeing (Simpson et al., 2016b), including the economic case (Simpson et al., 2016c).

For blue light services, the social prescribing vision is much more about public health interventions and prevention, by identifying the causes of social distress and acting early to mitigate their effects on wellbeing. This begs the question as to whether health and care leaders similarly have the capacity and the cultural agility to do likewise.

Good and Bad Help

So far we have looked at the mechanics of signposting people to community assets to support their wellbeing and the actual competencies of social prescribing link workers that are set out nationally. But there is a subtlety to the form of help that is effective. In 2018, the social innovation think tank NESTA published guidance on what 'good help' looks like.

Some help—what we call 'good help'—supports people to feel hopeful, identify their own purpose and confidently take action. Other help—which we call 'bad help'—does the opposite, undermining people's confidence, sense of purpose and independence.

Good and bad help: How purpose and confidence transform lives

(Wilson et al., 2018)

'Bad' help is determined by others, who tell you what to do, who undermine your own agency. When we look at Felicity Thomas' description of how people with mental distress are supported in general practice (Chapter 22), this is an example of bad help—not being listened to and being offered a prescription for anti-depressants. Another example comes from Rhian Monteith's account (Chapter 25) of how high-intensity users can be treated with punishments, deterrence and shaming.

NESTA identifies three critical factors that enable people to take action:

1) Identifying and achieving a sense of purpose
2) Having the confidence to act by witnessing the success of others, or by personally achieving some success, being supported and encouraged and feeling positive when you feel yourself moving forward
3) Overcoming barriers in our life circumstances

They also identify seven characteristics of good help:

1) Power sharing rather than directing people
2) Having enabling conversations about what matters to the person

3) Helping people to identify their own personal goals
4) Offering a scaffold where practitioners gradually step back to enable people to build their own confidence
5) Offering role models who can offer peer support
6) Making opportunities for people to take action—facilitating introductions or bringing in external sources of help
7) Professionals sharing information about the people that they are helping with those people rather than gatekeeping it.

Many of these characteristics overlap with not only link worker competencies but also with many of the ideas previously identified, such as community power (Chapter 9) health creation (Chapter 11) and relational welfare (Chapter 12).

Self-Managing Teams

Much of this bad help stems from the current pressures on primary care, acknowledged by health professionals and citizens alike (Chapter 22). The Buurtzorg model of Dutch district nursing, identified by Brendan Martin in Chapter 23, gives us hope that, by empowering staff to be self-managing and to take their own decisions, this can be great for wellbeing as well as great for the public purse. By employing experienced nurses, the higher care costs per hour per patient is offset by fewer hours needed in total—a reduction of up to 50%. Overhead costs are halved, and client satisfaction is more than doubled (Nandram, 2014).

There have been many places across the UK that have tried to implement the Buurtzorg model, most notably Guy's and St. Thomas' NHS Foundation Trust (Hamm and Glynn-Jones, 2019). But there are reports that Buurtzorg is a poor cultural fit within a UK NHS context. The model relies on trust in staff and goes against the hierarchy 'written in the DNA' of UK nursing (Maybin, 2019; Taylor, 2021). Perhaps this is why Buurtzorg has struggled to succeed so far. But if social prescribing can be the start of a pivot in the NHS as a whole, can Buurtzorg offer a model for a new cultural pivot within community nursing?

Kindness

The Carnegie Trust have for many years been working on how kindness represents a 'blind spot' in public policy because of the relentless focus on a rational, evidence-based approach. 'Fairness', for example, may clash with 'personal'. Social prescribing link workers require all the human, emotional and relational capabilities characterised by the kindness shown by a link worker descended from the Windrush generation (Chapter 21), neighbourhood nurses (Chapter 23), paramedics supporting high-intensity users (Chapter 25), arts officers and peer navigators in housing associations (Chapter 26) and a GP supporting an unloved coastal community (Chapter 27).

Julia Unwin, who conducted research into kindness in public policy for Carnegie UK (2018), says that there are two lexicons: the 'rational lexicon' of management and the 'relational lexicon' of connects and relationships. Kindness breaks down barriers and shows that you care. To be successful in overcoming society's challenges, says Unwin, we need to become 'bilingual' in both rationality and relationships. Perhaps the closest we get to the language of kindness in health policy is compassionate leadership, characterised by paying attention to another person, understanding their distress, having empathy and helping others in a thoughtful and appropriate way (Atkins and Parker, 2012).

Compassionate Communities

This leads us to the idea that social prescribing can benefit from the development of 'compassionate communities'; where community-led partnerships of local people and services work together to support people at the end of their lives, driven by an overriding ethos of compassion. This has now become a social movement, supported by a VCSE organisation called Compassionate Communities UK (https://compassionate-communitiesuk.co.uk/). This charity supports many communities across the UK, offering civic engagement and community development, public education and changes to the social and policy environment. In Inverclyde, for example, community members deliver 'back home boxes' to frail elderly people being discharged from hospital (Compassionate Inverclyde, online). This is the sort of civic initiative that might emerge after identifying a need for palliative care, as part of a community-enhanced social prescribing model.

Cultural Competency

Linked to this idea of kindness and good help is the ability of a link worker to understand and respond appropriately to community suffering. In Chapter 21, Gay Palmer eloquently explores the experience of the Caribbean and African community. She describes a community that has experienced trauma that has resulted in an alienation between citizens and the state and mirrors the one described by Darren McGarvey (2021) in his book, *The Social Distance Between Us*, where working-class Glaswegians were vilified and victimised by the police. Trauma and adversity are very common: almost half of children and young people living in the UK have experienced one or more forms of adversity (Young Minds, online). Thus is it important that health and care staff and relevant community organisations have knowledge of trauma-informed practice. In an interview with the Health Foundation (2022), Jacqui Dyer, a black community leader and councillor in London, said:

'I think some of my communities are very much aware of the systemic discrimination and systemic oppression that they are living through and would source some of that impact on their health, particularly in the context of mental health'.

The National Academy of Social Prescribing (NASP) commissioned research into why people from Black, Asian and ethnically diverse population groups are under-represented in social prescribing (Tierney et al., 2022). They concluded that there is very little evidence to explain it, but from the very limited evidence that they found, they discovered that it may be about:

- Communicating and building awareness of social prescribing
- Cultural expectations, such as that it may not be appropriate to ask for help outside the family
- Building connections and trust with community leaders
- Identifying with those providing social prescribing so they feel welcome and understood

- Reaching out into communities by offering local venues meeting the diverse needs of difference communities

Clearly there is a lot of work that needs to be done with some communities to rebuild trust, understanding and relationships so that social prescribing can succeed in some minority ethnic and hard-pressed communities. This begs the question of who the best people are to be employed as community link workers. It is perhaps those that understand the citizen experience and to whom citizens can relate. Palmer exudes cultural competency—that innate ability to understand, interpret and respond. This is an essential part of the job description and person specification developed by the NHS (NHS England, 2023). But it also requires that system leaders understand this alienation and the social history of the community that goes alongside it so that they can build it into their planning. Palmer not only addresses the social distance but is able to advise decision-makers on how to proceed. Another example here is Fleetwood GP Mark Spencer who goes out of his way to meet the community on their turf and listen to their experiences. This is a lesson to all—but one that may not be heeded unless frontline staff and the people they support have a way to express what they see and hear to system leaders.

Pressures on the VCSE Sector

The resourcing of social prescribing described by both Jopling (Chapter 18) and Coffey (Chapter 28) is described as 'precarious', and this of course has an impact on capacity and sustainability. Responsibility for funding is also unclear, meaning that many VCSE organisations are funded from multiple sources, with multiple timescales and the perennial risk of running out of funding entirely.

Academic partners working alongside NASP identified several funding models (Kimberlee et al., 2022):

- Single commissioner: mostly from the NHS, local authority or housing association
- Collaborative commissioning: NHS and local authority, working alongside the VCSE sector
- In-house joint delivery by the NHS and local authority
- Direct funding of the VCSE sector by the NHS

- The possibility of using personal health budgets or integrated personal health budgets
- Social impact bond; a 'payment by success' model of outcomes-based contracting

An important question arising from this list is where the community power and agency might lie within these funding models—to be able to adapt and change as communities change. And many VCSE organisations complain about their capacity to be able to respond to the bidding, monitoring or outcomes reporting process, which may crowd out smaller but more nimble and innovative organisations.

As well as funding, economic recession and the rising cost of living has added additional difficulties as charities, for example, face rising inflation and energy costs. And third-sector employers, wanting to recruit to meet demand, have found steep competition for staff and reducing rates of volunteering (Larkman and Mansoor, 2023).

Summary

In practice, the social prescribing models that have emerged so far have varied widely. Many professional groups such as AHPs and community nurses have a long history of working alongside communities and can be seen as assets whose experience can be drawn upon. To be successful, they need freedom to act, to offer good help and be compassionate, kind and culturally competent. Social history and an understanding of collective and individual trauma are important. The contribution of multiple sectors, such as housing and police as a preventative model, will add much. Shifting power and resources to the community itself and finding ways to 'commission' community building in ways that are equitable and sustainable remains vital.

REFERENCES

Allen, D., 2019. Men's Shed tackles social isolation. Royal College of Nursing Bulletin, 21st August. Available from: https://www.rcn.org.uk/magazines/bulletin/2019/september/mens-shed-tackles-social-isolation-in-scotland (Accessed 9 August 2023).

Atkins, P.W.B., Parker, S.K., 2012. Understanding individual compassion in organisations: the role of appraisals and psychological flexibility. Acad. Med. Rev. 37 (4), 542–546.

Barclay, P., 1982. Social Workers: Their Role and Tasks. Bedford Square Press, London.

Compassionate Inverclyde. Ardgowan Hospice (online) Compassionate Inverclyde. Available from: https://ardgowanhospice.org.uk/how-we-can-help/compassionate-inverclyde/ (Accessed 21 August 2023).

Elgot, J., 2023. Labour plans to embed career advisers in health services to help people into work. The guardian online. 11th January. Available from: https://www.theguardian.com/politics/2023/jan/11/labour-plans-to-embed-career-advisers-in-health-services-to-help-people-into-work (Accessed 9 August 2023).

Fell, G., 2022. The Voluntary and Community sector: from 'integrated care' to 'social prescribing' and into social value & social capital. https://gregfellpublichealth.wordpress.com/2022/06/15/the-voluntary-and-community-sector-the-secret-weapon-for-joining-up-care-for-people/ (Accessed 21 March 2024).

Hamm, C., Glynn-Jones, J., 2019. Implementing an adapted Buurtzorg model in an inner city NHS trust. Br. J. Community Nurs. 24 (11), 534–537.

Health Foundation, 2022. How the public thinks about health, and why it matters—with Dr JacquiDyer and JohnHume. Available from: https://www.health.org.uk/news-and-comment/podcast/what-the-public-thinks-about-health-and-why-it-matters-so-much-with-dr-jacqui-dyer-and-john-hume (Accessed 31 August 2023).

Henry, H., Howarth, M., 2018. An overview of using an asset-based approach to nursing. J. Gen. Pract. Nurs. 4 (4), 61–66.

Kimberlee, R.H., 2013. Developing a social prescribing approach for Bristol. University of the West of England, UK.

Kimberlee, R., Bertotti, M., Dayson, C., Elston, J., Polley, M., Burns, L., Husk, K., On behalf of the NASP Academic Partners Collaborative, 2022. (Sustainable) funding models for social prescribing. National Academy for Social Prescribing, London. Available from: https://www.shu.ac.uk/centre-regional-economic-social-research/publications/sustainable-funding-models-for-social-prescribing (Accessed 18 August 2023).

Larkman, J., Mansoor, M., 2023. Running hot, burning out: an analysis of the VCSE Sector Barometer, in partnership with Nottingham Trent University National VCSE Data and Insights Observatory. *Pro Bono Economics and Nottingham Business School.* https://www.probonoeconomics.com/running-hot-burning-out-the-state-of-the-charity-sector (Accessed 21 March 2024).

Lindsay, E., 2004. The Lindsay Leg Club Model: a model for evidence-based leg ulcer management. Br. J. Community Nurs. 9 (Sup2), S15–S20.

Maybin, J., 2019. Going Dutch in West Suffolk: learning from the Buurtzorg model of care. Available from: https://www.kingsfund.org.uk/blog/2019/09/buurtzorg-model-of-care (Accessed 18 August 2023).

McGarvey, D., 2021. The social distance between us: how remote politics has wrecked Britain. Ebury Press, London.

Nandram, S., 2014. Features and impact of the Buurtzorg approach. The Commonwealth Fund. Available from: https://www.commonwealthfund.org/sites/default/files/documents/___media_files_resources_2014_ihp_briefing_book_att_g15features_and_impact_of_the_buurtzorg_approach_netherlands112314.pdf (Accessed 18 August 2023).

Naylor, C., Wellings, D., 2019. A citizen-led approach to health and care: Lessons from the Wigan Deal. King's Fund. London.

NHS England, 2023. Social prescribing: reference guide and technical annex for primary care networks. Annex C Sample job description and person specification. Available from: https://www.england.nhs.uk/publication/social-prescribing-reference-guide-and-technical-annex-for-primary-care-networks/#annex-c (Accessed 18 August 2023).

Oster, C., Skelton, C., Leibbrandt, R., Hines, S., Bonevski, B., 2023. Models of social prescribing to address non-medical needs in adults: a scoping review. BMC Health Serv. Res. 23, 642. https://doi.org/10.1186/s12913-023-09650-x.

Simpson, M., Buck, D., Ross, S., 2016. Health professionals' attitudes to evidence and the influence it has on decision-making. New NHS Alliance and The King's Fund. Available from: https://thehealthcreationalliance.org/wp-content/uploads/2018/11/Health-professionals-attitudes-to-evidence-and-the-influence-it-has-on-decision-making.pdf (Accessed 9 August 2023).

Simpson, M., Buck, D., Ross, S., 2016. Developing a business case for health—what does good look like? New NHS Alliance and The King's Fund. Available from: https://thehealthcreationalliance.org/wp-content/uploads/2018/11/Developing-a-business-case-for-health-what-does-good-look-like.pdf (Accessed 9 August 2023).

Simpson, M., Buck, D., Ross, S., 2016. The economics of housing and health: the role of housing associations. New NHS Alliance and The King's Fund. Available from: https://www.kingsfund.org.uk/publications/economics-housing-health (Accessed 9 August 2023).

Taylor, D., 2021. The ICS case for the Buurtzorg nursing community care model. The Good Governance Institute. Available from: https://www.good-governance.org.uk/publications/insights/the-ics-case-for-the-buurtzorg-nursing-community-care-model (Accessed 18 August 2023).

Tierney, S., Cartwright, L., Akinyemi, O., Carder-Gilbert, H., Burns, L., Dayson, C., Chatterjee, H. On behalf of the NASP Academic Partners Collaborative, 2022. What does the evidence tell us about accessibility of social prescribing schemes in England to people from black and ethnic minority backgrounds? National Academy for Social Prescribing, London. Available from: https://socialprescribingacademy.org.uk/read-the-evidence/accessibility-of-social prescribing-schemes-in-england-to-people-from-black-asian-and-ethnically-diverse-population-groups/ (Accessed 18 August 2023).

Unwin, J., 2018. Kindness emotions and human relationships: The blind spot in public policy. Carnegie UK. Available from: https://carnegieuktrust.org.uk/publications/kindness-emotions-and-human-relationships-the-blind-spot-in-public-policy/ (Accessed 21 March 2024).

Wigan Council, 2016. Wigan council: shaping demand through engagement and insight. Available from: https://www.local.gov.uk/sites/default/files/documents/find-out-more-information-566.pdf#:~:text=This%20approach%20focuses%20upon%20supporting%20our%20workforce%20to,their%20strengths%20rather%20than%20their%20needs%20and%20problems (Accessed 9 August 2023).

Wilson, R., Cornwell, C., Flanagan, E., Khan, H., 2018. *Good and bad help: how purpose and confidence transform lives.* Available from: https://www.nesta.org.uk/report/good-and-bad-help-how-purpose-and-confidence-transform-lives/ (Accessed 9 August 2023).

Young Minds, 2021. Understanding trauma and adversity. Available from: https://www.youngminds.org.uk/professional/resources/understanding-trauma-and-adversity/ (Accessed 5 September 2023).

Chapter 30

Conclusion

Heather Henry

Social prescribing represents a significant change in the mindset of health services leaders and practitioners across the UK and beyond. It has taken a bunch of determined people—senior clinicians and community leaders—several years to get this far. It is notable that social prescribing came from the grassroots and from the realisation that the current system is broken. It has been built on the testing and learning of pioneers across many different communities and generations.

Solving the Right Problem

After more than 70 years of the NHS, what has caused leaders to break with its weddedness to a biomedical model? Commentators such as Kimberlee (2013) have pointed to the crisis of rising demand and complexity in primary care and the realisation that much of this is driven by social issues. This also suggests that the problem being solved is the problem of NHS demand rather than, as Cottam (2018) suggests, of how we can enable people to flourish. Perhaps it can be argued that the current design of the system does both, and that the flourishing part is encapsulated in the shift from 'what's the matter with me' to 'what matters to me'. However, this is an individualistic view, and contributors argue that there is a lack of emphasis on community building.

From Sickness to Wellbeing

No longer is the NHS a national health service (some would argue that it has become a sickness service) but, at its best, it can also actively support wellbeing. Contributors such as Nancy Hey and Gus O'Donnell help us to understand what makes

us well and how to measure wellbeing more clearly. This evidence is beginning to shift into practice.

From my own perspective as a nurse working in the VCSE sector, I sometimes see a depth of understanding of what wellbeing actually means, and with it, the concept of human flourishing—and sometimes the latters is markedly absent. Others such as Russell view social prescribing as an extension of a 'service' that 'makes people better' by salaried strangers 'fixing' their problems—a deficit- rather than an asset-based approach. Russell also writes about first inviting people to contribute their 'gifts' to their community (often described as the assets of 'head, heart and hands'; Rippon and Hopkins, 2015) rather than starting with a focus on needs. The term 'prescribing' can underline this for some—and for others this term represents an understandable starting point for patients and a health system so wedded to a medical model.

Social prescribing may be about telling people what to do (bad help) or it may be about helping people to find their purpose, give them confidence to act and build their capabilities (good help). It may be about defining a pathway of action, or it may be about getting out of the way and enabling community building.

Does It Work?

This simple question is far from simple. Firstly, the variation of social prescribing models makes its evaluation tricky. Secondly, there are levels of sophistication in the standards of evidence, with an (expensive) randomised control trial being the gold standard, and at the other end a logic model explaining causes and effects. Since social prescribing is a relatively new intervention (although it emanates from long-standing asset-based community development approaches), the evidence base is still catching up. But there is an additional issue of how we evaluate social models of care compared to medical ones, because it is difficult to apply a linear cause-and-effect logic to social models, where there are many confounding factors.

Some commentators have called for a level playing field in terms of measuring the outcomes of social prescribing compared to clinical interventions. They point to the amount of evaluation that small community organisations are often required to undertake compared to big NHS organisations (Fell, 2020).

Despite all this, we must consider the hard-nosed politics of investing in social prescribing. It is enough to be obviously a good thing, or to survive; does it need that detailed evidence that finance directors and treasuries require? Polley et al.'s (2017) research indicates that social prescribing does have a protective effect on health service usage, but that value for money would increase if it was targeted at those that 'complete and respond' to it. And there's the rub. How to identify those people: the alienated/hard to reach/easy to ignore such as Gypsy Romany Travellers, men who delay coming forward to discuss their mental or physical health and those stigmatised or written off by society, such as former offenders or so-called 'troubled families'. And people don't come with a label saying, 'I will save your precious NHS resources' like the obese young man attending his GP who played computer games all day, described by Bethan Griffith.

As I write, the NHS has chosen to evaluate social prescribing against the ONS4 model, developed by O'Donnell and others, of measuring life satisfaction, happiness, a worthwhile life and anxiety (ONS, 2018). Maltby (2019) suggests that we count the number of friends a person has, which correlates well with the Vaillant's (2012) longitudinal student study that found that it was the warmth and quality of the men's long-term relationships that lead to better life satisfaction and longer lives.

Resources

Just as the models for social prescribing itself vary, so do the options and the opinions for resourcing it.

The Sheffield director of public health Greg Fell has been speaking out about the inequalities in funding health care versus public health and preventative work for many years. He blogs about social prescribing:

'Imagine if there were a tariff for the activity that people are enabled to access [social prescribing] in the same way there is a tariff for a rheumatology outpatient appointment. Imagine a big scheme to incentivise referrals to dermatologists but without any investment in dermatologists The Brit[ish] Assoc[iation] of Dermatology would go ballistic…'

(Fell, 2020)

The government in England has invested in establishing the National Academy for Social Prescribing and offered £1.8 million for a Thriving Communities Fund and £3.6 million in mental health support (HM Government, 2022). The evaluation of investments arising from these funds will aid learning, but compared to the investment in drugs, NHS equipment and staff, or in the set-up of the social prescribing system (quoted by Fell at £500 million over 5 years), these amounts are just a drop in the ocean. There are also gaps in the evidence base requiring funded research.

Gus O'Donnell has pointed us towards the recommendations from the Law Commission for Civil Society (2023) that he chaired. The report calls for:

'strategic investment from funders, this government and the next, in the productivity of the social sector, the data available to and about it, and in the changes needed to unlock philanthropy. This must be accompanied by a dramatic acceleration in the partnership between civil society and business, and a reset of the relationship between civil society and government.'

The integrated planning of social prescribing requires the full support and resources of local authorities, and yet there is a decline in local government resource allocation and a geographic inequality in how resources are distributed, leading to a gap between promises and reality on levelling up (Webb et al., 2022).

What contributors call for in this book is strategic planning for community investment and, alongside this, a thinking through of the mechanisms: contracts, grants, social impact bonds, trading, philanthropy and more. Monitoring of spend and measurement of outcomes go alongside this, to be commensurate with the level of investment and size of the organisations themselves, so that community groups can overcome the barriers to market entry and get on with the day job rather than develop a bigger back office. Whether or not to develop some shared markers of value and impact of the VCSE sector may benefit from discussion (Fell, 2022). The Law Family Commission on Civil Society and Pro Bono Economics (2023) recommends that monitoring should focus on outcomes, but others may still want further reassurance of money well spent, such as activity. High-profile reviews point to evidence saying that for certain interventions, such as art therapy (All-Party Parliamentary Group on Arts, Health and Wellbeing, 2017), further testing is no longer required, meaning that we should stop asking VCSE organisations to evaluate these interventions over and over again.

Economics

As Hey explained in Section 1, personal finance and the economy are strongly linked to wellbeing. So how can social prescribing help? A narrow focus might be on supporting individuals with benefits or with employment. But a more strategic focus would be for integrated care systems to take action on community wealth building: public procurement, developing a fairer local labour market and offering local people jobs, a living wage, inclusive ownership of land and buildings, microfinancing of community businesses and local businesses and supporting wider social entrepreneurship.

A healthier, happier nation is more productive. At governmental level, there is a growing movement towards wellbeing economics. This prioritises human and planetary needs rather than treating economic growth as an end in itself. It is where rules and incentives support all sections of society to feel safe, comfortable and happy.

Health Inequalities

As Sir Michael Marmot has indicated, social prescribing or indeed the Universal Model of Personalised Care is not going to tackle the real drivers of health inequalities, but it will help people and communities to tackle the effects of them. Meantime, Marmot is hopeful about the increasing understanding of the various Royal Colleges about the structural issues required to tackle health inequalities and how they as clinical bodies might be able to help. This is genuine progress.

Marmot also advises that action on health inequalities and levelling up requires not only great policy documents but also political will at all levels, plus genuine investment. It requires joined-up government, whereby each department considers the impact of policy on inequality and how variations in wellbeing might link to the economic success of the country as a whole. Should we be measuring, as Lord Gus O'Donnell states, 'gross domestic wellbeing'?

Power and Culture

In some cases, social prescribing leaders are sensitive to the agency of the community itself and will seek to use their abilities as system convenors and 'proscribers' to enable community-building, backed by levers such as the Social Value Act and asset transfers as well as much-needed resources.

Awareness is rising that to be successful, the colonial instinct of the NHS and its partners to see community assets as part of *their* system must be resisted. The pressure on the NHS to reduce demand and meet targets is vast. Yet communities cannot be led into activities that are not a cultural fit. Asking for citizens' help as well as offering it, giving away power and control to communities and enabling community building are equally important to social prescribing. Contributors have offered us clear reasons why it is important to be humble, to test, fail and learn. The NHS is now recognising and supporting the gifts and talents of even the most oppressed and stigmatised. To give away power means nurturing relationships, healing wounds and understanding culture so that there is mutual trust and respect.

A civil society that has grown up with a consumer culture was jolted by COVID-19 into the reality that the sources of wellbeing primarily lie in the power of people helping people. Our foremost reserves, according to Russell and DeWolfe (2023), exist in our neighbourhoods, and for everything else there are services, not the other way around. Cottam (2019) advises that 'the 5th Social Revolution' is about creating and making with each other and to build our capabilities of learning, work, health, relationships and community.

Systems Leadership

Social prescribing has influenced not only the NHS but also leaders across the social determinants of health. As I write, it has now entered NHS policy, strategy and practice and has become embedded in integrated care systems. Our partners in local authorities, education, housing, criminal justice, business, faith, employment, voluntary, community and social enterprise have joined in enthusiastically with the concept. However, some partners such as fire and rescue and policing understand and interpret social prescribing differently. Here, there is much more emphasis on the prevention of issues that negatively impact wellbeing. There is also a variable recognition amongst ICS leaders of how sectors such as business and housing might contribute to social prescribing, with some working in partnership and others in parallel.

Much has been written about systems leadership and complexity science in this book. The bottom line is that it will be difficult to standardise an approach to social prescribing, as every community is its own complex system, and standardisation may mean loss of community control. This may present a confusing national picture and may result in difficulties in comparing and evaluating social prescribing between Bangor and Bognor.

Communication

Social prescribing is such a significant shift that it is not surprising that frontline teams may be confused about it. Griffith explains in her contribution that the overall ethos may not be clear in primary care, and several contributors have recognised that feedback loops between referrers and social prescribing link workers may not yet be happening.

Palmer expands on this to talk about the advocacy role of the link worker to offer the community experience to PCNs and ICSs. So in order to test and learn there needs to be feedback loops at grassroots and at system levels.

At city and governmental level contributors talk about 'health in all policies' and an inter-departmental

government approach to tackling the social determinants of health.

There are also issues about how we communicate the concept of social prescribing to the public. We discovered in Chapter 12 that it is important that we explain or 'frame' this conversation as well as we can. For this we need to understand that the public thinks of health and wellbeing as a personal matter influenced by their choices and has difficulty understanding the impact of structural inequalities (Health Foundation, 2022).

Beliefs and Behaviours

Part of managing complexity is about understanding people's health beliefs and behaviours. Over the past few years, the Behavioural Insight Team has done much to analyse behaviour change theories and to make them accessible to the public sector. Now we can move from *understanding* human behaviour to an ability to use a range of tools to *take action* too.

Workforce Development

As the system pivots towards a social model of health and wellbeing, education and workforce development pivot too. This is recognised by universities, NHS training hubs and organisations such as the College of Medicine, which are all testing out new ways to align staff towards social prescribing.

Yet to come is the battle with, amongst others, regulators of nursing, midwifery and medical registration and education. They need persuading that educational standards and learning outcomes may need to be revised so that students are prepared upon registration for a new world that recognises and supports community assets as equal partners. Undergraduate learning placements in VCSE organisations, supported by VCSE placement supervisors, also need consideration. At the post-graduate level, public health leaders such as Fell (2022) suggested that senior VCSE leaders offer peer mentorship to health and care leaders.

The skills of systems leadership have been promoted for several years now (see the NHS Leadership Academy, www.leadershipacademy.nhs.uk). Recognition has been gained that power and control may be hard to cede until relationships build trust. But how we get the community-enhanced social prescribing vision to Gladwell's (2002) 'tipping point' by engaging mavens, salesmen and the like may need further workforce development. Some leaders have already recognised that the VCSE sector is a source of data and insights, influencers, communication partners, researchers, key policy shapers and strategic thinkers and not just providers of services—and some still need to discover this.

There are new roles and skills still to embed: system convenors or connectors, gappers, a wider understanding of wellbeing economics and community wealth building. Workforce development may need to target specific communities that could benefit from specialised social prescribing initiatives such as children and young people, families and carers, people with mental health issues and rural and coastal communities (Chapters 14, 22, 23, 27 and Emmins et al., 2023).

There are behaviours to be unlearnt by the workforce too, such as the desire to care for and protect people rather than build their capabilities. Some may need to overcome an addiction to caring—that great feeling that you have when you have helped someone. Being a cheerleader may not feel quite the same as being a leader.

We also need to invest in VCSE workforce development. 10GM is a joint venture by local VCSE infrastructure support organisations in Greater Manchester. It has set up a workforce development project to address issues such as recruitment, nurturing new talent, diversity and inclusion, leadership and wellbeing (https://10gm.org.uk/vcseworkforce.html).

Final Words: Cherish Humanity

When I first became interested in asset-based working around 2010, I was listening to a lecture at the University of Wrexham from the only professor of salutogenesis in the world, Bengt Linstrom of the Nordic School of Public Health, Gothenburg. I asked him why salutogenic approaches were not well understood or represented in public policy. He sighed and said simply, 'People do not bring themselves to work'.

When I explained to a group of fellow nurses how I was enabling a group of fathers in one of the hardest-pressed communities in England to find their own solutions to improve their wellbeing, all they said was, 'But do you do any *proper nursing*?' Empowering citizens to build their capabilities takes time and may take second place to more urgent 'proper' clinical work. Yet the work of those fathers may have interrupted intergenerational inequalities, because their improved wellbeing positively impacted their children's wellbeing (Robertson et al., 2015). Empowering health and care staff to bring themselves to work and carving out time for them to empower local people is important. Many clinicians I know do just that. Some get into trouble for it: I know I did. But it is important to be present and to listen and see what goes on and not to leave it just to link workers.

Contributors throughout this book have talked about listening, about kindness, about good help that doesn't try to control or tell people what to do. They call for a level playing field between statutory and community sectors. They describe connecting or reconnecting people to each other, about helping people to find meaning and purpose in their lives and about building relationships—particularly with communities experiencing disadvantage, who have felt alienated for generations. Where I work in Greater Manchester I see this shift to a more human system. It is my hope that politicians don't kill off social prescribing before we've learnt how to do things—and learnt to fail—and before that 10-year public health shift comes to reveal itself in our morbidity and mortality data.

Being human is not being weak; it is the journey that we must undertake to rebuild the wellbeing of the nation.

Social prescribing is now part of the NHS Long Term Plan. For many it is only the beginning of a journey and what happens next is important. Throughout this book I have attempted to curate contributions from a range of perspectives to assist you in your thinking. I leave the rest up to you.

REFERENCES

All-Party Parliamentary Group on Arts, Health and Wellbeing, 2017. Creative health: the arts for health and wellbeing. Available from: https://www.culturehealthandwellbeing.org.uk/appg-inquiry/ (Accessed 1 September 2023).

Cottam, H., 2018. Radical Help: How We Can Remake the Relationships Between Us and Revolutionise the Welfare State. Virago Little Brown, London.

Cottam, H., 2019. Revolution 5.0: a social manifesto. Available from: https://www.hilarycottam.com/wp-content/uploads/2019/12/Social-Revolution-5.0-_dec19.pdf (Accessed 4 September 2023).

Emmins, N., Leckie, C., Monro, R., Pragnall, M., 2023. Communities on the edge: a report for the Coastal Communities Alliance and Partners. Pragmatix Advisory Ltd. Available from: https://www.coastalcommunities.co.uk/knowledge-base/category/reports/communities-on-the-edge (Accessed 4 September 2023).

Fell, G., 2020. Blog: is there any actual evidence for social prescribing yet? Available from. https://gregfellpublichealth.wordpress.com/2020/01/20/is-there-any-actual-evidence-for-social-prescribing-yet/ (Accessed 24 August 2023).

Fell, G., 2022. The Voluntary and Community Sector: from 'integrated care' to 'social prescribing' and into social value & social capital, https://gregfellpublichealth.wordpress.com/2022/06/15/the-voluntary-and-community-sector-the-secret-weapon-for-joining-up-care-for-people/ (Accessed 27 March 2024).

Gladwell, M., 2002. The Tipping Point. Back Bay Books, New York.

Health Foundation, 2022. How the public thinks about health, and why it matters—with Dr JacquiDyer and JohnHume. Available from: https://www.health.org.uk/news-and-comment/podcast/what-the-public-thinks-about-health-and-why-it-matters-so-much-with-dr-jacqui-dyer-and-john-hume (Accessed 1 September 2023).

HM Government, 2022. £3.6 million social prescribing funding for mental health support. Available from: https://www.gov.uk/government/news/36-million-social-prescribing-funding-to-bolster-mental-health-support-and-ease-pressure-on-gps (Accessed 25 August 2023).

Kimberlee, R.H., 2013. Developing a Social Prescribing Approach for Bristol. University of the West of England, UK.

The Law Family Commission on Civil Society and Pro Bono Economics, 2023. The Law Family Commission on Civil Society. Available from: https://civilsocietycommission.org/ (Accessed 10 March 2023).

Maltby, B., 2019. Blog: an asset based approach to health—the 3 things you should know about social prescribing. Available from: https://beckymalby.wordpress.com/2019/10/09/an-asset-based-approach-to-health-the-3-things-you-should-know-about-social-prescribing/ (Accessed 24 August 2023).

Office for National Statistics ONS, 2018. Personal well-being user guidance. Available from: https://www.ons.gov.uk/peoplepopulationandcommunity/wellbeing/methodologies/personalwellbeingsurveyuserguide (Accessed 24 August 2023).

Polley, M., Bertotti, M., Kimberlee, R., Pilkington, K., Refsum, C., 2017. A review of the evidence assessing impact of social prescribing on healthcare demand and cost implications. https://www.researchgate.net/publication/318861473.

Rippon, S., Hopkins, T., 2015. Head, hands and heart: asset-based approaches in health care: a review of the conceptual evidence and case studies of asset-based approaches in health, care and wellbeing. Health Foundation. Available from: https://www.health.org.uk/sites/default/files/HeadHandsAndHeartAssetBasedApproachesInHealthCare.pdf (Accessed 4 September 2023).

Robertson, S., Woodall, J., Hanna, E., Rowlands, S., Long, T., Livesley, J., 2015. Salford Dadz: year 2 external evaluation. Project Report. Unlimited Potential. Available from: https://eprints.leedsbeckett.ac.uk/id/eprint/1728/ (Accessed 10 July 2023).

Russell, C., DeWolfe, S., 2023. Podcast: the connected community. Available from: https://podcastindex.org/podcast/6595618 (Accessed 4 September 2023).

Vaillant, G. 2012. Triumphs of experience, The men of the Harvard Grant Study. The Belknap Press of Harvard University. Cambridge, MA.

Webb, J., Johns, M., Roscoe, E., Giovannini, A., Qureshi, A., Baldini, R., 2022. State of the North 2021/22; Powering Northern Excellence. IPPR. Available from http://www.ippr.org/research/publications/state-of-the-north-2021-22-powering-northern-excellence (Accessed 29 December 2022).

Glossary

ADDER: (Project) Addiction, Diversion, Disruption, Enforcement and Recovery
ASBO: Antisocial Behaviour Order
C2: Connecting Communities
CFOA: Chief Fire Officers Association
FRS: Fire and Rescue Service
GDP: Gross Domestic Product
GM: Greater Manchester
GMCA: Greater Manchester Combined Authority
GMHP: Greater Manchester Housing Providers
GP: General Practitioner
GSPA: Global Social Prescribing Alliance
HP: Housing Providers
ICS: Integrated Care System
ISPPA: International Social Prescribing Pharmacy Association
NASP: National Academy for Social Prescribing
NCCH: National Centre for Creative Health
NFCC: National Fire Chiefs Council
NHS: National Health Service

NVQ: National Vocational Qualification
OECD: Organisation for Economic Co-operation and Development
ONS: Office for National Statistics
PCF: Person-Centred Framework
PCN: Primary Care Network
PERMA: Positive Emotion, Engagement, Relationships, Meaning and Accomplishment
PHB: Personal Health Budget
PHE: Public Health England
SDG: Sustainable Development Goal
SPLW: Social Prescribing Link Worker
SPYN: Social Prescribing Youth Network
SRG: Self-Reliant Group
SWYPFT: South West Yorkshire Partnership Foundation Trust
UK: United Kingdom
WEMWBS: Warwick-Edinburgh Mental Well-Being Scale
WHO: World Health Organization

Index

Note: Page numbers followed by '*f*' indicate figures, '*t*' indicate tables, and '*b*' indicate boxes.